NEW DEVELOPMENTS IN MEDICAL RESEARCH

THE CRISIS IN CONTEMPORARY MEDICINE AND THE RISE OF THE REFLECTIVE PHYSICIAN, SECOND EDITION

NEW DEVELOPMENTS IN MEDICAL RESEARCH

Additional books in this series can be found on Nova's website
under the Series tab.

Additional e-books in this series can be found on Nova's website
under the e-book tab.

THE CRISIS IN CONTEMPORARY MEDICINE AND THE RISE OF THE REFLECTIVE PHYSICIAN, SECOND EDITION

IAN MCDONALD

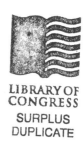

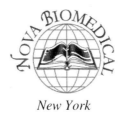

New York

NOTICE TO THE READER

The Publisher has taken reasonable care in the preparation of this book, but makes no expressed or implied warranty of any kind and assumes no responsibility for any errors or omissions. No liability is assumed for incidental or consequential damages in connection with or arising out of information contained in this book. The Publisher shall not be liable for any special, consequential, or exemplary damages resulting, in whole or in part, from the readers' use of, or reliance upon, this material. Any parts of this book based on government reports are so indicated and copyright is claimed for those parts to the extent applicable to compilations of such works.

Independent verification should be sought for any data, advice or recommendations contained in this book. In addition, no responsibility is assumed by the publisher for any injury and/or damage to persons or property arising from any methods, products, instructions, ideas or otherwise contained in this publication.

This publication is designed to provide accurate and authoritative information with regard to the subject matter covered herein. It is sold with the clear understanding that the Publisher is not engaged in rendering legal or any other professional services. If legal or any other expert assistance is required, the services of a competent person should be sought. FROM A DECLARATION OF PARTICIPANTS JOINTLY ADOPTED BY A COMMITTEE OF THE AMERICAN BAR ASSOCIATION AND A COMMITTEE OF PUBLISHERS.

Additional color graphics may be available in the e-book version of this book.

Library of Congress Cataloging-in-Publication Data

ISBN: 978-1-63484-256-3
Library of Congress Control Number: 2015956838

Published by Nova Science Publishers, Inc. † New York

Contents

'Preface'
to the Second Edition

The target of this book is primarily to examine the role of science in seeding widespread unrest in health care. Since this book was published in 2013 I have perceived a revolution in the important area of the influences of tacit knowledge and emotions in judgement and decision-making. I would have most definitely included this development had I realized its importance at the time. I believe that implications for the intellectual world and for the rehabilitation of clinical judgement are far reaching. The major changes which have occurred mainly over the past 20 years involve judgements and decisions in medicine, science and social sciences, and specifically the absolute necessity to include the influence of tacit knowledge and of emotions. Both subjects have been virtually taboo in medical and scientific research circles for a long. The time has come to review this attitude.

Both concepts are now seen as clearly crucial to decision-making, and this includes the much maligned 'clinical experience' about which many physicians feel an entirely unwarranted defensiveness. The forces driving what is a radical change has been a confluence of research in neurology, neuroanatomy, neurophysiology, psychology, economics, cognitive, computer and management sciences. Samson is already shaking the foundations! Despite the fundamental importance of this new thinking about judgement, I have not been able to locate a comprehensive concise account in the literature. This is probably because the relevant research has been undertaken in the various academic fields studying judgements made in medical care, medical science and science in general. In addition, there could be subtle resistance of the modern paradigm to such a threatening development in an area so central to clinical and scientific decision-making. The resultant growth spurt in understanding of decision-making has spawned a corresponding confusing proliferation of research methods based in advances in MRI and PET imaging of the brain, allowing localization of thought processes. Accompanying this surge has been a multitude of theories which are difficult to compare with one another or to describe, let alone to evaluate or reconcile as we clearly must.

The two areas of knowledge previously neglected have been the vital roles of tacit (subconscious) knowledge, and, somewhat surprisingly, the crucial influence of the emotions in making judgements. The proposal in this research is that purely rational decision-making is a myth, and that to exclude emotional influences and unconscious forces, as do current economic theories of decision-making (standard expected utility theory), is fallacious because these powerful factors simply can no longer be ignored. Indeed, the evolving perspective would also absolutely vindicate the place of "clinical judgement," so mercilessly pilloried by the clinician's arch enemy, namely "evidence-based medicine." This movement narrows the concept of evidence to 'scientific' empirical data from randomized clinical trials – a grotesque and simplistic distortion of medical decision-making, revealing at its core a revival of the discredited philosophies of 'scientism' and 'positivism.' This is covered in the earlier draft of the book. I have therefore done what I feel is a much needed synthesis of this rapidly advancing field as Chapters 13 and 14 of this new edition.

Acknowledgments

Thanks are due to Doctor Jeanne Daly of La Trobe University who provided sociological expertise. I thank also those members of St. Vincent's Hospital staff who have cooperated in our studies, and especially Dr. Michael Jelinek with whom I have enjoyed an ongoing dialogue. I am grateful to Doctor Michael Stanford, Chief Medical Officer and Doctor David Campbell, Chief Executive Officer of St. Vincent's Hospital at that time for trusting in my vision. Special thanks to Ms. Dianne Tanzer, the chief echocardiography technologist, who drew attention to a patient still anxious after explanation of a normal echocardiogram response and thereby prompted this project. Finally, I am indebted to the late Doctor Alvan Feinstein, formerly Professor of Medicine and Epidemiology at Yale University, pioneer of clinical epidemiology, acerbic critic and astute student of clinical practice, who opened the Centre.

The following provided valuable comment on drafts of the manuscript: Prof. A. Kellehear, Prof. E. Byrne, Prof. J. Best, Dr. K. Breen, Prof. M. Jelinek. Dr. G. Greenbaum, Prof. B. Collopy, Prof. N. Pride, Dr. B. Rush, Dr. J. O'Callaghan, Prof. C. Nettelbeck.

Chapter 1

Introduction

Medicine rode to fame on the coat-tails of science during the 19th and 20th centuries. Following the Renaissance, science transformed society with a series of triumphs. Particularly influential was the moon journey. Impressive for quite different reasons was detonation of the atomic bomb. But science was also targeted by those concerned by science and technological 'progress' culminating in global warming and the problem of industrialism. Science also impugned for the reign of technology, seen as colluding with the modern capital state. Its very basis, the adherence to complete 'objectivity' in research was seen as spurious by the emerging postmodern social paradigm. Scientific advance in medicine, gradual during and after the Renaissance, gathered pace with French Revolution, and during the course of the 19th century came into full flower. Not for six or seven decades did there seem to be any clouds on the horizon so far as medicine was concerned. Then, as we will see, this Golden Age suddenly evaporated in the face of an ill-defined public disquiet, backed by some bureaucratic rumblings. We suggest that this societal disillusionment with aspects of scientific medicine had probably simmered during the earlier decades of the 20th century because a catalyst was required to ignite inchoate dissatisfaction. That catalyst was Ivan Illich.

More recently, the public images of both science and medicine have become somewhat tarnished. McKeown showed that the steep decline in community mortality rate from the early 19th century was not due primarily to medical advances as many had assumed, rather it was attributable to improved social conditions. Yet there had been some brilliant medical scientific advances - to whit the use of autopsy to locate disease in specific body tissues, design of 'scopes to examine the heart and to peer into every body cavity and orifice, identification of the 'quid divinum' causing infectious disease - bacteria - and anaesthesia, surgery, and childbirth had become safer. Why then medicine's fall from grace?

Doctors who have achieved some outstanding successes in the treatment of disease, have reaped rewards in the form of social prestige and formidable political clout. Nevertheless, hardly had scientific medicine come into full flower after World War II than there were signs of a back-lash. This book is in no way intended to be an analysis of personal experience. Nevertheless, the author, practising in a hospital setting for just 40 years, did experience this turmoil from the inside in a country with a mixed public and private health system, roughly midway between those of Britain and the U.S. This experience does therefore offer an insider's perspective and a convenient starting point. These 40 years fall neatly into two halves. The first half, from 1958 to 1977 was a period of prosperity locally and of stability in health. Leading up to this period of prosperity was Burnham's Golden Age of Medicine when medicine in scientific garb had established its dominant position in the health system. It was experienced as a tranquil time of 'hegemonic harmony'. The medical profession enjoyed a position of dominance which was not seriously in dispute, indeed clinical practice was not a matter of public controversy nor a political issue. The second half, from 1978 to 1997, has been quite different. This has been a time of conflict, confusion and contention. This was a time of 'transitional conflict'.

In retrospect, the stability and apparent harmony of the earlier years reflected the extent to which medicine dominated the health system, and the lack of any perceived need for major change. In the modern world following the Second World War, medicine enjoyed success and social status, respect for medical science remained high there was general agreement that the mission of scientific medicine was the cure of disease. This was a credible commitment in the eyes of doctors since it reflected the thrust of the medical curriculum under which they had been trained since early in the 19th century. Memory of a traditional medicine with its primary commitment to the humanities was, however, growing dim. This mission was generously funded in the Western World. The great achievements of scientific medicine, crowned by wartime triumphs, had conferred the political capital which allowed the doctor to dominate the clinical consultation, and the medical profession to essentially write its own ticket in the public sector, free of external scrutiny and unencumbered by any calls for accountability.

During this period of stability, modern scientific medicine looked unassailable, and its dominant status in the health system was essentially unquestioned, indeed virtually invisible. The public were generally in awe of the repertoire of the scientifically trained doctor and the facilities of the modern hospital, appreciative of the doctor's key role as scientific diagnostician and eradicator of infectious disease. Patients were generally silent and uncomplaining, trusting and undemanding. Few, it seemed, had any wish to understand precisely what was going on, let alone hanker for a part in making the decisions. The achievements of medicine seemed to have conferred on doctors what seemed like unlimited credit with the community.

Belief in medicine was reinforced by the simple observation that many of our friends and family had so obviously benefited from it. Some would not have been still alive without it. After all, pregnancy and childbirth had become much safer, most of us and our children successfully negotiated the perils of infancy and early childhood. Most of us have remained free of serious disability and pain during adult life or could be helped, and many have avoided premature death. For those of us anxious about our health, there were scientific tests to help reassure us that most of the potentially worrying symptoms we suffered from time to time were not harbingers of serious disease. Most of the illness, compressed into the later years, would yield in part to palliative care so that we could often enjoy a more comfortable old age, and perhaps an easier passage to death even, in some countries, assisted death.

Hegemonic Harmony

During this time, hospital medicine was dominant, and specialisation was the road to higher professional status, community prestige, greater income and more secure knowledge.

The role of doctor as captain of the clinical ship was not controversial. It seemed that, by and large, nurses, other health providers and hospital administrators saw that their place was to provide support for the work of the doctor. General practitioners tended to be seen professionally as drop-outs but patients and families appreciated the continuity of care and home visits they offered. Research then meant biomedical research, even when conducted in a clinical setting, and the idea of evaluation of health care, let alone the scholarly study of clinical practice itself, was simply unthought of! Laboratory scientists were held in respect. Medical audit performed by colleagues in-house was not too threatening. Intrusive external review was out of the question. The health services research which was developing slowly in Britain and North America was still nowhere in sight. Socialised medicine had been successfully repelled in many Western countries so that private practice reigned supreme. In other countries, medicine still flourished as the key element of a nationalised system of health care. The very idea of corporate medicine was simply unthinkable. Medical education followed a formula which reflected the impact of science early in the century. The first half was devoted to laying the foundations of a medical scientist. The second half was a clinical apprenticeship - but in a teaching hospital dedicated to scientific education about more serious organic disease. However such disease is uncommon in general practice and functional illness common in the outpatient department and in general practice where the bulk of medicine is practised. The two approaches were not easily reconciled, resulting in divided loyalties whereby the science and the art could each damage the other. Clearly, science won this encounter.

Political tolerance of professional self-regulation was a reflection of public trust. Governments were pleased to accept the political kudos for provision of effective health services, and the professions generally had an intimate relationship with those responsible for public policy. Doctors were deployed as gate-keepers to the health system, a means for ensuring a healthy and compliant workforce, a role doctors at the time accepted without reflection. Social institutions such as the law and the welfare system reflected medical attitudes and sometimes definitions. Health care was synonymous with medical care. Neither home care nor alternative medicine was encouraged. Practitioners and researchers took for granted the largesse of the state which simply paid for what medical practitioners did or ordered for their patients. Big business exploited the skills of the biomedical scientists, kept practitioners informed about 'new advances,' and rewarded them in various ways for prescribing their products.

Transitional Conflict

The next 20 years, from about 1978 to 1997, were quite different. Indeed, from the point of view of those involved, it has felt as though modern medicine and health care were under siege. Medical war stories have become popular cocktail party patter. Health is a hot topic in the press. Medical breakthroughs still make good copy. Yet much that we read in the press and in magazines is critical. Beginning in the late 1970s, and well underway by the early 1980s, was a time of rapid change and political turbulence. It seems that latent tensions building up earlier had suddenly been released, taking medicine and the clinical world rather by surprise. There was clearly much underlying public disaffection. There has been criticism of medicine from all sides. One can scarcely open a newspaper without encountering sometimes lurid accounts of medical misadventure, of alleged negligence, of 'adverse events.' Patients now complain of lack of communication in the clinical consultation, often fail to take their treatment, delay seeking help, do not necessarily accept reassurance and often vote with their feet, spurning doctor for alternative health practitioner. Consumer groups often assume an antagonistic stance. Social critics had a field day and 'doctor bashing' as a popular blood sport was imbued with academic refinement in the social sciences. The chief focus was on medical dominance of the consultation and health system.

Even more confusing was that social conventions were changing in a way which threatened the clinician's foundational assumptions about their role in the medical consultation. Many could not or would not make necessary adjustments. There was also competition from other health professionals and healers. There was surprisingly little counter argument from the profession. Granted that some doctors had recognised these problems, most of the informed criticism came from without. Many doctors are now unhappy with their lot. Some have regretted their career choice, some have withdrawn from the public sector, some have retired early from practice. An optimistic interpretation of all of this is our conviction is that a major cultural change is at the root of this confusion controversy and conflict. Hence an optimist would see this second period as a time of 'transitional instability' on the way to a new postmodern paradigm in which the social sciences, in particular, will bring to medical education, practice and research the much needed skills of interpretive qualitative thinking. The future of medicine can only be seen for a short way ahead. The purpose of this book is to peer into the gloom and try to discern, no matter how vaguely, the shape of postmodern clinical medicine and the activities of its practitioners.

The grafting of science onto the ancient traditions of healing has led to the marvelous contributions of scientific medicine. However we will see later that it has also been paradoxically, at the root of public disaffection. The liaison of clinical medicine with science first began to bear fruit in the form of a vastly improved understanding of the body following the Renaissance, but it was only at the end of the 18th century Enlightenment, just after French Revolution, that science unveiled a deeper understanding of disease mechanism. It was this understanding which led to the beginnings of preventative and curative treatment of disease. The beginnings of scientific medicine were in France after the Revolution. It is said that the eminent British historian, Arnold Toynbee, upon being asked to comment on the impact of the French Revolution, remarked 'it is too soon to tell.' The same could be said of the impact of science on health care and clinical medicine. Thus, in historical terms, scientific medicine, an important organ of the democratic state, has been a recent development. In this sense, science is like a juicy piece of fillet steak which medicine has swallowed whole but not yet managed to digest. Many of the current complaints about consultation with doctors, and controversies over health services research and cost containment are a direct reflection of tensions between the old art and the new science of medicine, or a reaction to the profession's privileged relationship with the state, so-called 'medical dominance' which also owes much to science. But history has not waited for medicine to sort out its relationship with science. These are manifestations of yet another cultural tidal wave in the offing.

Impact of Postmodernism

Here is not the place for a dissertation on postmodernism. However, my belief is that one cannot avoid coming to grips with postmodernism if one is to understand events in health now and in the immediate future. The concept has permeated philosophy, art, literature and literary criticism, and architecture. Nevertheless, the very existence of postmodernism is controversial. Basically, postmodernism is a return to the Aristotelian ideas of organic complexity, emphasising uncertainty, contingency even radical scepticism. Central to postmodern thinking are a vision of both the natural and social worlds, and especially language, as highly complex dynamic and evolving systems. Determinism has made way for complexity theory, systems theory to chaos theory. Certainty and foundational belief characteristic of science have given way in some quarters even to ironic detachment. Science has therefore been widely challenged and has lost some public support as a result of its failure to solve basic social problems, by its contribution to environmental degradation, and by the rejection of some of its most fundamental beliefs - for example, its claim to complete objectivity - by the postmodern movement. There is no chance that the culture of medicine could avoid such a pervasive social revolution. Furthermore, part of the postmodern worldview is the insistence that science be seen as part of the broader culture, not value-free and apolitical as it has claimed to be. This is directly relevant to medicine which had rejected its traditional broad umbrella of the humanities in favour of science. We have used the term 'humanities' in this book to refer to social sciences and those disciplines most relevant to a doctor – particularly philosophy, literature and history. The current lack of teaching of these subjects in the medical curriculum has been well summarized by Macnaughton (2000). We have used the term 'humanistic' to refer to both the social sciences and humanities, as defined, especially to the hermeneutic interpretive perspective of qualitative sociology.

Social Upheaval

Since the rise of a counterculture and the student rebellion of the 1960s, it has become apparent that pervasive shifts have been occurring in the cultures of Western countries. Intellectuals dispute whether we are seeing manifestations of 'late capitalism' or of a new 'postmodern' era. Both appear to co-exist at present. It is inconceivable that medicine as a subsystem of the wider society would not reflect these changes. Both seem to be co-existing in a state of tension. 'Globalisation' is largely a product of the Information Age. A positive effect of the information revolution has been the acceleration of an earlier slow movement towards a more integrated system of health care driven by improved communications. A health system enhanced by modern developments in computer and communications technology could provide more efficient and equitable care by promoting better integration of primary medical care, social services and hospital care. Home care can be enhanced by provision of information which could support appropriate self care. Information technology could also enhance the care of the chronically ill, aged and homebound. Information technology has also made it possible to collect and analyse the vast amount of data which can be generated at the coal face in the course of routine clinical care. This could be exploited to provide unique information which will enhance the decision-making of doctors, of administrators and of policy-makers, to monitor the quality of care, to establish the effectiveness of interventions, to study the mechanism of disease and the natural history of illness, and its social and cultural context.

The globalising or integrating tendency which brought players in the health sector closer together has a downside however, acting as a force bringing together institutions and players previously independent, it has created a new complexity and a clash of paradigms or disciplinary perspectives. One of the central features of the postmodern world is an increase in the complexity of our social institutions. To the burgeoning complexity of medical science was added a new social complexity. The different basic perspectives, assumptions and agendas of clinicians, consumer groups, governments and health bureaucracies has inevitably lead to friction which hampers cooperative action and research. There are more voices to be heard in most debates, including those pertaining to health. In the case of health care, this once involved just three paradigms or sets of shared assumptions - those of the doctor or other healer, of the patient seeking help, and of the common societal culture they shared. Today the gap between the medical and lay discourses has widened, and many voices have been added - those of politician and bureaucrat, business and consumer bodies, and those of the wide range of professionals and academic disciplines engaged in research into and evaluation of health care. Differences between their perspectives are of particular importance at present in health care because paradigmatic incompatibility seriously threatens the unity of purpose required for cooperative effort and constructive change at a time of disorientation and turbulence.

Late capitalism refers to the struggle to maintain economic growth essential to the capitalist enterprise. A blow-out in health costs and the impact of economic rationalism have eroded government support of medicine and boosted managed care, so that there have been serious moves to constrain medical autonomy and cut health costs. The headlines now frequently reflect the fact that health care has become a political issue in the Western world because of claims of unsustainable cost, and of public concern about the quality of care when services are cut back or rationed. Economic rationalism includes an attempt to reduce welfare spending. In this atmosphere, governments, and not just those of the right, have targeted health care as a big spender. Health services are frequently a central election issue even a political football. Cost cutting measures have been implemented. The media highlights patients on trolleys for too long, dirt in hospitals, long waiting lists for surgery and delays in ambulance responses. Concerned to head off any perception that quality of care might have been impaired, the government reassures the public that all is well.

Wary of a profession with a track record of political muscle skillfully mobilised to protect vested interests, governments have encouraged public health professionals to go it alone in evaluating health. This often fails because of lack of expert clinical input. In any case doctors have been more interested in laboratory research than in evaluation needed to justify their own practice and to improve the care of patients, wherein resides their true expertise. The introduction of managed care has created a cockpit for conflict between government, consumers, professionals and corporate interests, and the introduction of corporate principles in the health systems of Britain and in New Zealand has sparked controversy. Of recent years health has loomed as an important election issue both in Britain and in the United States. At the same time a perceived crisis of capitalism has resulted in a contraction of welfare spending which has had a direct impact on health facilities in the public sphere, and a corresponding shift in the direction of managed care in which government has partially withdrawn from the funding of health care, and, especially in the U.S., the corporate sector is expanding its role in the form of managed care. Cost containment measures introduced in the name of scientific objectivity may be damaging to clinical standards and pose a threat to patients.

Opportunity on Offer?

Concentration on the downside suggests that we have to see ourselves as the passive victims of accelerated change. But there is also opportunity in the fact that the health system is currently in a more fluid state. Old rigidities can now be dispensed with more easily, old institutions are crumbling, entrenched vested interests, dated organisational structures and inappropriately conservative practices can be attacked. A thorough shake-up in the system of health care could allow us to exploit the skills of many disciplines in an ongoing study which provides new ideas and a rational basis for reform, and to forge new alliances for action between the key players in the health system. To be closely involved in monitoring and facilitating constructive change is a moral imperative for the profession. Only then can doctors react in such a way as to block the unfavourable trends and to opportunistically reinforce the favourable, and to plan institutional change which can support positive change. Thus clinicians have an ethical obligation to develop a better understanding of what they do, and to apply this understanding to the improvement of quality of both the art and the science of medicine, and to do so with a minimum of self-interest. By enhancing the trust of the public, they will then be able to undertake a vital watchdog function.

In Chapter 2 ("The Smoke") we take a closer look at the controversy surrounding medicine. First we consider the public debate then the criticisms from within the medical profession. This controversy we see as the smoke. Where then is the fire? The fire is generated by the friction between paradigms of the players in an increasingly complex more integrated health system. No longer is medicine a cottage industry free to make its decisions as it pleases. The prediction, made some 35 years ago, that medicine would disappear as a profession has obviously not materialised. Instead there has been some change, and the creation of a period of instability.

In Chapter 3 ("More Smoke") we identify more smoke in the public reaction and political fortunes of medicine The public seems ambivalent, valuing the offerings of scientific diagnosis and treatment, generally favourably disposed towards their personal physician but unhappy with the health system. Of recent times medicine has fallen out of political favour. The major issue is cost escalation at a time of economic rationalism. We outline the changing perceptions of the general public and the strained relationship with government. We consider the contrast between the U.S. and British experience as our illustrations. The major drivers of change are cost-containment, public dissatisfaction, and concerns over rationing and the quality of care.

In Chapter 4 (The fire – thought collective, paradigm or discourse) we begin the task of exploring the fire responsible for the smoke.) In undertaking this analysis, we need to call upon the idea that groups of people, be they doctors, scientists, social scientists, health workers or all of us in society, share common goals, ideological commitments, philosophies, beliefs which, in turn, powerfully influence their behaviour and mould their institutions. We justify the use of Thomas Kuhn's term 'paradigm' to characterise such tacit systems of belief and commitment which can cause serious division between the players in health care and concerned in its evaluation. We use this term to apply to professional and academic bodies. We also use the term to describe the collective beliefs of patients, and of health bureaucrats or politicians, accepting that this constitutes a looser usage of the term but one which fits the dictionary definition.

We also apply this term to analyse the subtle but intricate reciprocal interactions between our society, medicine, and our culture as a whole. The impact of science, seen as a shift to scientific explanations of the world, beginning at the Renaissance and continuing as the Enlightenment Project. This has come under fire as 'bureaucratic,' 'technocratic' and harmful to social interaction and institutions. In medicine we shall consider the impact on patient health care, the clinical consultation on medical education and research which have an impact on public satisfaction. Medical education leads to a perspective of the doctor as an applied scientist – a view which some readily accept. In research, science has led to a strong commitment of science, first biomedical then empirical statistical, currently led by the 'evidence-based medicine' movement. With the loss of the art of medicine with recent calls for a broader narrative-based people-centred orientation, and a biopsychosocial model.

We also introduce the notion of the influential research paradigms which permeate academic disciplines and professions, influencing in particular their approach to research and evaluation. These we call the 'scientific analytical' and the 'interpretive humanistic paradigms' respectively. Seen as opposing perspectives with very different methods of research, these are a common source of conflict. The scientific analytical paradigm is reductionistic, quantitative and universal. The interpretive humanistic paradigm is holistic, qualitative and contextual. Some health disciplines have a commitment to one or the other. Some such as sociology and clinical medicine are internally divided by a commitment to both paradigms. More recently 'systems thinking' has evolved as an instrument or tactic for understanding complexity, including that of the social world. Systems thinking is beginning to have an impact on clinical thinking, especially in the crucial area of continuous quality improvement. It is a useful tool for predicting the shape of postmodern medicine with the necessary compromises.

In Chapter 5 (The classical paradigm of medicine) we discuss in detail the classical paradigm of medicine dating from ancient Greece, which has evolved as it adapted to cultural change over more than two millennia. Our justification for devoting space to the history is that we can locate the roots of problems confronting us today - reliance on clinical experience to the exclusion of scientific evidence, medical authoritarianism, lack of communication, and tendency to intervention. The paradigm has been largely incorporated into the modern paradigm as the 'art of medicine.' Aspects of it have come into conflict with science and with the beliefs and attitudes of patients, as we have already asserted. Hence it is important to understand its scope and influence.

Chapter 6 (Modern paradigm of medicine) describes the shift from the ancient classical to the modern scientific paradigm. Medicine's commitment to the humanities has been largely replaced by an engagement to science. This paradigm shift, a societal and political sea change which occurred in the context of the French Revolution, was accompanied by a fundamental change in the clinical model of illness, and a shift of the centre of gravity of medical influence into the teaching hospital. It is important to understand these events because we can locate some of clinical medicine's problems today in the inappropriate subjugation of the art by the science, and equally inappropriate resistance of the clinical to appropriate scientific refinement.

Chapter 7 ("Paradigms Close to Medicine") is devoted to discussion of the paradigms of public health, the social sciences and humanities which are being brought into contact with the medical paradigm more and more in the context of public debate and the evaluation of clinical care. Medicine and public health have complementary perspectives representing the interests of the individual and of the population respectively. Medicine is now seen as having got too much credit for the decline in community mortality and morbidity in the late 19th and early 20th century. Public health was used as a political instrument to diminish the power of clinical medicine in the French Revolution; it is currently involved in the evaluation of clinical care and coming into conflict with medicine in this capacity. Sociology has provided much of the ammunition for criticism of medicine. However, cooperation with clinicians is essential if the perspectives of patients and doctors are to be reconciled. Economists too have been critical of doctors. They need to understand the complexity and uncertainty of clinical practice if they are to have a positive influence.

Chapter 8 (Alternative medicine – paradigmatic conflict) Here we consider the case of alternative medicine. There are several reasons for discussing this topic. The first is that alternative medicine is a classical example of a subjugated paradigm in our society. The second is the contention over how to evaluate its claims to efficacy, which raises the concrete problem of a clash of paradigms, with alternative medicine claiming patient satisfaction and Western medicine demanding randomized trials. The third is that such evaluations provide good training in a demanding area of research for reflective physicians in the centre for the study of clinical practice. The fourth is that there could be sufficient rapprochement for alternative medicine; thus increased attention paid to supportive care could at least prod medicine into lifting its game, faced by truly complementary medicine.

Chapter 9 ("Clinical Inefficiency") We next discuss 'clinical inefficiency,' a discussion of how a commitment to traditional thinking has limited the potential contributions of science to clinical practice - a clash of the art and science components of the paradigm of medicine. Clinicians have been slow to invoke science to minimise error which is ubiquitous in clinical practice. Unexplained variations in patient care and evidence of inappropriate intervention cast doubt on the validity of clinical judgements. Specific problems have been studied, particularly statistical misunderstandings. Common adverse events in hospital practice attract publicity and criticism. Almost all of the research in this area has been undertaken from the top-down, from the community perspective. However, there is doubt about the validity of the retrospective methods used, hence an urgent need for clinicians to mount their own prospective studies in clinical practice.

Chapter 10 (Consultation failure – genesis) introduces the notion of 'consultation failure' whereby a lack of communication and support can leave patients dissatisfied, and impair treatment and health outcome. We see how too strong a dose of scientific training can impair the function of the doctor in the clinical care of ambulant patients where most medicine is practised. The educational curriculum of modern medicine isolated the preliminary training in science from subsequent clinical training and socialisation. This set up a clash of paradigms within medicine. Modern doctors became bemused by dint of their commitment to science in the face of the complexities of practice in ambulant care which require also the skills of the art reinforced by the social sciences. The doctor trained in hospitals to detect and treat organic disease is in danger of being swamped by symptoms related to problems of living and psychological distress. This debate has recently been sharpened by conflict between physicians and the advocates of 'evidence-based medicine' which has been accused of denigrating the role of clinical judgement and the art of medicine.

Chapter 11 (Consultation failure - symptoms) explores in more detail the consequences of the failure of the clinical consultation to achieve its basic objectives resulting in the 'symptoms' of consultation failure - patient dissatisfaction, noncompliance with treatment, failure of reassurance of the 'worried well,' and the rise of patient advocacy and alternative medicine. Each of these problems has proved controversial and, especially in the case of non-compliance, refractory to attempts at better understanding and improvement. The reason is that we do not understand these problems from the patient's perspective, do not perceive the interaction of variables which underpins patient judgements as opposed to those of the physician. Studies involving interview of patients and qualitative data analysis are needed if we are to develop the better understanding required for successful solution of these 'wicked problems.'

Chapter 12 ("The Evaluation of Health Care"). The clash of paradigms, within medicine and between medicine and related disciplines, not only leads to friction, discontent and criticism. Medicine is nowadays subjected to external scrutiny. Its evaluation is also subject to conflict between disciplinary paradigms. Early medical audit based upon self regulation have been overtaken by the evaluation of clinical practice from above by health bureaucracies. This runs the risk of distortion and failure because the vital perspective of the medical paradigm which clinicians should bring to the debate is all too often missing. The disciplines of health technology assessment, effectiveness and health outcomes research all have, in the main, a policy perspective. Quality assurance was for a long time a medical discipline but is now of interest to health bureaucracy and managed care. Clinical epidemiology and evidence-based medicine had clinical origins but are now also central to health services research. The boundary fences between these disciplines are being lowered but each has a unique perspective to offer. The objective is a seamless cooperative form of multidisciplinary continuous clinical practice research linked to health services with a community perspective such as we outline in the last chapter.

Chapters 13 and 14 (The impact of which kind of science and with what effect). In the time of Hippocrates in ancient Greece, critical rational thinking extended to medicine, resulting in 'traditional Hippocratic western medicine' although the view of illness itself remained to some extent superstitious. Only 2000 years later, in the 19th century, following the French Revolution, did scientific thinking prevail to transform society and medicine. Progress in the 'basic' disciplines of anatomy and pathology had made some progress but the pace accelerated, bacteriology transformed traditional to 'modern' medicine via revealing the cause of disease – or so it seemed! Statistics allowed one pioneering clinical bedside clinical trial then evaluation lapsed, and epidemiology was picked up by public health. A branch of mathematics vital to the concept of disease and its treatment was 'taxonomy,' the scientific classification of species always part of clinical medicine but revived only last century. Another important change in scientific thinking was that the basic notion of 'evidence' was radically transformed and came to mean 'supported by empirical observation,' not by the opinion of ancient authorities.

An important adverse effect of the positivistic philosophy of 'scientism' was to rigidly follow philosopher Rene Descartes' separation of body and emotions for so long. As a result of his traditional total embrace of rationality with rejection of any impact of the emotions seen as either unimportant in decision making or as having an adverse effect. This idea dominated decision-making theory, and in the realm of academe, especially economics. This resulted in a theory – 'maximimisation of expected utility'- based on an extraordinarily narrow, totally rationalistic point of view which excluded potentially powerful emotional influences on decisions obvious enough to the thoughtful layperson! Subsequent research in a range of disciplines has thoroughly discredited such a myopic perspective but the stigma still seems to live on in some circles. There is surely no call for debate on the importance of the emotions which can dominate some important decisions.

Research has been impeded by rejection of the potential contribution of the social sciences, and especially by a narrow, excessively quantitative view of clinical research. The result has been truncation of the clinical research program to the detriment of the social and humanistic aspects of care. Importantly too, a lack of application of 'qualitative' research needed to understand the decisions of doctors and patients such as is necessary to tackle the basic problems of patient dissatisfaction, failure of cooperation with treatment and rise of alternative medicine - to mention but a few! The impact of medical education virtually to the quantitative analytical paradigm with marginalization of the interpretive contextual approach has also had obvious restrictive effects since the social sciences and humanities have been sidelined for most of a century. We discuss also the way in which governments and other bureaucracies can use numbers as an alternative to the often much more arduous task of obtaining community consensus. There has also been the recent burgeoning of 'evidence-based medicine' which has delivered some benefits but created much friction as well (Ch13).

Disagreement extends to the process of diagnosis seen as simply computation, a serious oversimplification of a complex iterative, dialectical process of interpretation reliant on the recognition of patterns of illness features. Clinicians use taxonomy and classification, 'the principal scientific basis of clinical medicine,' as a means of handling complexity. We shall see that the rise of science has also had a downside so far as the image of clinical practice was concerned, seen as a scientistic, analytical view of the diagnostic process, a distorted view of it as a computational exercise, whereas there is strong evidence that most expertise has an unconscious basis in the form of 'intuitive' or 'tacit' thinking. Thus iconic clinician William Osler likened the patient to a text which is read by the doctor (Hunter 1991), hence much closer to the humanities, and to the methods of qualitative research. It is time to stop worshipping what we, often erroneously, imagine science to be. In addition, trauma to the art of medicine is blamed with damage to the 'art' of supportive care.

For a long time, the 'mind-body split' ruled such that the conventional wisdom was that decision-making under conditions of uncertainty was an entirely rational affair. Much recent research too has thoroughly discredited this idea. The current view is that the emotions play a central role in decision-making with guidance from past experience. There are important implications here for clinical practice and research. The new data supports the clinician's contention that clinical judgement remains at the heart of rational management of patients.

Chapter 15 ("Evidence-Based Medicine – The Clash with Clinical Medicine") Largely because of its dismissive attitude to clinical evidence, especially the 'soft data,' and role in evaluation of health services, raising the bete noir of coercion, evidence-based medicine is at odds with clinicians. A healthy debate in a spirit of good will must eventually lead to rapprochement. Operations research for evaluations other fields has proved useful in constrained contexts but unsuccessful in the more complex fields of the evaluation of social institutions, social planning and political decision-making. The distraction of science has led to a charge of lack of humanistic supportive care; the scope of this reaction can be gauged from the appearance of so many movements to restore supportive patient care such as the biopsychosocial model and patient-centred clinical care.

The most serious criticism has been that evidence-based medicine espouses an unrealistically narrow definition of clinical 'evidence,' when in fact a large number of variables are clearly involved. Those factors carrying most weight in the judgement will obviously depend on the specifics of the particular patient and illness. Only a much broader perspective, a more inclusive and comprehensive 'postmodern' medical paradigm can rectify this deficiency. Evidence-based medicine promotes healthy scepticism about the efficacy of interventions. This has led critics to insist that it too is a technology which must be rigorously evaluated. Nonetheless, evidence-based' practice is surely the flavor of the month. Many disciplines claim that their practice is or should be 'evidence-based of medicine' but this leaves no room for tacit knowledge underpinning the art of a practice. A common error is to fail to clearly distinguish between two terms used for validity of evidence. The term 'internal validity' has been coined to mean approximation of evidence to the truth, applicable to a randomized trial.

'External validity,' the complementary concept, is used to describe the extent to which the experimental result can 'generalised' to similar situations or to individual patients. Important 'soft data' can be captured by converting qualitative information into quantitative indices. There is some hope that evidence-based and traditional medicine in the emerging 'postmodern paradigm, so that patients can benefit from both schools of thought or intellectual paradigms.

In Chapter 16 ("Postmodern Medicine"): What is ultimately needed is a major cultural shift to postmodern times. As a major organ of society, medicine will not be spared the pain of this transition. We will argue that the details of a new paradigm of medicine cannot be predicted. Because we cannot predict the unexpected, we emphasise instead the comprehensive ongoing program of truly clinical research which must guide progress, and the central role of the reflective physician in driving this process and interpreting its significance. In addition to trends already perceptible, like all complex dynamic systems, health care will throw up unanticipated oftentimes unanticipatable change for which we must at least be alert and prepared, striving to maintain a steady sense of direction. We can continue to create and reinforce favourable current trends. When major unexpected trends to the good emerge, as they will, we must move quickly to exploit and reinforce them, to turn them to the best advantage of patients, the community and clinicians. These will be the difficulties confronting those who would evaluate evidence-based medicine. There can be no more excuses. This new discipline must be subjected to a through iterative program of evaluation like any other complex technology. Information technology also provides a similar paradigm case of the approach to the evaluation of a complex clinical intervention, and warning of the intricacies and difficulties involved. These changes will also be catalysed by the impact of information technology on the organisation of health care in general. Essentially, the evaluation by clinical practice research and continuous quality improvement are the same evaluation process with simply a different focus.

Key tasks for clinicians are to engage in quality assurance, to evaluate medical technologies to develop a comprehensive clinical taxonomy and definitions of terms, apply clinical epidemiology, evidence based medicine and engage the insights of sociology and the humanities in multidisciplinary research – 'clinical practice research,' in order to research and evaluate the clinical process of diagnosis and management. Major changes include enhancement of quality of care, based upon scientific evidence and humanistic scholarship, focused on patient wishes and needs, with improved access and better coordination of care, facilitated by information technology.

Chapter 17 (The reflective practitioner, clinical practice research and the centre for the study of clinical practice): Here we wrap up our argument. The centrepiece is the reflective physician, a lifelong learner who engages in and coordinates clinical practice research, and teaches with university staff. The centre for the study of clinical practice, guided by a steering committee, will train these practitioners, provide leadership in clinical research, a forum for interdisciplinary discussion and a repository of research methods and statistical expertise. Its basic objectives are to bring to bear on the ongoing study of clinical practice the methods and skills of clinical epidemiology and evidence based medicine, of the behavioural and social sciences and of the humanities. Biomedical research will no doubt continue its successful trajectory.

This involves the hospital in setting up the centre, which strengthens its evaluative and research capabilities. The scope of the centre is intended to complement the university curriculum in encouraging study of the 'humanistic' aspects underpinning clinical care of patients. These are issues have been brought to the fore by the increasing success of alternative medicine, and the advent of patient-centred, humanistic and integrative medicine, all of which are predicated upon recovering what many see as the loss of the humanistic perspective, central to the art of medicine so important to patient satisfaction.

This book has two major themes. The first is that clinical medicine, and the health care system in which it is imbedded, are on the cusp of a shift from the modern to the postmodern. There will be opportunity for major reforms. This will, however, require clearer understanding of the genesis of medicine's current problems. The second proposition is that much of the current friction and turbulence surrounding health care is a consequence of tacit belief systems, and that we are part of a shift to a postmodern paradigm. After careful consideration of alternatives, we have used the Kuhnian concept of 'paradigm' to analyse these tensions. We begin our analysis in the next chapter by examining what critics within the profession and without have had to say of recent years - this can be seen as the 'smoke of battle.' In the following chapter, we examine the stocks of medicine with the public and government and find more smoke.

Chapter 2

The Smoke - Complaint, Criticism, Controversy, Conflict

A central point of our argument in this book is that the skills and insights of clinicians are an indispensable ingredient of any attempt to build a better and cheaper system of patient care. If the current welter of change can be understood, there will be opportunities presented by a system in flux grounded in the realities of day-to-day care in the doctor's office, outpatient clinic and at the bedside. Understanding of the processes of clinical care will be misleading or incomplete, reform will be impeded because of lack of the cooperation of those at the coal face which is needed for implementation of constructive change impossible to achieve in the earlier time of stability. Doctors must assume a leadership role in improving the quality of care and develop better channels of communication with the other key players. In order to do this, they must listen to the criticisms and interpret the controversies embroiling them. The key premise here is that strictures and regulation from without cannot alone improve the quality of health care nor constrain cost. The trick for containing costs is ultimately to improve the quality of care, especially that of clinical decision-making. This must be done by systematic research and evaluation which has the full support of the medical profession.

Smoke of Battle

On the other hand, reform of any kind will be unsuccessful if it does not address the basic concerns of those in the health system. Our objective in this chapter will therefore be to evaluate the criticisms, to locate the source of this 'smoke' which has been rising from the health care system. The rest of the book is devoted to locating the fire caused by continuing friction between art and science within the paradigm of medicine, and between those of other players in the health system squeezed ever closer together by the integrating pressures of the information society. Each has a distinctive collective worldview, a perspective, a 'paradigm' which acts as a grid to powerfully shape beliefs, objectives, intellectual activity and power relations (Chapter 4). From the public critics, I have selected some voices which have been especially influential or prescient.

The Debate Goes Public

Controversy has been politically damaging to the profession with medical dominance seen as allowing distortion of the health system, promotion of vested interests, alienation of patients and unacceptable cost escalation as the key issues among the intellectual critics. So far the cogent criticisms of health care and of the medical profession's part had been in house or confined to the cloisters of academe but this all changed with the beginning of public criticism in the mid-1970s.

Prior to the 1960s, however, scientific medicine was generally seen as a jewel in the crown of society. Doctors were becoming increasingly aware, of course, of the two-edged nature of powerful therapy, especially of the potential of the new drugs to engender side-effects, and surgical misadventure was an occasional topic of conversation. The toxicity of ionizing radiation was known, but the idea of patient harm arising from artifact or misinterpretation of an unnecessary test was almost never considered; indeed its importance is still underestimated today. The broad-ranging critiques of the medical profession and of health care which I have considered had their roots in the counterculture movement of the late 1960s and in questions of inequality and injustice raised mainly by Marxist critics. This raised two basic issues in health care. One was the idea of social control, with medicine seen as a dominant influence in society responsible for the medicalization of daily life. The second was renewed interest in the important role of social problems and of psychological factors in illness.

Nemesis or Phoenix? - The Prophesy of Ivan Illich

Ivan Illich (1974) did for health care what Nader did for the automobile industry. The specific catalyst for global criticism of medicine was his pungent polemic. Illich's attack on medicine was a landmark. The Lancet described the first three chapters as 'a volley of grapeshot across the bows of our mechanistic philosophy of health care' (Lancet review of Medical Nemesis). Despite the fact that he pilloried medicine in what is widely regarded as an intemperate analysis, Illich nevertheless gained some acknowledgement from those who replied on the part of the profession. Illich's voice was heard not only because his vitriolic attack was highly articulate and supported by impressive historical scholarship, but also because he drew together so many issues into a comprehensive critique which clearly struck a resonant chord in the community. Thus he called on the evidence for the greater effectiveness of social and public health measures vis a vis biomedical science and clinical cure, reviewed the literature on iatrogenic clinical harm and, above all, castigated the medical profession for taking advantage of its dominant position in society to extend its influence.

A Catholic priest and academic with a background in history, Illich had an axe to grind since his political agenda extended well beyond health care. He was involved in the establishment of the 'Center for Intercultural Documentation' in Mexico which held seminars on alternatives to major societal institutions. Essentially then he was concerned with the evils of over-industrialisation of which organized medicine was but one - along with education and other social institutions. As a critic of the control exerted by the modern state on the individual, he advocated 'deprofessionalization' in education, in health and in industry. He began with education (Illich 1971); following this came his foray into health.

Thus Illich accused medicine of following the technocratic imperative of the modern industrial state thereby creating problems in the form of adverse events, imposing its concepts too widely in society, and of disempowering the people by discouraging self-help and community involvement in health matters. In castigating modern medicine for inflating its role in making society healthier, thereby raising the expectations of the public, Illich drew on the earlier ideas including those of Dubos (1960). He went further, however, by claiming that the net impact of modern scientific medicine has been harmful. Since 'deinstitutionalization' was necessary to allow the individual greater autonomy, he saw medicine as beyond reform hence made few constructive criticisms. In fact he predicted its 'nemesis'!

At the outset, we note that Illich's analysis makes more sense if we do what he failed to do - to first acknowledge the value of certain highly effective technical interventions which, as we discussed above, are the legacy of scientific medicine which are obvious to all. He also fails to address the old chestnut of preventing exploitation of the ill by charlatans, a problem which has plagued the state in past centuries, in Britain, in France and in the United States. In France it was one of the stimuli for the very reforms which spawned scientific medicine. Illich emphasised 'iatrogenesis', broadly defined as harm induced by medicine, and divided it into 'clinical,' 'social' and 'cultural' varieties.

Clinical iatrogenesis reflected the conventional medical usage of the term to describe the side-effects of medical treatment, now commonly referred to as adverse events, most commonly arising from the use of drugs or surgery. In this, Illich simply drew attention to what is now acknowledged to be an important problem of scientific medicine as well as a potent issue for litigation. In retrospect his focus on the problems of clinical practice was actually far too narrow. Patient dissatisfaction and harm can, in fact, arise as a result of a wide variety of adverse consequences. Harmful side-effects of drugs and patently ill-advised or demonstrably unnecessary surgery are one thing. Serious harm can arise in more subtle ways, including the unnecessary use of diagnostic tests and misinterpretation of normal findings. By identifying 'clinical iatrogenesis' in the form of side-effects of treatment, Illich recognized only the tip of the iceberg.

We should note that most patients suffer no such ill-effects of a physical or psychological nature. They are often simply dissatisfied because they have been at cross purposes with their doctor. The modern doctor, lacking the necessary communication skills and preoccupied with organic disease and technology, is often singularly ill-equipped for dealing with the symptoms arising from problems of living, and for distinguishing these from the effects of organic disease with which they feel more at home. Yet the need for this kind of supportive care has got greater not less. The upshot is pervasive 'clinical inefficiency' contingent upon faulty clinical decisions and unwarranted interventions (Chapter 9), and mismatch between the expectations of the patient and the objectives of the doctor - 'consultation failure,' (Chapters 10 and 11). This in turn translates also into lack of cooperation with treatment which can damage health. If he had been aware of the extent of these problems, Illich might have required less rhetoric to convince the public of some of the more serious problems of medicine.

Illich's social iatrogenesis refers to harm attributable to the social and political influence of the medical profession which is even less direct. This includes the intrusion of medical influence and ideas into the affairs of daily living. This phenomenon covers a multitude of sins which we have already discussed as part of the sociological critique. One of the most important is the crucial function of acting as gatekeeper to the sick role. Related phenomena are the bureaucratic definition of illness and labelling of patients with disease diagnoses. Also singled out were population screening and routine physical examinations, of unproven effectiveness and prone to diagnostic error and its consequences, the medicalization of old age and of dying. Inappropriate treatment of the terminally ill was a special target, vividly encapsulated by his statement that 'dying has become the ultimate form of consumer resistance' (Illich 1974).

Finally, his cultural iatrogenesis, a more metaphorical usage, referred to a process whereby self-reliance is discouraged and an unhealthy dependence on the medical profession is promoted instead, with the result that lay people become disempowered and deskilled, robbed of their capacity for self-help and of the satisfaction of autonomous coping. Illich went even further by implying that submission to pain has value in itself as ascetic self-purification!

It is surprising that Illich did not accuse medicine of being in breach of its responsibilities by failing to draw attention to the overriding importance of social class in predisposition to illness and premature death. Over the years since Medical Nemesis was written, there has been some adaptive change in response to criticism. Thus there has been much discussion at least of a more cooperative doctor-patient relationship with 'patient-centred' clinical consultations, calls for a broader 'biopsychosocial model' for medicine, pressures for changes in medical education, even some evidence of ebbing of the dominance of the doctor in clinical care with a trend towards teamwork. There is evidence too of some loosening of the ties between medicine and the state. But there has not been anything resembling 'deprofessionalization' or of 'proletarianization' of the profession. Medicine has not met its Nemesis, as Illich predicted - scarcely surprising given that it is difficult to imagine such radical change occurring in isolation from major social and cultural upheaval.

We could perhaps draw an analogy between Illich's gloomy prognosis for medicine and Karl Marx's grim predictions of revolution in capitalist industrial society. Just as adaptive responses of the corporate state and industry have deflected some criticism of capitalism by correcting more glaring inequities and excesses, so too have numerous small and scarcely revolutionary changes in medicine and health care have had a similar effect by muting the voices demanding change. This should not be taken to imply that Illich's broadside was without effect any more than we could say this of Das Kapital!

However, perhaps detailed criticism of his position misses the point. Surely his intention was to be provocative. Illich essentially spoke as a social revolutionary. He dismissed, as unlikely to succeed, major reform measures such as regulation of standards, control over professional organization, measures to ensure equitable distribution of care, derestriction of alternative medicine, and a broader social and environmental focus of health. In fact, less radical reforms than the abolition of medicine, especially 'band-aid' reforms initiated from within, Illich might well have seen as blunting the revolutionary drive while leaving control in the hands of medicine. That he believed that this is so is suggested by his subsequent comments. He now was more critical of the 'superstitious reshaping of society and culture through the internalisation of medicine's myths' (Illich 1995). He no longer blamed medicalisation for the 'lifelong concern with self-diagnosis, self-regulation, and anxiously prognostic self-treatment,' and for the inability to accept death. He therefore shifted most of the blame to Western culture and the technical slant of its social construction of health.

Navarro and Waitzkin

Illich's synthesis of earlier criticisms and research crystallized the issues, stimulated public debate and was a catalyst for change. Criticisms of his work have generated further insights. Two medically trained health sociologists, Navarro and Waitzkin replied publicly to Illich. Navarro spelt out the differences between Illich's critique based on the problems of industrialism and the Marxist position which identifies class and the capitalist system as the culprit. For the industrialist ideology, the bureaucracy is the new elite and the values served are 'productivity, efficiency, progress and modernization' (Navarro 1976). The bureaucrat is heir to the capitalist's leadership. The capitalist and socialist state converge on the industrial model. Illich subscribed to the view that society can be debureaucratized and deprofessionalized, with a return to individual autonomy. The conflict is then one between the medical bureaucracy and the patients who have had their work alienation defined as illness, and been robbed of their independence and autonomy in matters of health.

In Navarro's view, liberal and socialist solutions would be counterproductive since they simply provide more of the same medical care more widely distributed (Navarro 1976). The alternative view is that it is the consumerism inculcated in the capitalist country, which is at the root of patient dependence on medicine, is also in a position to define its 'needs.' The hierarchical structure of society is determined mainly by class and sex roles, so that medicine and the other professions are essentially technologies administered by bureaucracies operating according to these rules. In this sense, to attack the bureaucratic distortions attributed to medicine by attempts at deprofessionalization would tackle the symptom not the disease. Debureaucratization cannot therefore be the answer. Nonetheless, the anti-industrialist creed has attractions for the state and for the medical profession. By locating problems in personal behaviour of autonomous individuals, important social issues can be evaded and behavior modification substituted for political action. Waitzkin (1976) too saw Illich's position as focusing too much on the individual. This diverts attention from the social factors in health and to this extent limits the responsibility of the state and encourages cutbacks in social programs.

Horrobin

Apart from the reviews of his book, the initial response from the medical profession to Illich's challenge was silence. Few practising doctors appear to have read the book; some have dismissed it as the ravings of a radical. Two doctors, Horrobin (1977) and Dollery (1978), did mount a response. Neither could be seen as simply 'defenders of the faith.' Not surprisingly, neither agreed with Illich's major thesis that the medical profession should be abolished, but each saw the need for reform and accepted some of his argument. The debate here has hinged on specific criticisms of medicine and of health care, and on the extent that the medical profession should be held as blameworthy for the problems raised. As might be expected, the broader sociological issues of industrialism and of Marxist interpretation did not feature in the medical debate.

Horrobin, a psychiatrist, accepted Illich's contribution as a 'brilliant polemic,' conceding its importance as a critique of medicine likely to influence politics, and recognizing its broader target of the excesses of industrialized society. However, the argument he saw as 'over-dramatic,' sometimes in breach of commonsense and experience, the suggested solutions impractical. He noted the lack of empirical evidence to suggest that the public wants less medical care rather than more, or that there is a willingness to take more personal responsibility for health and to enjoy it, or to submit to pain and derive spiritual benefit from it. The author he describes as 'one of Plato's Guardians, a clever, good man who knows what the people need but is unwilling to take undue notice of what they might want.' (Horrobin 1977).

Horrobin concedes too that health care has been inequitably delivered, that medicine should confine its activities to those areas 'where its effectiveness is genuine,' and that people should enjoy more autonomy in health care but insisted that a modern democracy does promote better health than in the past and that most people enjoy 'a reasonable state of well-being.' Horrobin disputes that people are capable of handling much of their illness by themselves and that they wish to return to some primitive arrangement. The loss of the holistic approach to clinical care is regrettable but is a problem which has been at least acknowledged by the profession. Some medical contributions to public health should have been acknowledged, and some iatrogenic effects were grossly exaggerated. He agrees that there has been undue reliance on technology, some of dubious benefit, and that there is a need for its evaluation. Illich's attitude to relief of pain Horrobin regarded as highly philosophical and rather impractical.

Horrobin accepts Illich's version of the dominant position of medicine with respect to the definition of illness and its ramifications vis a vis the claim of alienation in an over-industrialized society. However, he saw this dominance as the result of cultural change brought about by the perception that death could be postponed by medical intervention as well, as respect for science and the obvious effectiveness of some treatment. While conceding the problems of medical dominance he exonerates the profession of the charge of having sought this, rather the power was acquired 'in a fit of absent mindedness' (Horrobin 1977). Horrobin's most fundamental disagreement with Illich is that he rejected the inevitability of 'nemesis,' believing that the most important reform is only feasible from within, and likely to be piecemeal and evolutionary rather than radical bureaucratization.

Dollery

Another physician drawn into the fray was Dollery, Professor of Clinical Pharmacology, Royal Postgraduate School, The University of London, an academic clinician and biomedical scientist (Dollery 1978). His mandate as Rock Carling Fellow of the Nuffield Provincial Hospitals Trust was to address criticisms of medical science by Illich and by other critics of scientific medicine. The major charges he addressed were of conspiracy against the public, unethical research, inflated claims of improving community health, inhuman application of medical technology, failure to evaluate its effectiveness, and of neglecting research into the application of health care in the community. The problem of iatrogenic illness he accepted, but Illich's charge of conspiracy, he deplored as overstatement and irrational, and he highlighted the positives - the curative achievements of medicine and capacity for self criticism. Dollery did not, however, come to grips with the underlying issue of the dominance of medicine in the health care system, its consequences of social and cultural iatrogenesis, and the resentment it has engendered. In answer to earlier charges of a callous lack of ethics in medical research, especially of failure to obtain adequate informed consent, Dollery acknowledged some past sins, accepted the problem of 'technological inhumanity' but emphasized the more recent development of ethics committees. He also accepted Cochrane's call for the formal evaluation of health technology, attributing failure to do so in the past to medical credulity together with a dash of deceitfulness.

By suggesting improved epidemiological training of medical scientists as an appropriate response, Dollery anticipates the impending blossoming of interest in 'clinical epidemiology' and 'evidence-based medicine,' and the rise of the new discipline of 'technology assessment' in North America. On the other hand, taking exception to the condemnation of technology by both Illich and Horrobin, he makes a particular point of extolling the virtues of modern imaging technology, and took issue with the position of Thomas McKeown (1962) which contested the importance of the contribution of clinical medicine to improvements in community health and longevity. The overriding problem of the relationship of illness to social class, age, handicap and deprivation receives oblique mention only as a problem of drug non-compliance.

Le Fanu

A physician and journalist, in his monograph 'The Rise and Fall of Modern Medicine,' Le Fanu makes a case for a progressive decline in medicine which, he believes, reached a peak around 1970. In particular he draws attention to a slowing of clinical research, stalling of technological innovation, the iatrogenic effects of much epidemiological research, and to exaggerated claims made for genetic research "a relentless catalogue of failed aspirations." (Le Fanu 2013). Having completed a demolition job, not surprisingly he does not attempt to propose cure on such a broad front.

Taylor

Perhaps the best summary of the problems of medicine as seen from within the profession but with a broad public health perspective can be found in Taylor (1979). Writing some 5 years later than Illich, the lurid title notwithstanding – 'Medicine Out Of Control: The Anatomy Of A Malignant Technology' - Taylor took a measured critical attitude towards the medical profession. He saw medicine as a microcosm of the wider society, suggesting that change will be evolutionary rather than revolutionary. He summarised evidence for the importance of social and environmental factors in illness which should be recognized by clinicians when treating patients and public health doctors when planning health promotion and disease prevention.

He traced the current dominance of individual care to evolution from the earlier practice of 'physik' by the university-trained doctor providing care for the rich to modern scientific medicine which created an insatiable need for medical care. The emphasis on science and technology was, however, an important factor in 'medicalization' which drew the minor ailment and social problem into the orbit of medicine and of general practice in particular, which encouraged excessive use of drugs including 'pills for personal problems.' As an insider, he was aware of the more subtle problems of inappropriate use of tests creating problems of labelling, and the creation of 'non-disease.'

Just as war has been said to be too important to leave the generals, Taylor was correct in his prediction that pressures for change would come from many quarters, from government and political parties, from health insurers and departments of social and preventive medicine, from social scientists including economists, from systems analysts and from patients' rights groups. Reforms would be based on increased emphasis on prevention, correction of maldistribution of doctors and of facilities, abolition of fee-for-service practice, together with the containment of therapeutic medicine to handle the biomedical problems which it handles best but subject to scientific evaluation.

Carlson

There were other critics who explored the significance of Illich's critique for the health system as a whole. One who advocated radical change in health care was Carlson, an attorney (Carlson 1975). The Preface of the book was written by Illich, and like that author, he believed that 'the end of medicine is near.' His net of criticism is widely spread and encompasses much of the territory covered by Illich. His motivation for writing the book appears to have been the assumption that the establishment of some kind of National Health Service in the United States was imminent and his strong attack was therefore directed toward exerting some influence on events. Carlson advocates a broader paradigm of health care comprising an ecological approach with more emphasis on disease prevention and environmental improvements, backed up by increasing research on the relationship between health and lifestyle and better definitions of health.

However, like Illich, Carlson does not address the thorny issues of poverty, propensity to illness and politics. He openly acknowledges the positive contributions of medicine and incorporates what he sees as the best of medical science into his suggestions for reform. These hinge upon increased patient autonomy contingent on health education, wider availability of certain drugs and simple medical equipment, and deprofessionalization to the extent of allowing certification but not licensure for practice. Scientific medicine would be retained to cater for the acutely ill and appropriate illness, coexisting with alternative practices. A hierarchical system of neighborhood hospitals cum education centres, regional health centres and accommodation for the elderly would be served by health teams. Indeed this appears to be the first global and radical criticism which has even attempted to propose solutions.

Kennedy

A widely quoted critique was that of Ian Kennedy, a lawyer and ethicist who delivered the BBC Reith lectures subsequently published under the title 'The Unmasking of Medicine' (Kennedy, 1981). The territory he covered was similar to that of Illich and Carlson but his tone was much more moderate, his perception largely ethical. His major focus was on the need for medicine's greater accountability to the individual patient as consumer and especially to the wider society. Nevertheless, perhaps because of sensitization attributable to Illich's earlier charges, perhaps because of the wide public exposure given a BBC production, he did receive a lot of criticism. Kennedy identified the root metaphor of mechanism which underpins the reductionist approach of biomedical sciences as the fundamental cause of underestimation of the importance of social and environmental factors in the genesis of illness.

Kennedy thought that doctors who saw themselves as scientists would therefore be unwilling to tackle the problems, so that corrective political action would be needed. He addressed a wide range of other issues, most of which had been raised by earlier critics. These included medicalization of life, the emphasis on behaviour modification which risks blaming the victim, the need to integrate individual with community care, unemployment as a risk factor for illness, problems of definition and handling of mental illness, the problems of technology. Kennedy's suggestions for improvement, less than radical, were that people should take more responsibility in health matters and expect greater public accountability from the medical profession.

Shorter and Reiser

Several historians, one of them medically trained, have analysed the problems of modern medicine. Physician historian Reiser (1978) documented in detail the impact of technology on the culture, the clinical techniques and research orientation. He also documents the reactions of clinicians to the growth of influence of science and technology. Historian Edward Shorter (1985) documented the drift of modern internal medicine from its reliance on the therapeutic effects of the clinical consultation to preoccupation with technology. Most people value a good relationship with their own doctor. The medical profession also places great stress on this relationship, sometimes to protect its own interest, but also recognizing that faith in the doctor is a crucial element in the art of medicine allowing effective support, often improving symptoms, even hastening cure.

Shorter concluded that medicine in a technological age had increasingly lost sight of the power of the medical consultation as an important therapeutic weapon. With the advent of the welfare state and health insurance, there has been a massive expansion in the proportion of the population seeking medical care for less pressing symptoms, with functional illness. This is precisely the kind of patient for whom the consultation and the support of the ancient art of medicine has most therapeutic benefit to offer. Ironically, the success of medicine and opening the gates of individual medical care to the population at large has coincided with a decline in the very tool that the doctor most needs in dealing with the common functional symptoms, and in the general management of any patient whatever the disease might be.

Odegaard

Charles Odegaard (1986), historian, addresses the split between the humanities, to which medicine owed its allegiance for two thousand years, and science with which it has been seen to increasingly throw in its lot during the last two centuries. His historical account provides a strong counter-argument to those who believe that rigorous thinking is synonymous with the natural and biological sciences. Modern intellectual rigour grew out of a revolution in universities in Germany. Strict rules for acceptance of evidence as valid and similar rules for interpretation of written texts, part of the Graeco-Roman heritage, blossoming during the Renaissance, was developed in Prussian universities early in the 19th century. Indeed the research imperative involved the humanities before the natural sciences. This division between the natural and biological sciences on the one hand and the humanities on the other is more profound in Britain and Australia, in the United States and Canada than in Europe. French and German usage, on the other hand, applies a definition of 'science' which can be applied to all domains of knowledge, nature and of man.

Odegaard argues that modern scientific medicine is based on silent assumptions whereby disease seen as a specific biological entity with a specific aetiology, and the doctor is seen as a bioscientist (Odegaard 1986). This conception, of course, totally ignores the social nature of medicine and its involvement in the political sphere, emphasized by Virchow and which are obvious enough to anyone who cares to look. Odegaard shows just how deep this cleavage runs. Not only are the natural and biological sciences split off from the humanities but the social sciences, in turn, have themselves split partly off from the humanities in an attempt to emulate the success of classical science. The strong early education of the doctor in the basic biomedical sciences according to the Flexnerian medical curriculum tends to diminish the importance of the social sciences and humanities, and to engender prejudice against their methods. And this in spite of the fact that the disciplined reasoning and rules of evidence generally thought of as the hallmarks of 'scientific thinking' were actually developed first in the humanities!

Katz

Freedom of communication between doctor and patient is crucial to the success of the clinical interview, to the cause of 'humanistic' medicine, to medical ethics and to the public image of the profession. Katz (1984), a medically trained legal academic, has shown how the debate over informed consent has actually probed to the heart of the doctor-patient relationship, exposing powerful historical forces extending way back to Hippocrates - who advised that treatment should normally be conducted 'concealing most things from the patient while you are attending him.' The legal challenge to medicine in the form of patient rights and informed consent have therefore come into conflict with tacit assumptions of clinical practice which have deep roots. Katz's thesis is that doctors have been socialized by their training to oppose free exchange of information with patients and sharing of medical decisions. This ideology he attributes to the strongly held belief that faith and trust in the doctor, central to the art of medicine, is an important part of the healing process and certainly not conducive to the idea of joint decisions sought in the name of patient rights.

Jacob

Jacob, a sociologist, offers further interesting insights into the way in which the law has flushed out the incompatibility between the traditional ethical stance of medicine on disclosure of information and ideas of patient autonomy (Jacob 1987). These ideas were derived from Kant's Categorical Imperative which states that the fundamental consideration in such a social transaction is the worth of the individual person. This emphasis on individual autonomy is in some conflict with the paternalistic stance of Hippocratic ethics with the traditional emphasis on trust as the central requirement for healing. This, of course, has also been challenged by the technocratic social context and the rise of scientific medicine which defines cure simply as successful treatment of disease or injury.

Jacob saw the need for the excesses of the medical profession in this regard to be curbed without destroying the essence of the profession by reducing doctors to the role of mere experts which would indeed be their fate after 'deprofessionalization.' Jacob believed, however, that 'the rules governing medical practice can only be drawn up by those who have a sense in depth of what the functions of the profession are.'(Jacob 1987). The radical sociological critique which sees a deal between government and profession as simply involving mutual self-interest is therefore a serious oversimplification of an outsider who does not recognize the 'internal normative order.' Jacob advocates that medicine be refurbished and restored rather than an attempt made to rebuild its paradigm by external pressure. Hence excessive government intervention and legislation could result in the baby being thrown out with the bath water.

Osler, Cabot, Mackenzie

While sociological, historical and economic analyses have generally provided a sharp focus for criticism of the handling of health matters in society as well as ammunition for the critics, when it came to recognition of these side-effects of scientific and technological progress, however, it was the perceptive clinicians who led the way. There were physicians such as Osler and Peabody and also Cabot, one of the 'Holistic Elite' in 1920s North America who were worried about the decline in the art of medicine during the first decade of this century well before the new biomedical paradigm had become fully established their concerns included about the excessively technological face of modern medicine and the neglect of the psychological and social perspective on illness (Reiser 1978). Mackenzie in Britain, whose experience in general practice and as pioneer specialist had taught him about the gap between the physical signs of disease and his patient's symptoms, between biomedical explanation and human understanding. Late in his career, he established his Institute for Medical Research with the objective of investigating the natural history of minor symptoms and maladies so common in general practice (Mackenzie 1919). Much later, Bernard Lown put it elegantly when he said: 'Healing is best accomplished when art and science are conjoined, when body and spirit are probed together.'(Lown 1996).

Winternitz

Beginning in the 1920s, Winternitz planned to set up a multidisciplinary Institute of Human Relations at Yale (Visiltear 1984) which was to provide courses in sociology, economics, psychology, religion, law and government for medical students, as well as promoting interdisciplinary research. Arguably well before its time, the experiment failed. Nonetheless, his plan was evidence of incisive insight into perceived deficiencies in the medical curriculum at about the same time that Flexner had expressed his concern at the deficiency of the 'human dimension' in the curriculum.

Magraw and Magraw

Among the earliest to appreciate the full magnitude and extent of the problems facing medicine were Magraw and Magraw (1966). What they wrote was perceptive and, in some cases, prescient. They would be probably be surprised and disappointed to know that their concerns have, in the main, remained just that. Their major objective was to restate the mission of medicine in the face of what they saw as a loss of faith by patients, of a decline in the doctors' autonomy and prestige, and in the face of a cloud gathering over medicine in the form of forces for change. The doctor-patient relationship, at the heart of medical practice, involved a contract which gave the physician authority to treat and required trust in the patient in the context of an honest exchange. The Magraws recognized the doctor as a therapeutic agent, provided this was not used as a refuge for ignorance. The Magraws were aware of the complexities of patient presentation before this had become fashionable in the context of sociological study of 'illness behaviour.'

The Magraws saw the need to develop a better balance between biological science and humanism, to develop team work between workers in the Greater Medical Profession as well as with managers, and to overcome the problems inherent in medical specialisation. The hospital was therefore to be seen as a community resource and not simply a bastion of biomedical science such as has been the tendency since the impact of German science on U.S. medicine and the Flexner Report. Related was dominance of the biomedical model, burgeoning expenditure on research, and specialisation which he regarded as having had a negative effect on medical practice and education. They also anticipated the move back to general practice. Concerned about the general lack of awareness of impending crisis and the lack of social and political leadership by physicians, the Magraws concluded that their book was a plea for action to fill this leadership vacuum in the profession at a time of need.

White

One of the most constructive critics of medicine and public health has been Kerr White who noted that '(v)irtually all of the problems and issues discussed and much of the evidence had been voiced in medical circles for a long time - for at least a generation' (White 1988). He attributes medicine's difficulty handling the bulk of medical problems encountered in medical practice - variously categorized as trivial, amorphous, self-limited, functional, incurable, intractable or chronic - to the conflict between science and humanities as described by Odegaarde. Even worse is the tendency to attach pejorative and demeaning labels - pills, crazies, neurotics - to patients disabled by anxiety or problems of living. This White sees as essentially a device to cover ignorance and as one of the scandals of the system. Lack of integration of health services with concentration of so much endeavour in the university teaching hospital is a reflection of clinical medicine's disarticulation from the interests in the community which is thereby aggravated. Hope for the future is the development of a broader concept of medicine based on the systems idea, on multidisciplinary research and reform of medical education stressing the importance of the clinical interview, the direct therapeutic impact of the doctor via the placebo effect and related mechanisms, doctor-patient communication, better knowledge of the humanities and on the skills required for primary care practice. He also stressed the need to develop a suitable nosography to allow adequate classification of the patterns of patient presentation to general practitioners.

Barondess

Barondess (1991) raised similar issues, focusing his attention on the shortcomings of the U.S. Academic Health Center. This he portrayed as the 'tower' of excellence in the American Health Care System, the bastion of biomedical science, of experimental research and the main venue for teaching. Barondess summarizes its development, emphasizing the heavy financial support for these centres following the Second World War which profoundly influenced medical practice in the United States and world wide because of U.S. leadership and training of overseas graduates. He too deplored the negative impact on treatment and particularly upon teachers of 'perceived devaluation of clinical care,' 'disease-based instruction' and 'technology-intensive clinical style' which distracts from bedside observation and communication with the sick person. He also singled out for blame the ill-effects of subspecialization. As the priorities of medicine are seen to diverge more and more from the public interest, he warned of a backlash comprising loss of autonomy with increased federal intervention, more pressure for cost-containment and evaluation of the quality of care, and pressure to attend to its 'human elements.' Just as the Magraws had done 25 years earlier, Barondess called for leadership with regard to concerns about equity of health care and access to it. Failure to act in accordance with the wishes of society, to make education of physicians more relevant to practice requirements, to extend research to the clinical process itself, to take heed of public policy. In short he appealed to doctors to observe the social contract of medicine which will otherwise result in action by government and others to reduce its mandate.

Szasz

There have been other cogent criticisms of medicine. One of these is aimed at the status of psychiatry, another at the relationship with the pharmaceutical industry. Leader of the critics of psychiatry has been Thomas Szasz. He claims that the entire notion of mental illness is flawed, and generated by the doctors. In this regard, he sees it as an abrogation of people's freedom and tantamount to waging a witch-hunt (Szasz 1974). He referred to 'drogophobia' to describe those people who do not conform to norms of drug taking. Needless to say, this view is not widely accepted. A comprehensive critique of the role of the drug companies in manufacturing disease sees many doctors as complicit (Moynihan and Cassels 2005).

Engel

The contribution of Engel was to highlight the deficiencies of such a narrow biomedical paradigm. He saw the need to return emphasis to the psychological and social aspects of illness which had become overshadowed by preoccupation with science. Drawing on the systems theory of Weiss and von Bertalanffy, this was an early expression of more recent patient-centred and humanistic care movements in current clinical care. (Engel 1977).

Angell

Marcia Angell MD, associate editor for many years of the prestigious New England Journal of Medicine, published 'The Truth About the Drug Companies. How They Deceive Us and What to Do About It' (Angell 2007). This was a stinging indictment of malpractice by drug companies. Most concerned the conduct and reporting of randomized clinical trials to the extent that their shortcomings were concealed and drugs made to look more efficacious. This, in turn has lead to a loss of credibility among clinicians, and to exacerbation of disagreement between them and 'evidence-based medicine' advocates who have canonized randomized clinical trials as the scientific 'gold standard' for clinical evidence. This has resulted in some observers to call this claim 'scientism,' with its inappropriate claim to 'truth.'

Conclusion: Imminent Nemesis or Phoenix Rising?

In light of all of this criticism and reaction, it would naturally be assumed that medicine would have lost a great deal of influence in the community and in the health system in particular. The title of Illich's book suggests an imminent fall, the medical profession in a state of crisis, such that the only answer is the disappearance of the profession. The feeling of a physician who practised during this period is that doctors have indeed lost power to other health professionals, to hospital administrators, and on committees feeding into health policy, especially in the light of a move back to broader public health concerns. They are certainly less autonomous and more accountable. On the other hand, this does not mean that medicine has lost its control over its specialist knowledge, and it has retained the bulk of its social status and public respect.

Illich foresaw 'medical nemesis,' others a social downgrading - 'deprofessionalisation' or 'proletarianisation.' On closer examination therefore the impact of the 'transitional instability' and controversy so far turns out to be a difficult, contested and largely unresolved question. There are a number of reasons for this. An important one is that it is necessary to distinguish between power exercised at a political level, within the health system by subordinating other health professionals, and power over patients in clinical consultations. Secondly, there may be loss of power within an organisation with retention of crucial areas of control which depend upon specific medical expertise. Thirdly, a change of power relations cannot necessarily be extrapolated into the future. There may be cyclic changes, hence times of transition when matters between public, government, corporate sector and medical profession are contentious with renegotiation of medicine's privileges.

The revolution for which Illich and Carlson called has clearly not materialized. The profession has been neither deprofessionalised nor proletarianised. The paradigm has so far given little ground. Surely this must reflect both the extent to which the biomedical model has become entrenched intellectually, the power of the vested interests of the medical-industrial complex which keep it in place, and the adaptive or homeostatic capacity of the paradigm of medicine, historically a great survivor. Nevertheless we postulate that we are now in a confusing stage of 'paradigmatic instability', a phenomenon which Kuhn recognized as preceding the main paradigm shift, variously described as 'ferment,' 'identity crisis' and, as a cliché, as 'crisis.'

Broadly, the 'smoke' discussed in this chapter arises from the 'fire' caused by friction between within and between the paradigms of interest groups in health at a time of major re-alignment. We examine the attitudes of the public and the government in the next chapter. The social forces which have impacted to cause instability are, as we have suggested, those of postmodernism with an enhanced appreciation of complexity in natural and social worlds, and globalisation as a vehicle of capitalist power. To understand these changes requires that we look more deeply into philosophical perspective, the attitudes, beliefs, commitments, objectives and priorities and language of the major players – their 'paradigm' or their 'discourse.' We discuss the choice of the most suitable concept further in Chapter 4.

The assumption is that, in a fluid state of transition, opportunity for change presents to those who can first read what is going on, and that clear understanding of goals and obstacles is necessary for effective improvement of health services.

References

Angell M., The Truth About the Drug Companies: How They Deceive Us and What to Do About It. *Random.* 2004.

Anon., Review of Limits to Medicine - Medical Nemesis: The expropriation of health. London, Calder and Boyars. *Lancet.* 1974.

Burnham J. C., American medicine's golden age. What happened to it? *Science* 215: 1474-9, 1982.

Barondess J. A., The academic health centre and the public agenda: whose three-legged stool? *Ann Intern Med* 115:9; 1991.

Carlson R. J., The End of Medicine. *John Wiley and Sons,* New York, 1975.

Dollery C., The End of An Age of Optimism: Medical science in retrospect and prospect. *The Nuffield Hospitals Provincial Trust.* 1978.

Dubos R., Mirage of Health. Allen and Unwin, London, 1960.

Engel G. L., Science. ;196:129-36. The need for a new medical model: a challenge for biomedicine. 1977.

Horrobin D. F., Medical Hubris: a reply to Ivan Illich. *Eden Press,* Quebec, 1977, p. 117.

Illich I., Death undefeated. *BMJ* 311: 1652-3. 1995.

Illich I., Deschooling Society, Harper and Row, New York, 1971.

Illich I., Limits to Medicine - Medical Nemesis: The expropriation of health. London, *Calder and Boyars,* 1974.

Illich I., Limits to Medicine - Medical Nemesis: The expropriation of health. London, *Calder and Boyars,* 1974, p. 210.

Jacob J. M., Doctors and Rules: A sociology of professional values. *Routledge,* London, 1987.

Jacob J. M., Doctors and Rules: A sociology of professional values. *Routledge,* London, 1987, p. 131.

Katz J., The Silent World of Doctors and Patients. *Free Press,* New York, 1984.

Katz J., The Silent World of Doctors and Patients. *Free Press,* New York, 1984, p. 4.

Kennedy I., The Unmasking of Medicine. *Allen and Unwin,* Boston, 1981.

Lown B., The lost art of healing. *Houghton Mifflin,* New York, 1996.

Magraw R. M., Magraw D. B., Ferment in medicine: a study of the essence of medical practice and of its new dilemmas. *W.B. Saunders,* Philadelphia, 1966.

McKenzie J., The Future of Medicine. *Oxford University Press,* London, 1919, pp. 61-5.

McKeown T., Record RG Reasons for the decline in mortality in England and Wales during the nineteenth century. *Popul. Stud.* 16: 94-122, 1962.

Moynihan R., Cassels A., Selling Sickness. How drug companies are turning us all into patients. *Allen and Unwin, Crow's Nest,* NSW. 2005.

Navarro V., Medicine Under Capitalism. *Prodist,* New York, 1976. p352. New York, (Prodist, Neale Watson).

Navarro V., The industrialization of fetishism or the fetishism of industrialization: a critique of Ivan Illich. *Soc Sci Med* 1975;9;351-63.

Odegaard C., Dear Doctor: a personal letter to a physician. *The Henry J Kaiser Foundation, Menlo Park*, 1986.

Reiser S., Medicine and the Reign of Technology. *Cambridge University Press.* New York, 1978.

Reiser S. J., Medicine and the Reign of Technology. *Cambridge University Press.* New York, 1978, p. 178.

Szasz T., The Myth of Mental Illness. Foundations of a theory of personal conduct. *Harper and Row.* 1977.

Shorter E., Doctors and Their Patients: a social history. *Simon and Schuster,* New Jersey, 1991.

Taylor R., Medicine Out of control: The anatomy of a malignant technology. *Sun Books,* South Melbourne, 1979.

Visiltear A. J., Milton C., Winternitz and the Yale Institute of human relations: A brief chapter in the history of social medicine. *Yale J Biol Med* 57; 869-89:1984.

Waitzkin H., Book review- Illich I. Limits to Medicine - Medical Nemesis: The expropriation of health. *Contemp Sociol* 1976;5:401-5.

White K. L., The Task of Medicine: dialogue at Wickenburg. The Henry J Kaiser Foundation. *Menlo Park,* 1988, p. 3.

Chapter 3

The Public Perspective - More Smoke

The public at large, consumer groups, health bureaucracies and politicians have made their contribution to the smoke of battle currently hanging over health care. We will discuss further the tensions between the lay paradigm and perspective on illness and the medical paradigm, and their consequences for individual patients later. The cumulative effect of these is also evident in the reaction of the general public to medicine. The responses of health bureaucracies to medicine are also influenced by the politics of public opinion and perceptions of the quality of care. However, the escalating cost of health care has emerged as the major political driving force for demands for the evaluation of health care. All of these interactions are important stimuli for change in medicine, hence we need to look at them in more detail.

The General Public

The current public reaction to medical care shows signs of ambivalence. The medical 'breakthrough' still makes good press copy. Yet much of what we read in the press and in magazines is critical. Patients complain of lack of communication in the clinical consultation. This is related to the fact that a substantial proportion of patients are 'non-compliant,' failing to take treatment as ordered, and sometimes unwilling to uncritically accept medical reassurance after disease has been ruled out. Katz places these problems in a broader perspective since he sees the 'silence,' the failure of communication, as having therapeutic and self protective functions as part of what we will identify later as the modern paradigm of medicine (Chapter 4). More patients now demand a say in their own treatment or, at least, a clear understanding of the implications of their illness. Dissatisfied patients often vote with their feet, spurning doctor for alternative health practitioner, and consumer groups often assume an adversarial posture.

Patient satisfaction must be the central objective of health care. It is obviously a worthy primary aim in itself. It is, however, doubly important because satisfaction has been found to be related to the success of the medical consultation, crucial to therapeutic cooperation between doctor and patient, therefore an important influence on health outcome in its own right. How patients react to their doctors will obviously depend on both the attention they receive and on their expectations. According to Katz, patients have, in general, invested sufficient trust in the medical practitioner to allow successful treatment, but historically have been unwilling to accord them monopoly rights over such care. Moreover, the skills and motivations doctors have been the target of innumerable criticisms and witticisms over the centuries. Scepticism concerning the value of medical ministrations has not been lacking in the past. Following the Renaissance, William Petty, pioneer of health statistics had his doubts (White 1991) and Proust later claimed that belief in medicine was 'the height of folly' (Katz 1984). Voltaire's contribution was '(T) he art of medicine is to amuse the patient while nature cures the disease.' Then there was the honest self-appraisal of De Sorbiere, physician, priest and philosopher who confessed 'the more enlightened only feel their way groping amid a thick gloom' (Katz 1984). Medicine's reliance upon the vix mediatrix naturae, the healing power of nature had been known from antiquity and was reaffirmed by in the 19th century. Bigelow of Harvard University stated that 'the amount of death and disaster in the world would be less if all disease were left to itself.' (Starr 1982). The sceptical views of Oliver Wendell Holmes are also well documented (Illich 1978).

Certainly the doctor was not held in high regard in the United States even in the nineteenth century. This was not surprising in view of Henderson's claim that not until around 1910 or 1912 would a patient stand more than a 50-50 chance of deriving benefit from a random medical encounter (Freidson 1989). In addition, some of the ministrations of the 19th century doctor seemed as likely to kill as to cure. But times have changed dramatically. As Houston has pointed out 'the placebo has always been the norm of medical practice' (Katz 1984) and drugs with specific action were extremely few until well into this century. These criticisms referred, of course, to the nostrums and potions of prescientific internal medicine, of physik. However, following the boom in scientific medicine just before, during and after the Second World War, this could no longer be said.

Trite as the observation may seem, we simply cannot ignore the fact that most of us owe an obvious and substantial debt to modern medicine which most of the time we take for granted. Illich was disparaging on this point, claiming that '(a)lthough almost everyone believes that at least one of his friends would not be alive and well except for the skill of a doctor, there is, in fact, no evidence of any relationship between this mutation of sickness and the so-called progress of medicine' (Illich 1976). Nonetheless the perception remains strong. Many of us are aware of the high infant mortalities in our grandparents' families, and of the substantial increase in longevity. Moreover, an impacted gallstone would have almost certainly accounted for the author, and pneumonia to his infant sister in premodern days. Anecdotal it may be but such direct evidence is compelling, at least to the prospective victim! Together with media coverage of 'breakthroughs,' it obviously continues to shape public opinion. Medicine's reputation as a life saver tends to mute criticism of defects of the health care system - but perhaps sharpens the edge of criticism when the doctor disappoints. On the other hand, despite the trend to more alternative medicine consultations, there is certainly no evidence to suggest that the patient is demanding less health care, demanding to revert to self-help on a large scale or seeking low tech solutions to their problems, as Illich recommended. All the evidence is to the contrary.

There has, nevertheless, been a pervasive feeling at community level that, despite the occasional important medical scientific breakthrough, investment in biomedical research and scientific medicine has yielded diminishing returns at the margin. As developments in the new basic medical sciences rapidly augmented understanding of the structure and function of the body, new diagnostic techniques and new treatments continued to raise new questions which were solved by new developments. Thus success fed upon success to create a snowballing effect in the last half of the 18th and first half of the 19th centuries. For example, Laennec's discovery of the stethoscope opened the door to the accurate diagnosis of heart disease, and Lister's antisepsis to more aggressive surgery; together with a concatenation of further discoveries, these lead in an essentially unpredictable fashion to the development of open heart surgery. Similarly, Beeson reviewed the therapeutic recommendations of the 1st and 14th editions of the textbook of which he was an editor. He identified major therapeutic benefits from scientific internal medicine between 1925 and 1975 (Beeson 1980).

However, through the retrospectoscope, we see that the initial rapid progress comprising immunization for bacterial infection, surgical asepsis, anaesthesia, improved treatment of trauma and safer childbirth, insulin for diabetes and correction of vitamin deficiency, antibiotics for bacterial infection and suppression of inflammation, provision of safer childbirth, life-saving as these advances were - still represented relatively 'easy pickings' compared with the residual pool of more refractory problems. The replacement of infection by chronic illness as the major health challenge, the so-called 'Second Epidemiological Revolution' has meant that progress has slowed dramatically in the face of such problems as less tractable residue of chronic diseases such as arteriosclerotic heart disease and stroke, diabetes, cancer, obstructive lung disease, arthritis, cirrhosis of the liver and mental illness, all common in an aging population, and inherently more complex involving multiple causal factors and intricate pathogenesis. This phenomenon has been labelled 'the failures of success' (Gruenberg 1977). Thus diseases which were easier to treat have been 'conquered' leaving a residue of illness and disability which is more complex and less medically tractable, including the biological effects of aging, and the effects of stress and problems of living.

The Big Picture

Dubos (1960) saw mankind as frustrated by having to face new hazards in response to his own social evolution. Burnett (1971) picked up this theme when he foresaw diminishing returns in the treatment of chronic diseases, in the diseases of civilization and intractable social and ecological problems associated with industrialization and war. This feeling was reinforced by the downgrading of the claims of curative medicine to reduction of community mortality by McKeown (1979), although this claim has been disputed. The theme has also been picked up in community polls (Blendon and Donnellan 1988). In addition some of the early gains proved to be, in part, illusory. The emergence of serious viral infections and of antibiotic resistance have shown that not even infectious disease has been finally conquered. In retrospect, on the broadest canvas, this can be seen to be a special case of the S-shaped or logistic curve of gain. If we look at open heart surgery as a specific example, we find that surgery is now performed on an older and sicker population, and that the problem of post-operative infection has re-emerged in the form of bacterial resistant to most or all antibiotics.

Since the 1960's, however, there was a distinct plateau in the graph relating gain of life expectancy plotted against time, and an even more striking reduction in the ratio of such gain to financial expenditure. Since that time, there have been modest gains attributable to a substantial fall in mortality due to ischaemic heart disease and stroke but the role of medicine or public health in this decline, if any, has yet to be defined. Fuchs summarized the current situation succinctly when he said: 'In developed countries, the marginal contribution of medical care to life expectancy is very small' (Fuchs 1974). It would be churlish and misleading not to acknowledge that life-saving progress has continued in some important areas including the cure of childhood leukaemia and of lymphatic tumours (lymphoma) by chemotherapy, radiation and bone marrow transplantation, successful drug treatment for peptic ulcer, treatment of angina pectoris by surgery or balloon (angioplasty), non-surgical destruction of kidney stones, less painful and disabling endoscopic surgery undertaken through small incisions, replacement of joints and transplantation of the kidney, heart and liver. In addition, we have to acknowledge the likelihood of further important developments but, at present, there is no sign that progress will ever again occur on such a wide front or at such a rapid rate as was characteristic of the early gains. This is why apportioning large sums of money for 'fighting' cancer and ischaemic heart disease in the 1960's has yielded a disappointing overall result in terms of prevention and cure. Epidemiologists and sociologists have also engaged in community surveillance activities which have exposed much unreported illness amongst the elderly and disadvantaged. However, attempts to address the detection and treatment of occult disease in the community runs into a problem of what is to be regarded as normal, especially problematic if defined in statistical terms and in the aged.

The problem of aging provides yet another way of looking at how medicine has become a victim of its own success. In the United States, disease prevention and successful treatment of previously fatal illness or injury appears to have successfully eliminated approximately 80% of premature deaths (Freis 1980). Even the conquest of cancer would now only prolong average life expectancy by a matter of months. The earlier medical triumphs have therefore had the effect of compressing most illness, and expenditure on illness, into the declining years. The biological basis of this observation is that each species has a specific life span. If premature death due to disease or injury is avoided, old age brings with it decline in the function of individual organs, approximately linear during the middle years but accelerating in old age. Poorly understood cellular changes so weaken a system that its capacity for maintaining homeostatic adjustment and equilibrium, and capacity for self-healing becomes progressively compromised. Hence chronic illness becomes common, and the risk of death doubles every 8 years. Eventually, at an advanced age, the bodily system can collapse so that death can result from what begins as quite a minor challenge; a fall causing confinement to bed can result in fatal pneumonia or pulmonary embolism. Hygienic measures and regular exercise can slow this process only to a limited extent, even assuming that social conditions and distribution of appropriate community facilities would permit their widespread and optimal application.

The 'Symptom Epidemic'

The result of the decline in organic disease, the increase in symptoms associated with problems and anxieties of daily living, of increasing work pressure, and lower threshold for seeking medical care has greatly increased the number of people attending doctors. Uncommon organic disease is notoriously difficult to differentiate in patients complaining of chest or abdominal pain, headache or tiredness. However only a small proportion have the organic disease that doctors have been trained to seek out and treat with scientific interventions. In this situation, there is an ever present risk that the powerful products of scientific and technological progress, the drugs, the diagnostic tests particularly expensive imaging investigations, and the new treatments including developments in surgery such as coronary artery grafting will be used to excess. Non-invasive alternatives to surgery, especially such interventions as lithotripsy or coronary angioplasty, are more likely to be used in doubtful circumstances.

Here is where the root causes of most of the excessive and rising costs of health care are to be found, an impression confirmed by the fact that physicians generate about three quarters of health care costs, exceeding the direct cost of doctors' fees by a factor of four (Welch and Fisher 1992). The doctor's training has often cultivated little appreciation of subtleties of psychological or of social context. Clinical uncertainties have multiplied, decision-making has become more complex, and the stakes for error are higher for such potent interventions, a problem compounded by the lack of evaluation of medical technologies. In the absence of good evidence and firm guidelines, diagnostic and therapeutic interventions are commonly used outside that 'window' within which they are cost-effective and clinically useful. The risk of iatrogenic illness is then high and so too is the economic cost.

This situation therefore poses the twin hazards of overdiagnosis of organic disease and overinvestigation, and failure to recognise the manifestations of anxiety and depression. The result is often iatrogenic illness caused by aggravation of anxiety or an inappropriate intervention, or a dissatisfied patient who feels that the real problem has not been addressed. Finally, the medical culture tends to see death of a patient as failure, and fear of litigation; fear of the accusation of euthanasia, pressure from relatives and religious beliefs can all encourage what has described as 'futile care' or 'rescue,' the inappropriate application of high cost medical technology particularly inappropriate resuscitation and life-support.

Paradox of Health

More subtle but no less important than the changes in the burden of disease and in life expectancy have been the effects of altered public perception of and fears about illness, and attitudes towards use of medical care. Barsky (1988) captured the spirit of changing public perceptions and their effects on health care when he wrote of the 'paradox of health'. Thus, people are reporting more illness, more restriction of activity due to illness, having more medical consultations. There is also evidence of greater expectation of medical 'cure.' A similar observation was made by Wildavsky (1972) who argued that the general public is 'doing better and feeling worse.' This combination of lowered threshold for illness and increased expectation, Barsky attributes to the problem of 'medicalization' of all aspects of life which has been the subject of much sociological study as well as forming a central part of Illich's attack.

Hazards of Everyday Life

There has been a barrage of epidemiological case control studies which have purported to show relationships between a wide variety of daily activities and environmental agents on the one hand and risk of serious disease like heart disease or cancer on the other - what Feinstein has called 'the hazards of everyday life' (Feinstein 1988). The harmful effects of excessive sunshine, of our diet, of our indolence, of our coffee breaks, of sexual activity have been the subjects of warnings by the health authorities. Contradictory results are confusing, and such studies are prone to generate false associations. In a similar vein was the plaintive plea of Mark Twain that 'everything I like is illegal, immoral or fattening.'. His complaint could now be extended by adding 'or a risk factor for disease.' At the same time, self-interested parties capitalize on public fears. All of this in a society inclined towards narcissism (Lasch 1980) must encourage morbid introspection.

Key organs are constantly scrutinized for signs of impending malfunction, and minor symptoms, including those attributable to life's stress are often attributed to them, a major contributor to the number of medical consultations. Spending one's days looking over one's shoulder in this way and is surely in conflict with the wise counsel offered by Montaigne that '(t)he wise man knows what he should know, not what he can know.' A lower threshold for considering oneself ill, together with easier access to medical care and other cultural changes have encouraged medical consultation for minor but very common illnesses such as respiratory infections, legal requirements covering absence from work and involving another common problem of back pain; in particular, changed attitudes to illness in women and children have increased their rate of medical attendance.

The Old Fashioned Doctor

The reactions of some older people to doctors still seems to be coloured by fond memories of the 'old fashioned doctor' whose home visit was an occasion for clean sheets, a bowl of hot water, a clean towel and a fresh cake of soap; when in doubt, he consulted with 'a specialist,' usually a dignified and authoritative figure. This seems to have been an evanescent phenomenon. As Freidson has put it: 'The image of the old-fashioned family doctor who was all things to all people is based on that fleeting period when folk medicine had declined but medical practice was still incipient' (Freidson 1989). The accuracy of the perception can also be contested. Thus Eisenman and Kleinman (1988) disputed the evidence that the doctor of earlier times was, in fact, more sensitive in the absence of technology and effective treatment. By way of contrast, the stereotype frequently presented today is of a brusque impersonal, apparently uncaring doctor, excessively orientated towards technology, non-communicative, insensitive to the patient's need for personal support and explanation, all too often hurried and with an unhealthy interest in personal remuneration.

To the dismay of the American Medical Association, these kinds of criticism were voiced by patients in a survey which they commissioned (Nelson 1989). A majority thought that doctors were 'too interested in making money, and that they don't care about people as much as they used to' (Harvey and Shubat 1989). So concerned was the Association that it set up a Subcommittee on Evaluation on Humanistic Qualities in the Internist to address what were seen as important developments in medicine – 'greater expectations for satisfactory clinical outcomes, and the concomitant desires for personalized care and for the advantages of the type of care are provided by the large medical center.' The report went on to discuss those factors which the committee believed to be related to public perceptions; these included the distraction of high technology, the impersonal atmosphere of large institutions, the preoccupation of faculty with objectives not conducive to providing a good role model for residents, diffusion of medical responsibility and the negative side-effects of subspecialization.

Its results led to action to improve the humanistic skills of physicians (Nelson 1989). Given that patients reported dissatisfaction with explanation provided by doctors, with lack of time allocated, with excessive waiting time, it would be difficult to imagine that major changes in 'humanistic' attitudes could be effected by simply changing selection criteria for admission to medical training or developing guidelines for residency training. These are surely problems deeply rooted in medical culture and education, therefore likely to change only with a sea change in attitudes in the context of a shift of paradigm.

One would hardly expect the general public to be especially well informed on medical technicalities, nor to be in a good position to critically evaluate the level of skill deployed in the interventional care they have received. As one might expect, their criteria of quality of care will be based on their own experience of facilities, setting, reputation and service, including waiting time and duration of the consultation, as they have done since antiquity. Not surprisingly, they defer to expert opinion in matters technical or concerned with safety. They cannot easily detect medical error and, even if they do, few suspect negligence. Few would be aware of the inherent uncertainty of clinical medicine. Just as doctors have done over the centuries, they are likely to resort to post-hoc, propter-hoc reasoning, attributing spontaneous improvement to the last treatment or to blaming the doctor for a chance occurrence. Few would be aware of the statistical risk of iatrogenic injury, of the possibility of an unnecessary operation, or of a hazardous diagnostic procedure to which they might have been unnecessarily exposed. The psychological and social trauma of a false-positive or doubtful result arising from a community screening program, cholesterol testing or mammography, may raise doubts about the wisdom of having such checks. Most, however, will accept the vigilance of modern medicine in the spirit of such homely aphorisms as: 'a stitch in time saves nine,' 'an ounce of prevention is worth a ton of cure,' or 'better to be sure than sorry.' The protracted death of a loved one in an intensive care unit may occasionally raise questions about meddlesome intervention or ill-advised zeal, but more often the family are grateful for the effort.

Despite their ignorance of technical detail, gullibility with regard to benefit, and inability to apply a scientific standard of criticism, the evidence is that many patients are more sceptical about medical treatment than doctors think. Most doctors are only dimly aware of the network of family and friends which plays a major part in the patient's evaluation of medical care and their opinions exert a strong influence on whether or not the patient follows medical advice. Lay theories of illness have been resilient in the face of scientific medical evidence which conflict with them. A patient is unlikely to follow a course of treatment the rationale for which conflicts with their own beliefs. Rather than complain, many will make a silent protest by not complying with treatment, or vote with their feet by turning to alternative medicine, even sue the doctor.

Freidson

It is also common knowledge in the health professions that the doctor's bed-side manner and professional style do not correlate well with other aspects of competence but is much more easily judged and often more highly regarded. Moreover, in the United States, middle class patients are relatively well informed, especially those with chronic disease who often learn a good deal about their illness and their management. In pediatrics and obstetrics too, consultations also involve consumers who are often knowledgable. Freidson suggests that of the gap between the knowledge of doctor and patient is narrowing, and that the economic pressures are turning patients into the 'rationally calculating consumers dear to the hearts of economists' (Freidson 1989). However, in general, all they have to go on is their own experience on what they hear from their friends and what they read about in newspapers and magazines.

Opinion Polls

There has been further evidence from opinion polls and surveys in the United States and from Britain that public image of the profession is declining (Blendon 1988), and that two-thirds of the American public now believe that people are beginning to lose faith in doctors (Mechanic 1986). Possible reasons for this include to public reactions against the politically powerful, and the modern tendency to suspect the expert, and abuses of public trust by some in the professions. A common and consistent complaint, arguably the most important source of patient dissatisfaction, is of lack of information and of poor communication. However Freidson has argued that, although surveys have shown a decline in public confidence in all major professions, most confidence has been retained by doctors (Freidson 1989). He claimed that there was in the 1980s no evidence of widespread dissatisfaction with medical care in the United States. Despite complaints about practical matters such as cost, availability and waiting time, the American public as of 1982 appeared to be still 'overwhelmingly' satisfied with the quality of their medical care. Cartwright and Anderson (1981) in Britain reported that 90% of their sample were satisfied with their care, 30% of patients were critical of lack of explanation, and 23% of waiting room facilities. In Australia, surveys have documented satisfaction or qualified satisfaction in over 90% of medical consultations (Committee of Inquiry into Medical education and Medical Workforce, 1988). The conclusion was that there was not widespread dissatisfaction about medical care in this country. However the submissions included some strong criticism of handling of patients with specific problems such as epilepsy, chronic pain and terminal illness; complaints were also voiced by disadvantaged groups including women, the disabled and aboriginals (Committee of Inquiry into Medical Education and Medical Workforce 2004).

Not *My* Doctor

An intriguing ambiguity is that while patients are quite critical of local facilities and of the system in general, it seems that most cannot bring themselves to complain about the overall care that they obtain from their own doctor. Perhaps it is too uncomfortable to even contemplate the possibility of such foibles applying to one in whom they must trust. Hence if the patient decides to stick with a doctor, any perception of lack of competence or unworthy motivation might well be rationalised away in the interests of maintaining that trust. In such sensitive areas, however, the truth might not come out in a questionnaire when it might well be elicited by in-depth interviews. There are of course, various consumer groups which agitate for patient rights, along with a variety of specific lobbies and pressure groups including those representing the women's movement, racial groups, the aged, the handicapped and those suffering from specific diseases such as multiple sclerosis. Criticism emanating from these quarters is frequently well-informed, focused, trenchant and effective and sometimes backed up by sociological study.

The reservoir of public goodwill will be drained by self-interested behavior and failure to reform and self-regulate, and loss of the reputation for integrity, like the consequences of Humpty Dumpty's accident, may not be reversible. Since trust is essential to care and an important contributor to the effectiveness of much treatment, its loss will not only damage the profession but also seriously compromise therapeutic effectiveness. This is no small thing since dissatisfaction is not only harmful to the image of the profession, it is also related to failure of compliance with advice and treatment.

The level of public satisfaction expressed with individual doctors is not reflected in opinion polls with regard to the health care system as a whole (Blendon 1988). Blendon's analysis of the results of 75 national opinion polls conducted in the United States between 1966 and 1987 confirmed the ambiguous public attitude towards doctors. Although people generally expressed satisfaction with their own doctor, they were nevertheless critical of the health care system, agreeing that the personal expense incurred is too high, perceiving cost increases as unmatched by better care, and related rather to the desire of the providers for profit.

There has been evidence of international dissatisfaction to the point of opting for either 'fundamental changes,' even a 'completely rebuilt system' according to a poll conducted in 1988 and 1989 (Smith 1990). In 9 of the 10 western democratic countries polled, a majority wanted such major change rather than 'minor changes.' The exception was Canada (44%). The greatest discontent was expressed for the United States (89%), the country with the highest per capita expenditure on health ($2051). The level was intermediate for Britain (69%) with the lowest per capita expenditure ($758).). This level of discontent means that government and managed care bureaucracies have to tread especially carefully lest they be seen to cut costs at the expense of quality of care.

The Bureaucracies: Government and Managed Care

Since the modern sovereign state replaced feudalism in the western world, the health of society has been seen as a responsibility of the society as a whole. In post-revolutionary France, health was seen as 'a task for the nation.' This concept was formalised in Germany in the late 19th century, as part of in Bismarck's system of social insurance, introduced some 70 years later (Rosen 1993). This has been seen as a part of those rights and entitlements of the individual often seen as a 'social wage,' a necessary compromise with workers in the capitalist state. Russia established its rural public health system in 1861 which included the auxiliary health workers known as 'feldshers' (Rosen 1993). The motivations for these developments were undoubtedly complex. In addition to philanthropy, compassion, and desire for social order during the Enlightenment, there was fear of epidemic disease in Europe. Another force was economic. Even less worthy was the wish to alleviate the high cost of supporting the poor as proposed by Chadwick in Britain.

The details of health systems vary depending on the vagaries of cultural philosophy, ideology and social system, as would be expected. Thus the problem of designing a comprehensive health system is one of political feasibility rather than of practicality. There is obvious variation today in the extent to which governments have control over health care and its expenditures. Of course, they are fully responsible for health under a Communist regime. At the other extreme, the United States has avoided any form of National Health Insurance, confining its direct funding of patient care to interventions covering the aged, the very poor and the war veteran. Britain and the Scandinavian countries have opted for socialised medicine and National Health Services. Much of Europe, Australia, Canada and Japan have retained a mixed system comprising government-sponsored insurance cover as well as private activity.

The background to government action following the French Revolution was the earlier belief, naively optimistic in retrospect, that provision of more and better health care would result in less illness, hence less demand. This idea was linked to the idea of the health of man in the natural state uncorrupted by civilization, the idea of the 'noble savage.' Such ideas were part of the Romantic ideas popular at the very time that the foundations of modern clinical medicine and health care delivery were being laid. This same 'finite need model' also led to the expectation that the annual cost of providing the health service in Britain would decline as treatment reduced the burden of morbidity in the community. What transpired instead could be described as a 'bottomless pit model.' This kind of thinking is also based on mechanistic ideas, on a simple cause and effect model. This would suggest that scientific advance would eventually eliminate disease as a problem so that cost to the community would decline.

However the real world of health is a complex dynamic system if ever there was one. As discussed above, chronic disease did not yield to magic bullets like acute infection. The consequences of an aging population become manifest, and chronic disease increases with age. The major cause of symptoms in the community is minor illness, anxiety and problems of living, and the evidence is that these are on the increase. This expansion of ambulant medical care has comprised problems that doctors have not been well trained to handle. This has contributed to patient dissatisfaction, to iatrogenic illness and escalating cost.

Health and Social Class

Public health has from time to time drawn attention to the relationship between poverty and ill health but since this issue was raised by Virchow in the last century, it has been avoided as far as is possible. The conditions of the modern welfare state can hardly be compared with those of the industrialising city of the last century. However the problem presents now in a more subtle form. There is now overwhelming evidence that it is still a higher standard of living, related to national and personal wealth, which is the most effective protection against ill-health, an intensely political issue only indirectly and partially related to clinical care, even to the delivery of health care. The theory of 'trickle down,' based on the capacity of increased growth and market competition to increase Gross National Product and reduce poverty, has not materialized. The thrust of economic rationalism, based on the economics of the supply side, emphasizes market forces abstracted from consideration of the influence of social factors. This too has focused concentration on cost rather than on such political betes noires as redistribution of income or feuding with the medical profession.

Certainly no government has been able to face up to the political consequences of any major attempt to redistribute wealth. Indeed with economic rationalism and globalisation, class differentials of both wealth and health have widened. The problem has been further aggravated by cyclic recession which increases the rate of morbidity, especially that due to cardiovascular disease, and mortality. The repetitive and unfulfilling nature of work has been blamed for 'alienation' of working people and manifest as anxiety and depression. There is evidence that longer working hours and job insecurity associated with economic rationalism and micro-economic reform of the work place has aggravated this problem.

Clinicians have been largely silent on this issue, perhaps partly to avoid conflict with government. The evaluation of technology has focused on the choices between medical interventions. A politically broader view sees medical care as in competition with the funding of social services and of initiatives to address social problems such as unemployment (Evans and Stoddart 1990). Public health in the form of health promotion has been been accused of fostering an excessive focus on modification of individual behaviour and reduction of risk factors for disease, thereby reinforcing the role of curative medicine as well as of public health but diverting the focus from the much more crucial issue of the gradient of illness and premature mortality related to lower social class and income.

The problem of the cost of medical care had surfaced as early as the 1920s (Starr). It is at centre stage at present, coming to a head with the more recent pressure to cut back on welfare spending. Evans and Stoddart (1990) have noted that the 'crisis' of cost has been pronounced in various countries in which health cost as a proportion of G.D.P. has ranged from less than 5% to more than 10%, almost a threefold difference. The problem is to a large extent ideological rather than practical. Of recent years the tendency has been for costs to escalate rapidly through piecemeal yet comprehensive reform of health care. This is a painfully slow process.

Direct administrative intervention in the procedures of care and bureaucratic micromanagement uniformed by clinical expertise cannot address the basic problems. There is the risk too of serious distortion of patient care by rigid protocols and ill-advised interventions which will not improve patient satisfaction, and which will strangle the practitioner with red tape. The recent emphasis has been on health services research. This activity has been seized upon as a means of improving the quality of care, of reining in the medical profession and of constraining costs. We will examine this movement in detail later (Chapter 11). The same charge has been levelled at evidence-based medicine more recently, which emphasizes randomized trials as the proper 'scientific' evidence' to be used for patient treatment, especially in the form of clinical guidelines. For the present I record our conviction that what is required is much more than top-down evaluation and research conducted by public health or managed care professionals. An essential ingredient is the cooperation and active participation of clinicians in 'clinical practice research' (Chapter 16).

What is required is grassroots evolutionary reform of medical practice and education, informed by the experience of clinicians, represented in the future by the reflective physicians (Chapter 15). This should be conducted as an on-going multidisciplinary research and evaluation program in the environment of primary care and hospital practice. This 'clinical practice research' should be led by a centre for the study of clinical practice doctors well versed in the myriad problems (chapter 15). These will be the reflective physicians, discussed in the last chapter. Like all evaluation research, this must linked to health care policy generation, to public health and to health services research at the community level, as an-going iterative program. This program must include primary care. Improved clinical decisions and supportive care will not only improve patient health outcomes and improve patient satisfaction, in the long haul it is the only way to control costs and ensure value for money.

What governments have relied upon so far has been concentrated instead on cost-containment through regulation, clinical guidelines, capping of expenditure, rationing or reliance on 'free market' competition, supplemented by a quick technological fix through evaluation from a top-down and predominantly economic perspective, aiming to reduce the autonomy of clinicians and to standardise clinical care and restrict patient options. To undertake the necessary program of research and evaluation of 'clinical practice research' will mean a commitment which runs counter to political pressures predicated on the public perception of action before the next election.

The cultural characteristics of each of the Western countries have resulted in a health care story which is unique to each. Let us briefly illustrate some of these matters in the case of the ideological poles of health care in the capitalist Western world - The United States and Britain. Of the developed countries, the United States has led the way not only in basic medical research but also in encountering some of the most intractable problems of health care, eliciting the most vituperative criticism. Here the forces are relatively easy to see even if the events are caricatures by comparison with other countries. For this purpose of illustration we have therefore chosen to emphasise the events as they unfolded in United States.

The United States

It would be unwise to accept public opinion in the U.S. as representing that of other countries. However, it has been well documented by Blendon (1988) in his review of trends over a period of more than 20 years. These he has summarized as follows: Most Americans are satisfied with individual medical care, and believe that they spend too little overall on health with the caveat that there is no economic crisis, do not wish to see budget cuts in this area, and are opposed to reduction in allocation to the care of the elderly and to rationing of high-cost interventions. They are, however, concerned at the rate of increase in their own health costs which a majority cannot justify in terms of improved quality of care. In this country, there has also been dissatisfaction with the commercial orientation of medicine. Since that time there has been further public unease about managed care in the U.S. and concerns over rationing in Britain.

The idea of health as a right and of expenditure as part of the social wage has never been unequivocally acknowledged in the United States. Although the specific events in the evolution of health care are, in this sense and others, not typical of experience in other Western countries, yet the way in which medicine has achieved its special relationship with the state and dominance over its rivals reflect the same basic forces as in other countries. The responses of government and of the business sector, although perhaps written in bolder script in America, still provide a useful guide to changing attitudes towards medicine, especially during the 1960s when social welfare activities of the state were coming under increasing scrutiny in many countries. This whole process was a fertile ground for the academic sociologist and for the more thoughtful economist as will be seen.

The story of the tensions between medicine, alternative medicine, public health and government during the evolution of the system of health care in the U.S. is a long and complex one. The powerful influence of culture and politics on medicine's path to pride of place in the health care system has been well documented by Starr (1982). The chaos of entrepreneurial traditional medicine in the last century with a plethora of training facilities but overall poor standards, in competition with a variety of healers over whom there was no public control, drew much criticism. The free enterprise response was for the philanthropic Carnegie foundation to commission a report which established science as the foundation of orthodox medicine and which recommended more stringent standards. This Flexner Report (Flexner 1910) set the standard not only for the U.S. but for the world for most of this century. The emphasis of the report and its acceptance reflected the powerful influence of German laboratory science on a generation of American physicians, and on the health care system in general.

This view of clinical care as predominantly applied natural and biological science not only set the tone for medical education and clinical practice, it also proved to be an invaluable ally in the successful conquest of the paradigm of alternative medicine by that of orthodox 'allopathic' medicine. According pride of place to the basic medical sciences over clinical experience later received substantial vindication with the achievements of scientific medicine during the Second World War. Thus there was acceleration of scientific progress leading to development of antibiotics, improved treatment of trauma as well as technological gains leading to accelerated progress in diagnosis. This is well illustrated by of the outstanding success of imaging techniques such as diagnostic ultrasound which was a direct spin-off from radar technology. Afterwards the success of the academic medical center and of hospital practice was guaranteed by subsequent heavy financial support.

The problem of cost of medical care and need for health insurance had become an issue early in this century (Starr 1986) and the first proposals for compulsory health insurance came soon afterwards. Popular feeling and an anti-German sentiment during and after the First World War conspired against it, and labour opposed it too. The medical profession was initially in favour but soon recanted. In 1917 the American Medical Association proposed a national health insurance but subsequently overturned the decision. The College of physicians more recently regarded reform as 'imperative' (Maddrey et al. 1992) and proposed universal coverage based on combined private and public insurance. Following the Second World War, the idea became enmeshed in cold war rhetoric and fears of socialism, and despite further attempts has not succeeded in gaining sufficient support. Thus the United States remains the epitome of the laissez-faire capitalist state with regard to health, placing fewest constraints on medical practice, on the so-called medical-industrial complex, and avoiding government intervention as far as possible. The problems of control of the use of technology and of cost are complicated by the lack of primary care physicians in a gatekeeper role. The National Leadership Commission on Health Care, comprising prominent US citizens summarized the major problems of health care in that country as escalating cost, inequities of access and uneven quality.

The critiques of medicine at this time can be classified into two categories. The first is the political liberal 'more of the same' argument which essentially assumes the essential effectiveness of the current health care system so that it focuses on the problems of organization of health care, with the objectives of ensuring appropriate public health and access to medical care. The validity of this approach has been called into question by the doubts cast on the effectiveness of medical care and by evidence of more deep-seated inequalities. The second, more radical critique saw the need for major restructuring including a socialist reform which would see as important the redistribution of income, the 'decommodification' of medicine, reduction in the power of the medical profession, the empowerment of individuals and the community in health matters. The moves to assert civil rights in the 1960s also threw up some direct challenges for medicine with moves for greater patient autonomy in general, as well as specific attacks by the women's movement and on behalf of disadvantaged minorities.

American medicine's honeymoon with government came to an abrupt halt in the 1970s. Concerns about rising costs on the part of business interests and public, and crimping of government political options by rising medical costs in the face of economic stagflation became the driving force behind political manoeuvring, and also linked up with the moves to submit health care to evaluation. These concerns, in turn, became the thin edge of the wedge for the much more fundamental question discussed above - could better community health be achieved by more medical care? The earlier debate had been about providing more and better health care and ensuring equitable access. The political left were sceptical about the value of social services, seen as a means of social control; the right or economic rationalist view saw them as unwarranted burden on the economy and as a government intrusion. At the same time, there was public scepticism as to whether or not the medical profession could or would lead the way to worthwhile reform.

In the late 1970s, the Nixon administration and the subsequent Reagan regime encouraged the economic rationalist options of incentive and competition which has encouraged the process of corporatization in the health field which has culminated in a system dominated by managed care. As a result of this vast uncontrolled experiment in health care delivery, the United States has often led the way by encountering most of the serious current health care problems first or in their most extreme form. The annual cost of health care in the U.S.A. passed one trillion dollars in 1995. A wide variety of regulations and incentives have been aimed at of cost-containment listed above have been tried - to little avail. Thus when the physicians income is reduced, there have been documented 'compensatory' changes which would enhance income. Thus when prices were frozen in California in 1971 during the Economic Stabilization Program, there was an increase in services and change in mix in response to this bureaucratic intervention (Eisenberg, 1981).

Placing a constraint on hospital expenditure as part of the DRG prospective payment plans has resulted in arrangements for high technology investigations to be performed as outpatients, thus simply shifting the expense from one pocket to the other. The unexpected effect is well illustrated by the very history of health care in the welfare state. The expectation was that more and better scientific health care would reduce the burden of illness in society, resulting in less need and less expenditure. This was based on the assumption of the operation of simple cause-and-effect in a simple system. Instead, multiple interacting variables in a complex system resulting in increasing utilization of health services and rising costs, has been noted. Thus health decisions tend to be hard to influence since they represent a futile attempt to anticipate the outcome of many interacting system variables.

The 'Medical Industrial Complex' refers to the connections between doctors, medical schools, hospitals, health insurance companies, the drug and health technology industries and corporate medicine driven by the logic of power, profits and politics. This combination has been accused of the 'commodification' of health care, reducing it to just another product in the capitalist system, an effective political lobby and as a powerful influence bolstering a narrow biomedical model of disease against considerable pressure for a broader perspective taking account of social and economic factors in community distribution of illness, and in the genesis of illness in the individual. Employers and insurers have lobbied the government effectively in the direction of regulation and cost-containment. The logical extension of this activity has been the evolution of the health maintenance organisation into a vast managed care and health insurance industry. Thus the penalty U.S. doctors paid for insistence on fee-for-service, and implacable resistance to a national health service has been a takeover of medical care by private interests!

The dominant position of medicine in bureaucratic structures and institutions was also queried, cheaper alternatives such as nurse practitioners proposed, with calls for the deprofessionalization of medicine. Medicine was also seen as oppressive in its relations with patients, tending to conventionalize political factors in patient care, thereby supporting the status quo, and of dominating other health professionals and workers in a hierarchical institutional structure. During the 1970s, the effectiveness of clinical care was also challenged in the light of research which disclosed marked variations in rates of hospitalization and of surgical and obstetrical intervention which cast a spotlight on the uncertainties of clinical practice (Chapter 9). Neglect of primary care and preventive medicine were also highlighted. Criticism of psychiatry stimulated the notion of the social construction of disease whereby doctors not only dominated the handling of disease, they even defined it. A deepening ambivalence about medicine was abroad in the society. Nevertheless, whatever may have been the aspersions cast on the quality of practice by various critics, we have to keep in mind that in the eyes of government, '(f)irst and last, this was understood to be a crisis of money' (Starr 1982).

It might be said that the industrial revolution was completed when medicine went from a cottage industry to a corporate one. Thus managed care shares the government's commitment to containing costs by a range of manoeuvres which limit the choice of doctors, providing incentives to intervene less, restricting services, insisting upon second opinions. The government's primary weapon in the war on health costs was the support of managed care. The second was its formal evaluation which spawned medical technology assessment health outcomes and effectiveness research, and an interest in 'evidence-based' quality assurance. This evaluation movement will be discussed in detail in Chapter 11.

The Thorny Issue of Access to Care

The issue of access and equity does not bear thinking about in the U.S. context. Health insurance for those not covered by Medicare or Medicaid is provided through the employer. As a result, a substantial proportion of Americans, approximately 40 million of them, lack any form of health insurance cover. The debate over the relationship between social class and ill-health is not encouraged by the fact that U.S. is the only western country which does not collect and stratify mortality statistics by class, despite the fact that research has shown large differentials which are increasing. Even larger are the differentials in morbidity (Navarro 1990).

In the United States, the health debate centres on problems of insurance cover, need for rationing of facilities, evaluation of high cost technology, attempts to 'improve' medical practice from a distance, using standard protocols of care and survey methods of evaluating health outcomes. The combination of an ideology and positivist methods which favour a biomedical emphasis in public health research, public health education which discourages involvement in politics, sometimes regulation to prevent public health doctors from engaging in political comment and controversy, have conspired to focus public health measures on having individuals take responsibility for their own health. The likelihood of success of behavioural intervention with regard to conventional risk factors such as eating habits, smoking and alcohol is open to serious question. At worst, this approach is seen as 'blaming the victim' in the face of deep-rooted problems related to low income and social class.

Despite all of this, pressures have not built up to a level which makes political change mandatory, despite the fact that the U.S. public is strongly in favor of a national health service, even if this meant a tax increase (Blendon and Donnellan 1990). A bipartisan commission set up by the Congress (The Pepper Commission) reported in 1990 'in response to a rapidly growing health care crisis' recommended urgent action to build a system of health care based on mandated universal insurance. In the view of its chairman, a national health insurance scheme was 'simply not practical' on the grounds of cost and taxation burden (Rockefeller 1990, 1005). The editor of the influential New England Journal of Medicine supported its conclusions adding the riders that insurance would have to be based on the prepaid model since fee-for-service was no longer affordable in this context, and that evaluation of technology should be a high priority (Relman, 1990, 1991). There has since been a paralysis of leadership from other quarters and perhaps a need for a fundamentally different and less combative style of negotiation. (Welch and Fisher 1992).

Thus there has been a formidable backlash against the health care restrictions and crimping of physician autonomy (Mechanic 1996). There have also been calls for presidential leadership (Blumenthal 1991). Reform was attempted in 1996 by the Clinton administration but was defeated by strong corporate interests. Despite its compelling logic and promising support in polls, the Clinton reforms were ultimately not acceptable to the American public. Powerful though reactions to managed care have been, the American public was not prepared to embrace the proposed reforms. The political details of this issue is beyond our scope but has been addressed by Stocpol (1995). However it seems fair to say that a combination of rejection of socialism and opposition by the financially better off with health insurance casts a dark cloud over prospects for future reform. The poor are not likely to find a place at the table any time soon.

Proposals for change have ducked the key issue of income redistribution implicit in any reform. There has been for a long time a firm conviction that things simply cannot remain the same in the U.S., and the choice facing physicians were summarized as 'centralized government regulatory mechanisms, including global budgets, or individual incentives for cost control that operate in a pluralistic, privately dominated system. The status quo is not a viable option.' (Reinhardt 1992). The latter prevailed but it is not yet clear whether managed care can continue to control costs, and there has been considerable public backlash against some of the restrictions placed upon care.

And so, in the main, it has remained in the United States. Inevitably, the ethos of free enterprise and suspicion of state intervention led to successful resistance to 'socialist solutions,' particularly to the implementation of a national health service as a central plank of reform. Although there had been support for such a service between 1910 and 1920, ultimately the movement foundered on economic and ideological grounds (Starr 1982, p253). Reform has been mainly in the name of economic rationalism rather than a call for better health care. In the United States, failure to develop a public medical service left medicine vulnerable to take-over by the corporate sector. Privatization of health care and encouragement of competition have since become part of the conservative ideology in other countries, even now impinging on the British National Health Service. But the cost problem was the nidus around which other doubts crystallized. The United States system placed its stamp on medicine worldwide by virtue of its pre-eminence in research, its widely read journals, its postgraduate training programs for foreign graduates and, above all, through the influence of its scientifically oriented medical curriculum which was emulated by medical schools the world over.

Britain

The health system in Britain has also become a political issue (Dean 1991). From the Public Health Act of 1848 until the 1880s and 1890s public health was a major issue. Thereafter the focus shifted to curative medical care, reflecting the advancing prestige of biomedical science. However, the need for provision of adequate medical care for 'labouring poor' also developed in Britain and on the continent during the 18th and 19th centuries. The notion of unified state health service combining Poor Law medical provisions with public health activities is attributable to the influence of Beatrice Webb's report in 1909. This officially renounced the idea of poverty and its consequences as the natural lot of the indigent, and was the progenitor of the National Health Service established almost 40 years later (Stacey 1988). Navarro (1978) has interpreted this key event in terms of the class struggle.

The NHS has often been a cockpit of conflicting interests. The Service has continued to be seen as a success in terms of cost containment (Klein 1991). However a major challenge to the British system came in the form of the Black Report which raised the perennial problem of the relationship of illness and premature death to social class. Evidence of a direct causal link to poverty and environment, evidence that the gradient of risk has become steeper under the influence of economic rationalist policies (refer Chapter N), affirmation of its crucial importance by one of the pioneers of public health (Morris 1991) have all highlighted this problem. Evidence that the gradient of illness persists from the lowest social classes, through the middle class to the higher classes, and evidence that deprivation in early life can predispose to later illness have all kept the debate alive.

Events in Britain and United States provide an interesting contrast. While the system of health care has remained market oriented in the U.S., the British system has lurched from one based upon market forces to a planned one and back again. The severe problems of equity of access to health care encountered in the U.S. are, of course, not to be found in Britain. However, the pattern of neglect of the social and political aspects of illness is essentially the same, and this seems to be true of all of the western democratic states. Klein saw the two systems as a mirror image of each other - the former parsimonious and underfunded, rationing by queuing but providing comprehensive coverage, the latter as wasteful and profligate, rationing by exclusion (Klein 1991). Yet there is evidence of some convergence of aims with the U.S. struggling to find a comprehensive system involving a single payer, and Britain introducing competition in the form of a 'purchaser- provider' arrangement. However the emphasis on competition was replaced by cooperation with the advent of another labour government, and an emphasis on professional responsibility in the form of 'clinical governance.'

The history of moves to evaluate medical technology has also been different under the British system. Despite the pioneering of health services research by Morris (1957) and the call to arms over the need to evaluate medical technology by Cochrane (1971), until quite recently, there was no formal coordination of technology assessment in Britain. This might reflect the fact that global control over the NHS budget had the effect of controlling proliferation of technology. Similarly, the adaptation of epidemiological methods to the scientific study of clinical techniques, clinical epidemiology, which originated in North America did not take a firm hold in Britain until it forged closer links to health services research and to cost containment efforts in Britain as part of the evidence-based medicine movement (Chapter 15). The National Institute for Health and Clinical Excellence in Britain has been established to deal with regional differences in health care delivery, and to launch medical technology assessment.

The major advantages in Britain are the National Health Service which has eliminated the worst inequities and kept its cost at about half of the U.S., and retention of general practitioners as providers of primary care. The gradient of ill-health, a sloping relationship from the wealthiest down to the poorest, a major influence on community morbidity and mortality, remains as a persistent reminder of the impact of the industrial revolution (Black Report 1980, Exworthy et al. 2003). As Engels (1845) saw it: 'How is it possible ...for the lower class to be healthy and long lived? What else can be expected than an excessive mortality, an unbroken series of epidemics, and a progressive deterioration in the physique of the working population?' It is also worth noting that there is a gradient from those with the most occupational autonomy to those with least (Marmot and Wilkinson 1999).

Conclusion

The public does have concerns about medicine and the health care system. In general, they are satisfied with their own doctor but dissatisfied with the system. Issues are the quality of care, its cost and access. There is no suggestion that the public wants less medical care; the evidence is to the contrary. There has been a marked increase in the utilisation of health care, as opposed to naive expectations of reduced cost due to conquest of disease. There is also a sense of diminishing returns from expenditure on medicine, and doubt about medicine's capacity for reform. This dissatisfaction inevitably surfaces as political forces. In addition, governments are disturbed by the cost of care. Various measures have been introduced to control costs, including the evaluation of health care in the U.S., but opposition to any hint of socialism has resulted in a corporate takeover of medicine. Managed care has made inroads in other countries. Despite all of this, medicine has held most of its ground as a profession with no suggestion of 'proletarianisation.'

Revolutionary changes in health can only accompany revolution in society itself. In fact, the French Revolution brought about just such a change in the delivery of health care. Early in the 19th century the decision to break the monopoly of the traditional medical elite, and also to support the teaching hospital, together brought about the transformation of traditional into scientific medicine in France (Chapter 6). The French Revolution was also concerned with fundamental societal change with regard to class and distribution of wealth. In this regard, it is interesting to note how provocative is the World Health Organization's definition of health by stating that it is 'a state of complete physical, mental, and social well-being, not merely the absence of disease and infirmity' (Last 1988). This has therefore thrown the spotlight directly on the uneven distribution of income between and within countries which contributes most to ill-health under the present world order. Very little has been done to redistribute income to overcome the relationship between illness, premature death and low social class.

Radical reform according to current political structures would imply a socialist regime which would move to redistribute income, to reduce the dominance of the medical profession and increased lay control and involvement in decision-making. Those governments with a national health service like Britain and Sweden, and to a lesser extent those with a more mixed public and private system have successfully removed the grosser inequities of access. However, without the necessary reform of each of the organizations described above, they offer but access to more of the same. Resistance to the merest whiff of socialism appears to have effectively disabled any attempt to introduce a national health service in the United States. Here the alternative solution is in place - the progressive corporatisation of medicine.

References

Barsky A. J., The paradox of health. *New Engl J Med* 318: 414-8;1988.

Beeson P. B., Changes in medical therapy during the past half century. *Medicine* 59:79-99; 1980.

Black D., Inequalities in Health. *Penguin*, London, 1980.

Blendon R. J., The public's view of the future of health care. *JAMA* 259: 3587-93; 1988.

Blendon R. J., Donnelan K., The public and the emerging debate on national health insurance. *New Engl J Med* 323: 208-211; 19.

Blumenthal D., The timing and course of health care reform. *New Engl J Med* 325:198-200; 1992.

Burnett M., Genes, Dreams and Realities. Bucks Medical and Technical Publishing Co., *Aylesbury,* 1971, p. 226.

Bynum W., The McKeown Thesis. *Lancet* 371: 644-5, 2008.

Cartwright A., Andersen R., General Practice Revisited: a second study of patients and their doctors. *Tavistock,* London, 1981.

Cartwright A., Anderson R., General Practice Revisited: a second study of doctors and their patients. *Tavistock,* London, 1981. p. 162.

Cochrane A. L., Effectiveness and Efficiency: Random reflections on Health Services. *The Nuffield Hospitals Trust*, London, 1971.

Committee of Inquiry into Medical education and Medical Workforce Australian Medical Education and Workforce into the 21st Century. Australian Government Printing Service, Canberra, 1988, pp. 56,57.

Committee of Inquiry into Medical education and Medical Workforce Australian Medical Education and Workforce into the 21st Century. Australian Government Printing Service, Canberra, 1988, pp. 37-51.

Dean M., How voters boost health finance. *Lancet* 1991;338:1259-60.

Dubos R., Mirage of Health. Allen and Unwin, London, 1960.

Eisenberg J. M., Doctors' Decisions and the Cost of Medical Care. Health Administration Press perspectives, *Ann Arbor,* 1986, p. 31.

Eisenberg L., Kleinman., Clinical social science. In: The Relevance of Social Science for Medicine Eds Eisenberg L, Kleinman A. D Reidel, Dordrecht, Holland, 1981.

Exworthy M., Blane D., Marmot M., Tackling health inequalities in Britain: The progress and pitfalls of policy. *Health Serv Res* 105: 1905-1932.

Engels F., The condition of the working class in england. Stanford University Press, Stanford. 1845.

Feinstein A. R., Scientific standards of epidemiologic studies of the menace of everyday life. *Science* 242:1257-63; 1988.

Flexner A., The Flexner Report on Medical Education in the United States and Canada. Bulletin Number Four. A Report to the Carnegie Foundation for the Advancement of Teaching. New York, 1910.

Freidson E., Medical Work in America: essays on health care. *Yale University Press,* New Haven, 1989, p. 77.

Freidson E., Medical Work in America: essays on health care. *Yale University Press,* New Haven, 1989. p. 185.

Freidson E., Medical Work in America: essays on health care. *Yale University Press*, New Haven, 1989. p. 11.

Freis J. F., Aging, natural death, and the compression of morbidity. *New Engl J Med* 303:130-5; 1980.

Fuchs V. R., Shall Live? Health, Economics, and Social Choice. *Basic Books,* New York, 1974, p. 144.

Gruenberg E. M., The failures of success. *Milbank Memorial Fund Q* 55:3-24;1977.

Harvey L. K., Shubat S. C., Public Opinion on Health Care Issues 1989. Chicago Ill: American Medical Association, 1989.

Illich I., Limits to Medicine - Medical Nemesis: The Expropriation of Health, London, *Calder and Boyars,* 1974, p. 152-3.

Illich I., Limits to Medicine - Medical Nemesis: The Expropriation of Health, London, *Calder and Boyars*, 1974, p. 21.

Katz J., The Silent World of Doctors and Patients. *Free Press,* New York, 1984, p. 191.

Katz J., The Silent World of Doctors and Patients. *Free Press*, New York, 1984. p. 205.

Katz J., The Silent World of Doctors and Patients. *Free Press*, New York, 1984. p. 11.

Kerr D. J., Scott M., British lessons on health care reform. *N Engl J Med* 36: e21, 2009.

Klein R., The American health care predicament. *BMJ* 303: 259-60;1991.

Lasch C., Culture of Narcissism: American life in an age of diminishing expectations. *Abacus,* London, 1980, pp31-51.

Last J., A Dictionary of Epidemiology. 2nd edition. Oxford University Press, New York, 1988, p. 57.

Mackenzie J., (1909) Symptoms and their interpretation. London: Shaw and Sons.

Maddrey W. C., Gunnar R. M., Griner P. F., Cleaveland C. R., Ball J. R., Health care reform: an American imperative. *Ann Int Med* 117:513 – 519; 1992.

McKeown T., The Role of Medicine: Dream, Mirage or Nemesis ? Basil Blackwell, Oxford, 1979.

Marmot M., Wilkinson R. J., eds. Social Determinants of Health. Oxford University Press, Oxford. 1999.

Mechanic D., Public perceptions of medicine. *New Engl J Med* 312:181-3, 1986.

Mechanic D., Muddling through elegantly. Finding the proper balance in rationing. *Health Affairs.* 16: 83-92, 1997.

Morris J., Uses of Epidemiology. Williams and Wilkins, Baltimore, 1957.

Morris, J. N., Social inequalities in health. *Lancet:* 338:1337; 1991.

Navarro V., Medicine Under Capitalism. *Prodist*, New York, 1976.

Navarro V., Race or class versus race and class: mortality differentials in the United States. *Lancet* 336: 1238-1240; 1990.

Nelson A. R., Humanism and the art of medicine: our commitment to care. *JAMAb* 262:1228-30; 1989.

Reinhardt U., Commentary: politics and the health care system. *New Engl J Med* 327:809-811; 1992.

Relman A. S., Reforming the health care system. 1990;323: 991-2.

Rockefeller J. D., The Pepper Commission Report on comprehensive health care. *New Engl J Med:* 323:1005-7; 1990.

Rosen G., A History of Public Health. The Johns Hopkins University Press, Baltimore, 1993, p. 422.

Rosen G., A History of Public Health. The Johns Hopkins University Press, Baltimore, 1993, p. 421.

Smith R., Health Affairs p185, reported in, *BMJ* 1990; 301:358.

Stacey M., The Sociology of Health and Healing: a textbook. Unwin Hyman, London, 1988, pp. 116-132.

Starr P., The Social Transformation of American Medicine. the rise of a sovereign profession and the making of a vast industry. *Basic Books*, 1982, p. 55.

Starr P., The social Transformation of American Medicine. the rise of a sovereign profession and the making of a vast industry. *Basic Books*, 1982.

Starr P., The Social Transformation of American Medicine. the rise of a sovereign profession and the making of a vast industry. *Basic Books,* 1982. p. 381.

Starr P., The social Transformation of American Medicine. the rise of a sovereign profession and the making of a vast industry. *Basic Books*, 1982. p. 253.

Stoddart G. L., Evans R., G., Producing health, consuming health care. *Soc Sci Med* 31:1347-63; 1990.

Stocpol T., The rise and resounding demise of the Clinton plan. *Health Affairs* 16: 66-85, 1995.

Welch W.D., Fisher S., Let's make a deal: Negotiating a settlement between physicians and society. *New Engl J Med* 327:1312-5; 1992.

White K. W., Healing the Schism: epidemiology, medicine, and the public's health. *Springer-Verlag,* New York,1991.

Wildavsky A., Doing Better and Feeling Worse: the political pathology of health policy. Daedalus 1977 winter: 105-123.

Chapter 4

The Fire - Paradigm, Thought Collective or Discourse?

What Is at the Bottom of All of This?

We have committed ourselves to locating the fire generating the smoke which is currently engulfing health care. In general terms this is not difficult. Within medicine there is the traditional art which, at times, is in conflict with the much newer science. Within the clinical consultation, doctors and patients, long assumed to share the common objective of support and healing, find themselves at odds, and often for reasons they do not fully understand. Within the health care system, as we have seen, there are many more players who claim to have a stake in the quality and cost of health care than there used to be. The medical profession, proudly independent and long the ally of modern government, finds itself under increasing bureaucratic constraint and at risk of corporatization. Cogent criticisms also arise from public health, the social sciences, social critics and from within the profession. Common to these disagreements is the fact that groups of people have different beliefs, often strongly held and largely tacit, which can lead to serious misunderstanding and disagreement or to a clash of objectives. And this at a time when there is a special need for constructive dialogue in our health system at a time of change. Groupthink is the enemy of interdisciplinary cooperation, even of mutual understanding.

The successful transition to a more integrated and efficient system requires a level of accommodation and cooperation among the various players. Progress will be slow if there is dissonance between the various groups responsible for the clinical care and health care delivery, lack of common objectives, and if there is lack of guidance from cooperative research. We need therefore to understand how various group beliefs and commitments lead to dissonance. What problems can we sheet home to tension between the art and the science of medicine? What causes friction between doctors and patients? How do the basic assumptions of public health and social sciences differ from those of clinical medicine? What are the obstacles to cooperative research between an epidemiologist and a sociologist?

It is common knowledge that people are different and so are groups of people. The extent of these differences, and many of the implications, are not so obvious and have been the subject of much thought. Human groups share commitments, beliefs, ways of thinking and making judgements. In the case of professional and academic disciplines, there are different ways of conducting research, even different principles for deciding what is to be accepted as true or false. The basic idea which has been approached from a number of different perspectives is that all human groups socialize their members to see the world from a common perspective, to have similar goals, to think alike, to speak a common language, and to develop institutions which reflect their purposes and their thinking. People who flock together either are or become birds of a cognitive, intellectual and political feather! This is the central characteristic of Ludwik's Fleck's 'thought collective,' of Michel Foucault's 'discourse' and of Thomas Kuhn's 'paradigm.' Paradigm was developed with a focus on scientific disciplines; Foucault had his main focus on medicine. Ludwik Fleck's concept of 'thought collective has historical precedence, developed in the 1930s (Gillies,1996). Kuhn's 'paradigm has the advantage of wider understanding and usage. Foucault links his 'discourse' to 'power' considerations, important for our usage. Imre Lakatos' analogous concept of 'scientific research programme is also a candidate but has no particular advantages. We have chosen to merge 'paradigm' and 'discourse' as a hybrid concept which best expresses our thoughts in its application to the problems of the professions of clinical practice and health care delivery.

Fleck's 'Thought Collective'

The idea that social groups of people, commonly a profession or community interest group, share a framework of knowledge, belief, commitment and vocabulary was explored by the German physician and bacteriologist Ludwik Fleck in the 1930s. He spoke of a 'thought collective' and a 'thought style' which '(O)nce structurally complete and coded system of opinions consisting of many details and relations has been formed, it offers constant resistance to anything that contradicts it.' (Fleck 1973). The commitment was strong, ideological and largely tacit: 'Although the thought collective consists of individuals, it is not simply the aggregate sum of them. The individual within the collective is never, or hardly ever, conscious of the prevailing thought style which almost always exerts an absolutely compulsive force upon his thinking, and with which it is not possible to be at variance.' (Fleck 1930). The commitment could be a serious barrier to communication between social and professional groups: 'The greater the difference between two thought styles, the more inhibited will be the communication of ideas.' It could even be coercive: 'This social character inherent in the very nature of scientific activity is not without its substantive consequences. Words which formerly were simple terms become slogans. Sentences which were simple statements become calls to battle.' Such differences influence events over long periods and make dissent difficult: 'Whole eras will then be ruled by this thought constraint. Those who do not share this collective mood and are rated as criminals by the collectives will be burnt at the stake until a different mood creates a different thought style and different evaluation.' (Fleck 1973).

Kuhn's 'Paradigm'

Fleck's ideas did not gain much currency when first presented in the 1930s. However the reader is most likely to be already familiar with this idea in connection with Kuhn's concept of the scientific 'paradigm' (Kuhn 1970). This term describes the basic assumptions, the framework which guides the way in which the sciences conduct their research. Groups of scientists tacitly follow a consensus view in their area which operates as a framework for their beliefs and as a blueprint for research. This view of their world was inculcated as tacit knowledge during their education: 'For long periods, whole scientific disciplines or branches teach model solutions which dictate how they should be seen and solved. Periodically this orthodoxy shifts, stirring up conflict between old and new until a new consensus develops.' (Kuhn 1970). Thus discoveries by investigations which appear rigorous but do not fit the current paradigm tend to accumulate and cast doubt on the paradigm. The paradigm is then replaced by another - a 'scientific revolution' occurs. Thus Newtonian physics was replaced by quantum physics, or the old heliocentric universe by the solar system, scientific revolutions or paradigm shifts. So the medical paradigm underwent a paradigmatic revolution from the classical to the modern, and, as we see it, the modern one is now in the painful throes of a shift to the postmodern.

Kuhn's contribution to the debate, which scandalised many scientists because of the apparent challenge to scientific objectivity, was to emphasise the role of the social group of acknowledged experts whose consensus opinion was the arbiter of truth rather than some universal standard. In general, in any area of science, except for a brief period preceding a shift, only one paradigm at a time can prevail. 'One of the fundamental techniques by which members of a group, whether an entire culture or specialists' sub-community within it, learn to see the same things when confronted with the same stimuli is by being shown examples of situations that their predecessors in the group have already learned to see as like each other and as different from other sorts of situations.' (Kuhn 1970). Kuhn also stressed the problem of communication between disciplines. In extreme cases, proponents have no common ground for discussion so that they simply talk past each other: 'Since the vocabularies in which they discuss such situations consist, however, predominantly of the same terms, they must be attaching some of those terms to nature differently, and their communication is inevitably only partial. As a result, the superiority of one theory to another is something that cannot be proved in the debate. Instead, I have insisted, each party must try, by persuasion to convert the other.' (Kuhn 1970).

It is important to note that this notion of paradigm was introduced by Kuhn as theoretical underpinning for research in astronomy and the natural sciences. A basic attribute of science is the acceptance of certain universal rules where a single perspective characteristically prevails in a field for long periods. In most human groups and certainly in health care, however, plurality of social values and professional perspectives is the rule. Hence the concept, as originally proposed is more difficult to apply to the social sciences, to clinical medicine or to the culture at large where there are invariably multiple perspectives at any particular time.

Foucault's 'Discourse'

The most comprehensive treatment of this subject of 'group-think' for our purposes is the work of Michel Foucault which stems from a line of thought by Gaston Bachelard in French philosophy of science. Unfortunately, it is also the most obscure. His focus was on the relationship between the natural sciences and human sciences following the Renaissance, based on laws that evolved within an evolving culture. Foucault referred to the individual discipline or interest group as a 'discourse,' the framework of beliefs and attitudes as a 'discursive formation,' and used the term 'discursive breaks' to refer to the relatively sudden shifts of paradigm to which Kuhn had referred in his analysis.

A discourse is a domain of social communication which relates to language and social communication. It is characterised by shared group assumptions, attitudes, knowledge and beliefs, bound together and shaped by an invisible 'discursive framework.' It is characterised by commonality of outlook, goals and aspirations, shared attitudes, basic beliefs and commitments, a particular world view with regard to knowledge, its nature and its classification which, in turn, shapes its methods of practice, research and education. The framework of a discourse therefore constitutes a grid of interpretation determining what is true, which concepts offer valid interpretation and which do not. It also acts as a field of force which shapes the discourse's view of events and of history, moulds its social customs and institutions, determines who speaks with authority, what can be said and how, what is an issue, who is an ally, who an enemy, who is honoured, who is to be rejected.

Since it is socialisation into a group which underpins the thinking and communication of members, the ideas are as unobtrusive as our manner of dressing, our way of walking, our rules of conversation and our table manners. The influence of discourse on the individual is therefore both powerful but largely unappreciated, acting as an important, often a determining influence on every individual or group decision. An important feature of discourse is the extent to which it is taken for granted. Indeed the most basic assumptions of a discourse like physics or medicine may only be exposed when they are under serious challenge at a time of shift. At other times, such as when decisions are being taken on a day to day basis, these assumptions are tacit, assumed, unstated and invisible. As in the case of Kuhn's closely similar concept of 'paradigm' the influence of a discourse is largely tacit, so that related disagreement is often at the basic level of unexamined assumptions. This can lead to claims that someone else's beliefs are misguided, methods of research invalid, their practice lacking in rigour. Such fundamental differences can obviously be perceived as threatening, and a serious impediment to interdisciplinary communication. Hence the real basis of conflict may be unclear and such differences do not respond well to reasoned argument.

Foucault's concepts allow for plurality of commitments, overlapping discourses, and nesting of discourses within discourses. In medicine and public health, there is heterogeneity of thought with several discourses nested within each interwoven like the coloured threads of a tapestry. Co-existing within medicine in a state of some tension and competition are the main discourses of traditional clinical medicine, the biomedical, and the epidemiological. Within public health many threads of discourse are intertwined - that of social medicine, epidemiological, biostatistical, managerial, sociological, economic and more. Nesting within the medical paradigm are biomedical and statistical paradigms which are generally concordant, but which may disagree; this occurred as we shall see in the case of levels of clinical evidence proposed by the evidence-based medicine proponents. Similarly, within sociology there are two approaches to research, one based upon science, analytical and quantitative, and the other upon interpretion and hermeneutics.

The historical evolution of a paradigm proceeds within and is constrained by the culture, punctuated by intermittent 'discursive breaks' which are analogous to Kuhn's scientific revolutions. My belief is that most controversy in medicine can be traced to a paradigm shift from the modern with its major intellectual commitment to science favoured by our by our culture, to the emerging postmodern with a greater commitment to an interpretive paradigm based on the study of text. These paradigms are currently vying for supremacy but a balanced clinical research program must utilize both as appropriate. These group commitments inevitably create conditions for alliance or dissonance within clinical medicine and public health, as well as between them. For example, biomedical science and epidemiology are different in most respects but share a central commitment to the research methods of the natural sciences and to mathematical analysis.

Incompatible Beliefs

We all have multiple group commitments in our daily and professional lives, an important point noted by Fleck. This is clear in the case of the scientist who may subscribe to a realist and objective account of the world and at the same time harbour incompatible religious beliefs. Clinical medicine incorporates, in a state of tension, a variety of ideas and commitments related to the ancient clinical tradition, modern biomedical science and, more recently, epidemiology. Hence, in any single judgement, a modern clinician may have to juggle influences related to these discourses which are not always compatible with each other. Thus the logical compulsion of scientific intervention may clash with the patient's preferences or the social context. In addition, the clinician is asked to be at the one time a powerful advocate of individual patient rights as a doctor but also bound by a responsibility to society or equitable distribution of scarce resources in the community. Inevitably, therefore, there will be tensions within discourses, between discourses, and between ideas related to different discourses within individuals.

Paradigm Conflicts and the Exercise of Power

Another important issue mentioned by Fleck and alluded to by Kuhn, but central to Foucault's interpretation, is power. There is the obvious legitimated 'sovereign' power which exerted by the state. There is also 'capillary power' a more covert diffuse compulsion which follows from the socialisation of individuals in the culture and within discourses. Their tacit beliefs engendered by their education and initial socialisation, and reinforced by their peer contacts and institutions, ensure continuous unconscious self-monitoring and surveillance which can influence every judgement, decision and action. This power may be negative, coercive, subjugating. It then elicits resistance which is similarly diffuse and subtle. On the other hand, power can also be seen as the positive force which energises action, fuel for the engine of change which drives progress and innovation. So close is the link between knowledge and power that Foucault came to believe that they could not be separated.

Conflicts in society, more on the surface in times of change, are often about belief and knowledge but their resolution has much to do with the exhibition of power. There is therefore a balance of power between paradigms. What is the accepted point of view within a particular discipline and perhaps within the wider society is therefore to a large determined by the 'dominant paradigm.' This discipline is then clearly in a position of considerable power. Thus it was dominance of the scientific paradigm over the clinical in medicine's public face which explained the characteristics of the paradigm, and the dominance of the scientific medical discourse over public health and consumer interests which shaped the system of health care following World War II.

This leads to two important consequences. Different commitments of individuals may lead to conflict within or between groups. Conflicting attitudes in the individual may lead to faulty judgement and decision-making. We will encounter many examples of both. For example, a physician may recommend medical management of a patient while a surgeon favours surgery, a doctor committed to finding organic disease may undertake extensive investigation on a patient in need of counselling or treatment of depression. An epidemiologist may wish to conduct a survey to assess patient satisfaction when a sociologist believes that interview of patients with qualitative data analysis is more appropriate method. A general practitioner may feel that an ultrasound scan is the scientific way to investigate a stressed patient with abdominal pain, but is aware that a sound clinical opinion may actually be more accurate and less likely to generate a worrying false positive result or to turn up a confusing incidental finding.

These conflicts are therefore a basis of consensus or disagreement, cooperation or conflict between disciplines which will determine overall stability or dissonance in the delivery of health services, and also the direction and quality of research. At the same time, the interaction between paradigms in individual decision-makers can lead to unbalanced or distorted judgements made in patient management or in committee. The prevailing discourse shaping a discipline will therefore determine which other disciplines will easily communicate and cooperate within and without its borders, and those with which they are most likely to come into conflict. This is why the ideas of paradigm is so important in explaining the fire of controversy in health - the potential for clashes of paradigm enters into every interaction, every negotiation between the players in health care, and into every one of their judgements and decisions!

One of the central features of the postmodern world is an increase in the complexity of our social institutions so that many more discourses come into contact as a result of integrating forces, especially of the information revolution. There are more voices to be heard in most debates, including those pertaining to health. In the case of health care, this once involved just three paradigms - those of the doctor or other healer, of the patient seeking help, and the common social culture they shared. Today the gap between the medical and lay discourses has widened, and many voices have been added - those of politician and bureaucrat, business and consumer bodies, and those of the wide range of professionals and academic disciplines engaged in research and evaluation. Differences between discourses are of particular importance at present in health care because they threaten the unity of purpose required for constructive change. Moreover, since adherence to a paradigm revolves around tacit knowledge, beliefs mostly beyond the individual's conscious reach, reasoned even reasonable debate usually stays out of reach in most of these highly charged conflicts.

Which to Choose?

All of this leaves us with something of a dilemma. Foucault's concepts and terminology, analogous to Kuhn's, provide a better analytical framework for discussing medicine, public health and the social sciences. In particular, they allow for nesting of multiple paradigms as we have seen. On the other hand, Kuhn's ideas are much more familiar and more widely understood since they have entered the common lexicon, and 'paradigm' in this sense is now listed in the Oxford English Dictionary (2012). We intend to compromise. In our analysis, we will use the term 'paradigm' as defined in the dictionary, to refer to 'the goals, beliefs and practices of a group of 'like-minded individuals.'.'" We also apply this broader common usage of the term 'paradigm' to shared lay beliefs or to government commitments. The terms 'thought collective,' 'discourse' and 'paradigm' can for our purposes be considered interchangeable, and roughly equivalent to 'perspective' according to common usage. Thus modern doctors and consumers constitute a paradigm and a perspective, each with shared beliefs, attitudes, ways of thinking and objectives. We recognise paradigms of medicine, of public health, of sociology, of economics - all of which evolve over time. Before we discuss the evolution of the major paradigms in the health system we need to discuss two which are of overriding importance since the balance between them influences the culture and every intellectual professional and academic discipline.

Two Great Paradigms of Intellectual Enquiry

There is a pair of intellectual paradigms which nest within and are an integral part of many others including those of academic professions and health. They are derived from two major intellectual worldviews which have vied for supremacy since ancient times - mechanism with reductionism and organicism with holism. The former came to dominate when natural philosophy split off from the mainstream following the Renaissance and evolved into modern science. Research in science was laboratory based, positivistic, controlled and reductionist, and assumed the existence of universal truth towards which science converged ever closer. Research in the humanities was based on refinement of scholarship related to the study of ancient texts, a 'hermeneutic,' interpretive and contextual approach. This paradigm aims at understanding of meaning through iterative interpretation in context and is presented as a narrative argument.

There was reaction against the hegemony of scientific explanation of the world by thinkers who insisted on the ultimate primacy of human interpretation in a cultural context. Schliermacher in Germany had developed the rigour of biblical interpretation and this 'hermeneutics' was extended to the scholarly study of classical texts. Dilthey made a radical extension of these ideas by proposing that science with its explanation in terms of universal principles was appropriate within its realm but was not appropriate for the human sciences which always involved meaning and purpose, hence requiring a contextualised understanding which he called 'verstehen' (Dilthey1972). Kant had claimed that these categories filter and shape our understanding. Dilthey saw that this understanding was not static and inborn, rather that it evolved as the historical context evolved.

CP Snow (1964) brought again to public attention the tension, even antagonism which developed between what are really complementary approaches to knowledge. He referred to 'The Two Cultures.' This unfortunate and unnecessary division is alive and well in medicine and in the health system, reflecting the tension between the assumptions and methods of science and of the humanities. The social sciences and medicine straddle both. The scientific analytical and humanistic interpretive intellectual paradigms are entirely complementary, not in competition at all. When medicine shifted its allegiance from the humanities about 200 years ago, the false dichotomy between the art and science of medicine was created. Numbers and models can inform clinical judgement but not replace it or take primacy over it. This unfortunate ideological gulf distorts our understanding of the clinical consultation which is fundamentally interpretive in structure, although quantitative evidence is valuable and clinical techniques can undoubtedly be improved in some areas by scientific methods.

The various professional discourses tend to have a primary commitment to either the quantitative and analytical, or to the qualitative and interpretive, or to be internally split along these lines. In the analytical quantitative camp for which science is the guiding paradigm, the emphasis is on internal validity. This is an approach to an assumed truth, progressively approached by maximal exclusion of error. This, in turn, is ideally achieved by experimentation under conditions of laboratory control with mathematical analysis, yielding objective results allegedly independent of context and moral value. The analytical scientific paradigm is the dominant intellectual one in biomedical science, epidemiology, economics, one branch of sociology and in behavioural science.

Hard-liners from this camp tend to reject the results of interpretive qualitative research as subjective, soft, preliminary, descriptive or hypothesis-generating, even journalistic! This is, of course, the creed of 'scientism.' Eminent researchers, including immunologist Medawar (1984) and philosopher of science Kuhn (1970) have pointed out that qualitative data is also central to quantitative research. There may be quantitative results from a study. However the rationale for the study and the underlying hypothesis must be argued with qualitative argument. So too must its interpretation in light of relevant previous results in the scientific literature. Its objective is therefore to establish the 'meaning' of results in context. In fact, the very question as to whether or not a new paradigm has appeared is eventually decided by debate and conviction which has both qualitative and quantitative elements!

The interpretive tradition is based upon data collection by observation, interview and analysis of documents, and development of classifications. It is synthesised into an argument by employing appropriate theory to interpret rigorously defined evidence which is mostly qualitative. The argument mainly involves reasoning the meaning of factors in context, and is more flexible than decontextualized numbers. This interpretive camp includes some sociologists, also anthropologists, ethicists and historians, and - although few are aware of it – clinicians! Interestingly, despite pretensions to being an applied science and attempts to apply mathematical models, clinical practice itself is undeniably a form of iterative interpretive evaluation based on observation and interview, and analysis of mainly qualitative or semi-quantitative data. Those with primary allegiance to the interpretive tradition challenge the idea that universal laws apply in the social and human world, that context free and objective conclusions can be drawn, that knowledge can be value-free. It is tantamount to trying to fit a square peg into a square hole! Many are are also concerned that the scientific approach can dehumanise, and can be used to sidetrack public debate by inappropriately calling upon the authority of science to truncate public debate. Hard liners of both sides denigrate the methods of the other. At worst, these are like tribal allegiances which stir futile debates over who is scientific and who is not, whose claims to validity are superior and which methods are best. A useful account of the characteristics of qualitative research has been offered by Myers (2001), and a more comprehensive one by Avison et al. (2008).

Paradigmatic Conflict and Distortion of the Clinical Research Agenda

Conflict between the assumptions, methods and criteria of validity of science and of the humanities is a serious barrier to strategic multidisciplinary clinical research and evaluation, a barrier to communication which can also distort the research agenda when problems are chosen primarily to allow use of a familiar method. Yet a balanced program of clinical or health services research must call upon the methods of both paradigms in a flexible manner. Analytical quantitative methods are best for answering such questions as how many, how big and how much, and for making experimental comparisons between interventions. The interpretive paradigm includes qualitative information, and its concern is with interpretation of meaning, addressing questions such as who did what to whom, why, how, when and with what consequences. In a field as complex as health, it should be obvious that we need to ask all of these last questions and more. It should therefore be obvious that these two great intellectual paradigms, the analytical and the interpretive, are not at all in competition. Their contributions are complementary in the pursuit of flexibility, scientific expertise and the scholarship required to answer the infinity of questions thrown up by health care. Unfortunately, that is not the general view. As Confucius is alleged to have said 'the way out is through the door – what a pity more people don't use it..'

Systems Thinking - A Third Intellectual Paradigm

The philosophy of mechanism with its rigid causality, the basis of early science, ran into trouble even in 19th century laboratory research in the physical sciences. Hence Maxwell was obliged to introduce probability concepts into this theory of electromagnetic fields (Stewart 1991). Boltzmann did likewise in his efforts to develop a model of gas kinetics (Gillispie 1960). These were overt acknowledgments that strict scientific causality had its limits, and multivariate modelling became an important but limited way of handling the web of causality in a discipline such as epidemiology. The limitations of cause-and-effect thinking are even more obvious in ecology and biology. Here holism signaled its comeback. The response was to think in terms of the 'system,' initially a mathematical approach to a collection of mutually interacting variables introduced by Von Bertalanffy (1933) in an attempt to understand the intricate details of embryogenesis but later broadened to encompass 'systems thinking' which allowed for the complex interactions between many variables which cannot or should not be factored out by laboratory control. The world is composed of complex systems, some of which, a minority, yield to mathematics such as differential equations, but a majority which do not (Williams and Imam 2006).

The most important characteristic of a complex dynamic system is that it responds to change as a whole, so that simplifying explanations based upon cause and effect could be grossly misleading. Systems also typically resist change in a holistic way, a property known in biology as 'homeostasis' (Cannon 1926). This is certainly true of systems of belief such as a paradigm. However stimuli can also have an imperceptible but incremental effect which culminates in an unpredictable major re-orientation of the dynamic system which, in the case of scientific theory, we recognise as a paradigm shift or discursive break. The idea of hermeneutic interpretation in the humanities, and the rejection of science's claims to causal explanation in the human and social world can also be seen as an acknowledgement of its extreme complexity which cannot be adequately modelled solely in terms of cause and effect. Indeed a complex system can only be fully understood by documenting its behavior by observation of its behavior as a whole, including its response to external stimuli.

A central feature of the postmodern world is an emergent tolerance for uncertainty, for unpredictability, for ambiguity, for particularity, in short a willingness to acknowledge the typical holistic behaviour of the complex dynamic system of mutually interacting variables in nature and the social world. This trend is manifest in science as chaos theory and the complex dynamic system far from equilibrium characteristic of the living organism. It is evident in the humanities as poststructuralism, and in the recognition of language as a complex dynamic system of symbols which is our interface with 'reality' (De Sassure 1974). Conventional science could not handle complexity of this kind. Indeed it has meticulously avoided the problem by selection of tractable problems, that is simple systems with few variables, by laboratory control and by the use of differential equations. In a way, this resembles the somewhat misleading effect of the decontextualized evaluation of drugs by the randomized trial as we shall see.

Undoubtedly the most fundamental problem for medicine is the current tension between two paradigms, the art with its roots in the classical paradigm which underpinned medicine for over two thousand years, and the current scientific one establishing primacy from the Renaissance, achieving dominance in just 200 years. Systems thinking provides a useful model to express the anatomy of this highly complex conflict. Science has obviously shaped our modern society hence clinical practice, research and research in the modern era. But there is a major problem.

Foucault would postulate that this dominant scientific paradigm would inevitably have shaped medical practice, education and research – but he would undoubtedly pointed to an inevitable 'capillary resistance' in opposition to it. Hence there are powerful patient and political movements currently emerging calling for more 'patient-centred care,' longstanding calls for more social science and humanities in medical education, and our call for multidisciplinary program of 'continuous clinical practice research' lead by our postmodern 'reflective physicians,' and supported by 'centres for the study of clinical practice' (Chapter 16). The narrow scope of the medical curricular reform has also increasingly come under fire.

Science in medicine currently still dominates the art but the outcome of this formidable struggle should comprise, hopefully retaining the best of both worlds while jettisoning of the drawbacks of both. The virtues of biomedical science go without saying, and the positive contribution of 'evidence-based medicine' should not be gainsaid. However the warped view of 'clinical evidence,' postulated as synonymous with the empirical and statistical science, to the exclusion of clinical experience and evidence from biomedical science is simply untenable in light of research in cognitive science. Moreover, commonsense demands the inclusion of frequently numerous personal perspectives, social and other contextual variables which physicians know invariably impact upon clinical management decisions. Michel Foucault emphasized the positive side of such a paradigm driven power struggle as an important motive force for change. Yet the different perspectives of biomedical and empirical statistical science could remain in a balanced state of tension with a newly reinforced art without any achieving hegemony and completely satisfactory outcome, but generated the energy required for a shift of paradigm.

There are complex systems aplenty in health - in biomedical systems in health and disease, in human judgement and behaviour, in the interaction within and between paradigms in the social and cultural world. There are two important mechanisms for handling this uncertainty and complexity. The most obvious are to re-establish the important links of medicine with the humanities, and to exploit relevant research concepts and methods from sociology and anthropology. Sociology drew upon the experience of anthropology in developing field studies which could be used to explore the meaning of human decision and behaviour. This kind of qualitative research is necessary if we are to understand the judgements and decisions of doctors in planning treatment and how they communicate with patients, the way patients decide to seek or not to seek medical care, and how they respond to advice and treatment. In Chapter 16 we discuss the important contribution of interpretive (qualitative) methods to a balanced program of clinical research and evaluation. The process is basically an iterative learning process with online generation of theory and an ongoing adaption of methods of study in the face of changing circumstances.

Systems Thinking

'Systems thinking' uses the observed properties of complex systems to understand their observed behavior without necessarily invoking the mathematics. The second way in which the complexity of health care can be confronted is to cultivate such 'systems thinking' as a tool for deciphering complex events. To some extent this has already been done. The ability of the human body to maintain the constancy of the chemical context of cells was analysed as the 'milieu interieur,' the internal environment, by pioneer physiologist Claude Bernard. The mechanisms whereby this was achieved were described as 'homeostasis' by Walter B. Cannon early in this century. Following severe haemorrhage, for example, a cascade of compensatory mechanisms come into play as an attempt to maintain the output of the heart, and if this cannot be achieved, to maintain the blood pressure and divert blood from less essential organs like the muscle and gut to the brain and heart. The gradual decline in this ability due to progressive loss of reserve of the vital organs explains the frailty of old age in the face of challenges of trauma and infection compared to the enormous resilience of youth.

An observation with respect to a fundamental system unpredictability we have already noted in early bacteriology. The deadly diplococcus diphtheriae could be found in the throat of well people as well as those mortally afflicted by diphtheria. This complex interaction of seed and soil was well known to Pasteur and other early microbiologists who struggled to make fastidious organisms grow in the laboratory. Knowledge of the huge variety of different ways in which illness with a common biomedical mechanism can manifest themselves in different individuals is the basis of expert clinical experience.

Counterintuitive results with clinical interventions abound. Using effective drugs to prevent serious rhythm disturbances should save lives after a heart attack. It led to more deaths. A drain can be cleared by removing debris; the same kind of intervention is often followed by rapid recurrence of obstruction in the coronary arteries; an artery is part of a complex biological system. Routine physical examinations should, according to the 'stitch in time' logic, improve health but this has turned out not to be the case. Arguably even greater complexity is encountered in the behaviour of illness in the community. Early detection of cancer by screening should obviously lower community mortality - but it commonly does not. The rise and fall of coronary artery disease in the last century should be explicable in terms of our medical interventions but it is not. The reasons for the much higher risk of premature disability and death in the Western world is not to be found solely in the 'risk factors' defined by epidemiology and clinical science. There is clearly here a complex web of causality which extends to social circumstances and class, perhaps even to prenatal deprivation.

Humans and Complexity

The really complex systems in health care are the human transactions. L.J. Henderson, Professor of Biological Chemistry at Harvard Medical School pioneered understanding of the way in which the body maintains itself in balance with respect to acidity and alkalinity. He applied the same kind of thinking by applying the systems concept developed by Pareto in social science to the clinical consultation, affirming that 'a physician and a patient taken together make up a social system' (Henderson 1935). He was the first to explicitly apply the systems model to the medical encounter, thereby emphasizing the importance of the clinical context of illness: 'If physician and patient constitute a social system, it is almost a trivial one compared with the larger one in which the patient is a permanent member and in which he lives. This system, indeed, makes up the greater part of the environment in which he feels that he lives. I suggest that it is impossible to understand any man as a person without knowledge of this environment in which and especially of what he thinks and feels it is; which may be a very different thing.' (Henderson 1935). The unpredictability of human judgement reflecting the complex system interaction of a unique mix of technical, personal, social and cultural influences is well illustrated by variations in the clinical judgement of doctors, and in the puzzling and surprising variations in patient responses to medical advice, and in their differing behaviour in apparently similar circumstances even in the event of a life-threatening heart attack.

The introduction of a new technology was initially seen as a technical exercise. The problems of introducing and evaluating information systems, especially in clinical practice appears certain to put an end to the widespread tendency to ignore the clinical and social context. In the case of health care, new information technology will change the way clinicians practice medicine and, at the same time how the players in the health system communicate! Once again, the complex system approach is to develop understanding of the paradigms and work practices of those who will use the technology or have it used on them, and to iteratively merge the design of the technology to these requirements – a process of 'mutual re-engineering.' Even then, when it is introduced into practice, there is need for clear channels of communication, for adequate training of health professionals, for technical support, user back-up and much on-line trouble shooting if the project is to succeed.

What the introduction of IT into clinical practice taught us above all else is that the program of evaluation must be iterative evaluation loop if we are to detect problems, especially in the early stages (Chapter 14). Formal controlled methods of study based upon scientific principles, such as the randomised trial and cost-effectiveness analysis are 'top-down methods which can only be applied much later when the technology is in place and the practice established - when the worst of the problems are over. Before that, evaluation is done locally, on the ground and in the field, observing, interviewing staff, clinicians, patients, surveying, undertaking simple audit studies, compiling reports. This requires the operation of quality assurance. The health system itself is a gigantic highly complex system imbedded in the context of our even more complex society and culture. Hence its evolution over time cannot be predicted in detail. Rather, some general directions can be set, some rules proposed, and space created for innovation. This process must then be monitored, and interventions guided by an ongoing flexible program of research (Chapter 15). The same is true of the program of clinical practice research required for ongoing iterative improvement of bedside clinical practice which we advocate in the last chapter.

A practical lesson is that to bring about change in complex systems often requires multiple interventions at different levels. To successfully treat a heart attack, it is often necessary to treat pain, to use blood thinning and clot dissolving medication, to prevent rhythm disturbances, to use a balloon or to undertake surgery to relieve obstruction. Even then physical recovery may be complicated, and return to normal activities prevented by depression which requires psychological and social understanding and a range of tactics for its treatment. If, as is very common, a patient is not taking medication as described, it is often necessary to arrange reminders and facilitate the administration of treatment but it is also often necessary to explore problems of doctor-patient communication, to correct misunderstandings, to establish better rapport in order to achieve success. To have doctors change their practice habits is not a simple matter of providing good information either. Attention has to be paid to the clinical context of which they are a part. We have seen that the large reduction of community mortality in the Western World over the last 150 years cannot be explained solely by improved medical treatment, especially the conquest of infectious disease alone. There have been large contributions from improved nutrition, housing and improved hygiene through public health measures.

Conclusion

Differences in collective, largely tacit thinking, within and between groups of people with a stake in health care and its evaluation can be described in terms of disciplinary 'paradigms.' Such differences in thinking are a potent cause of misunderstanding and conflict, as we will see in the chapters to follow. Paradigmatic conflicts are particularly pernicious since they involve basic beliefs which are largely tacit, so tend to resist rational debate. The result is that the basis of disagreement is potent but often not obvious, and neither can speak the other's language enough to allow reasoned debate and a measure of tolerance. Two paradigms which influence the way in which all other paradigms think, work and research are the scientific analytical and the humanistic interpretive. 'Systems thinking' is a smaller third paradigm which has evolved to handle some highly complex problems especially in the biological and social worlds.

The problems of communication which divide those in health who have different paradigmatic commitments are powerful and subtle. As a first step, it has been our aim to make them more visible. Only then can we address them with understanding and hopefully in a spirit of good will. Since this idea is so central the problems of health, and to their understanding, it is important that the reader understand the concept of paradigm well. Kuhn's monograph is readily accessible to a reader. Foucault makes for some heavy lifting!

References

Avison D. E., Baskerville R., Myers M. D., Contemporary Hermeneutics as Method, Philosophy and Critique. Routledge, London, 2001.

Cannon, W. B., The Wisdom of the Body. New York: W. W. Norton & Company. pp. 177–201. 1932.

Saussure, F. de Course in General Linguistics, ed. C. Bally and A. Sechehaye in collaboration with A. Reidlinger, trans. W. Baskin, London, Peter Owen (rev. edn. 1974). First published in 1916.

Dilthey W., The rise of hermeneutics. New Literary history 3: 229-44; 1972.

Fleck L., Genesis and Development of a Scientific Fact. The University of Chicago Press, Chicago, 1979.

Fleck L., Genesis and Development of a Scientific Fact. The University of Chicago Press, Chicago, 1979. p. 109.

Fleck L., Genesis and Development of a Scientific Fact. The University of Chicago Press, Chicago, 1979. p. 43.

Fleck L., Genesis and Development of a Scientific Fact. The University of Chicago Press, Chicago, 1979. p. 99.

Fleck L., Genesis and Development of a Scientific Fact. The University of Chicago Press, Chicago, 1979. p. 41.

Foucault M., The Order of Things. An archaeology of the human sciences. Vintage, New York, 1994.

Gillispie C. C., The Edge of Objectivity: an essay in the history of ideas. Princeton University Press, Princeton, 1960, p. 361.

Henderson L. J., 1935. Quoted in Eisenberg L, Kleinman A. Eds The relevance of social science for medicine. D Reidel. Dordrecht, Holland 1987, p. 7.

Kuhn T. S., The Structure of Scientific Revolutions. University of Chicago Press. 2nd edition, 1970.

Kuhn T. S., The Structure of Scientific Revolutions. University of Chicago Press. 2nd edition, 1970, p. 193.

Kuhn T. S., The Structure of Scientific Revolutions. University of Chicago Press. 2nd edition, 1970, 198.

Chapter 5

The Traditional Paradigm of Medicine

The implications of tensions within the paradigm of medicine, and its interaction with the paradigm of those around it are is central to the thread of our argument. In this chapter, I consider the origins of the classical paradigm of medicine dating back to antiquity, and in the next chapter the paradigm shift to modern scientific medicine. The postmodern view of history is as a dynamic evolutionary process. Given the close links between medicine and the and culture of the society it serves, we would expect that the medical thought, that profile of basic beliefs and commitments which constitutes its professional paradigm, would differentiate with time by a process of evolutionary adaptation to its cultural context. In Chapter 4 we examined the now widely accepted idea, that the gradual evolution of cultures and of fields of specialized knowledge, even that of science, is punctuated by shorter periods of radical and rapid transformation of philosophy called 'paradigm shifts.' Thus we should be able to interpret the development of the paradigm of medicine as involving periods of gradual progress with the consolidation and orderly extension of knowledge, and shorter periods of revolutionary change. This has indeed been the case for medicine. But what has been superseded has by no means disappeared. Thus the classical paradigm of medicine still lives on in modified form as the modern 'art of medicine.' This justifies taking the history of the medical paradigm very seriously since it can often be identified in tacit and subliminal form in today's clinical practice and its many controversies.

The time of challenge to the current came at the time of the French Revolution, facilitated by fundamental changes in the social milieu of medical practice, its institutions and its customs. An abrupt change in the conception of disease accompanied the establishment of the teaching hospital. The modern biomedical paradigm which emerged initially in France became linked to rapid progress in science and reform of universities in Germany. This movement was exported to the rest of the Western World, in particular to the United States where it transformed medical practice and education. Here the new scientific modern paradigm was powerfully reinforced and exerted a worldwide influence by virtue of the ascendancy of American research achievements and prestige. From here, progress was evolutionary once more. Biomedical science gained strength, became dominant in research, the backbone of medical education, and had a strong influence on clinical attitudes. The modern scientific paradigm reached its peak soon after the Second World War.

No sooner was the paradigm stable and mature, however, than it began to show symptoms of the impact of yet another shift. We are still in the midst of this most recent shift which makes clarity of vision difficult. Postmodern 'reflective physicians' will be comfortable in both intellectual paradigms, art and science of medicine, seamlessly merged. If medicine and those with a stake in health care read the signs correctly, reform proposals are more likely to be well directed and received, and acted upon. This is our justification for subjecting the paradigm of medicine and its historical evolution to searching scrutiny in this chapter. The big historical picture must be well understood.

However, the resulting Enlightenment emphasis on the application of science for the benefit of mankind eventually had such a forceful impact that medicine became disarticulated from its traditional roots in the humanities. In a kind of Faustian bargain, there was a substantial price to be paid for spectacular technological progress in the skills of healing, and for the elevated status and professional power which science brought to medicine. Indeed, as I have already suggested, the tension between the traditional art and the new science is at the root of many of the problems of modern clinical medicine. Science has sometimes been used to oversimplify the complexities of diagnoses and lead to excessive technological intervention. The art has sometimes resisted the legitimate use of science to refine the techniques of clinical care. A narrow view of science has prevented enhancement of traditional clinical skills by the social sciences in particular. Moreover, the profession has continued to subscribe to the Hippocratic authoritarian stance which is no longer an appropriate model for patient care, indeed is simply not tolerated by many patients in our modern world. We now examine, in more detail, this remarkable paradigm which has managed to adapt and to survive for so long.

The Traditional Hippocratic Paradigm

The art and craft of medicine can be identified as far back as the dawn of recorded history. It was the transition of mankind from superstition to rationality which began in Classical Greek times (Louras 1968). In medicine this key event was accompanied by the emergence of physicians with a secular orientation as a distinct group in society. The individual treatment practised was in contrast to the cure of the primitive witch doctor whereby illness was seen as largely a spiritual problem relating to relations with others, so that the ritual of treatment was a social event. The Greek doctor's clientele was the aristocrat, his family and slaves. The dominant medical paradigm was the Hippocratic School which was established on the Island of Cos in the fifth century B.C. Its paradigm reflected the characteristics of the intellectual climate of the time. Hippocratic medicine was holistic, consistent with the philosophy of 'organicism,' based on the metaphor of the living organism. 'Mechanism,' the competing world-view later taken up by Newtonian science, was espoused as the 'atomism' of Democritus and Leucippus.

Balance was an important feature of the Pythagorean world order (Lyons 1987). Internal balance of four humours - blood, black and yellow bile, and phlegm, all in external equilibrium with the external environment was a requirement of good health. Illness was a manifestation of disturbance of this balance. Although obviously in error from the modern biomedical perspective, it is worth noting here that there has always been a strong holistic movement in biology and medicine despite the dominance of mechanism in the thinking of current biomedical science. It made a transient return to dominance in Germany in the 19th century as 'functionalism,' essentially a systems idea linked to philosophical idealism. Now it returns with a vengeance as part of postmodernism.

Patient care was rational in the sense that that disease had a natural rather than a supernatural explanation. The rationale of treatment was restoration of the posited disturbance of humoral equilibrium by interventions to restore equilibrium and to eliminate 'peccant humors' (Porter 1997). Hence the logic of procedures such as bloodletting, cupping, purging, puking and sweating used by generations of doctors and lay healers was the correction of plethora by the removal of fluid. This elaborate theory notwithstanding, Hippocratic medicine was conservative and generally non-interventionist, its therapies placing emphasis on rest, on hygiene and on diet (Porter 1997). The expectancy of natural cure (vis mediatix naturae) was accepted by Greek physicians. The Hippocratic physician appears also to have exploited the placebo effect; impressive ritual and ceremony was certainly a feature of the cures of the Asclepian.

The well-known clinical dictum 'primum non nocere' - the first thing is to do no harm - continues to be preached as an echo down through the ages of an ancient warning against meddlesome interference. Ironically, humoral theory was also the justification for aggressive bleeding and drastic purging with calomel, popular as late as the 19th century in the United States, which brought conventional medicine into disrepute and facilitated the educational reform which led to modern medicine. This dictum is still apposite as a warning to those who, in the modern era of technological intervention, are moved by the widespread compulsion to act when continued observation and a course of prudent inaction would be more appropriate.

Hippocratic Empirical Patterns of Illness

The Corpus Hippocraticum, a collection of writings claimed to have been written by Hippocrates and subsequently edited in Alexandria, may or may not have been the work of one man (Marinatos 1968). These case-histories were collected systematically and published as the Aphorisms, the first textbook of medicine, still in use until the eclipse of the humoral theory during the 19th century. These also included empirical disease descriptions, a keystone still of modern clinical diagnosis, and to be extended as the contribution of taxonomy to postmodern diagnosis. Public health was rudimentary (Lyons 1987) but ecological awareness was evident since among the many children of Asclepius were Panakia and Hygeia, patrons of clinical treatment and of disease prevention respectively.

Although scepticism was an intellectual virtue in ancient Greece, the methods of clinical examination of the time were nevertheless crude and uncritical. The accent of practice was on the patient as a whole and the focus of clinical inquiry and of the physician's education was bedside observation. The idea of description of the empirically observed patterns of illness was at the core of clinical practice (Porter 1997). Indeed, in Ancient Greece, with little to offer in the way of treatment, accurate prognosis was the key to the itinerant physician's reputation. In a culture with such emphasis on contemplation and observation, the manual craft (techne) was not highly regarded. Surgery remained a pragmatic craft sometimes practised by doctors, sometimes by other practitioners who generally had lower status (Porter

1997). Apart from the early biological studies of Aristotle, medical investigation was clinical, consisting of narrative case report and case series which remain an integral part of clinical research today.

These case-studies, systematic empirical clinical observations based on the evidence of the doctor's naked senses, represented the beginnings of nosographic clinical science, as revived by Feinstein's taxonomic classification of illness patterns last century. This thread was lost during the Middle Ages. The empirical clinical study of disease re-emerged with the bedside observational work of Thomas Sydenham in the 17th century. But this insight then disappeared again until it was resurrected three centuries later by physician and mathematician Feinstein who expressed these 'clinical patterns of illness attributes' in the form of the Venn diagrams of Boolean algebra.

The Oath of Apollo

Although science has come to dominate medical thinking and community attitudes have changed, the general Hippocratic ethos and ethics has been internalized, largely subconsciously, during the course of medical training and socialization by every doctor practising today. Hippocratic medicine was practised according to a strict code, traditionally according to the Oath of Opollo, which lay down strict guidelines for the behaviour of doctors in their relations with patients, and for the assumption of responsibility for the education of the next generation of physicians by apprenticeship (Lyons 1987). These ethics were derived from the beliefs of the school of Pythagoras who had founded such a loyal brotherhood. This code was associated at the time of the renaissance with the classical notion of the aristocratic 'gentleman' - benign, paternalistic and rational.

Hippocrates discouraged disclosure of information about illness to patients, reflecting an awareness of the importance of faith in the healing process, assuming that doctor and patient were pursuing a common objective, bound by the spirit of philia (brotherly love). Despite the fact that doctors were dealing with the aristocracy or with their slaves, their approach was authoritarian with no question of joint decision making. This has remained a powerful vestigial influence in modern medical practice as an authoritarian stance which was to bring modern doctors into conflict with modern patients with a different cultural perspective, and with government. It has been blamed for some serious problems of modern medicine, including patient dissatisfaction with doctor-patient communication, and dispute over the ethics of disclosure of information and related to the contentious issue of informed consent.

These principles and the humanistic ideals which underlay them were reaffirmed much later by Thomas Linacre during the Renaissance. A classical humanist scholar himself, he used his influence with Henry VIII to establish the Royal College of Physicians in Britain. This was an important symbol of the re-establishment of the medical profession as an aristocratic and influential body, emulating the image of the original Hippocratic doctor. Erudition in the humanities alone never did make a good doctor but a loss of the broad view of the patient and of the social world has now been clearly recognized as a problem in modern medicine, and a grounding in the humanities is certainly essential for understanding the interpretive tradition in particular and the philosophical and political underpinning of health care. Even Abraham Flexner, architect of scientific medical education early in this century in the United States, was aware of this and came to regret the narrow base of the curriculum he had designed. How to regain the humanistic skills has been a problem which has recently taxed medical educators. (Macnaughton 2000). So we note that the physician had been recognized by the King and had acquired 'royal' status several centuries before the major impact of science after the French Revolution.

Our justification for emphasizing the Hippocratic school is because it survived and became the dominant medical paradigm for so long. Nevertheless in no culture, including our own, has a single agency of health care been dominant outside of the home. Modern medicine had to fight off its competitors during the nineteenth century. Hippocratic medicine certainly did not have the field of care of illness to itself. In ancient Greece, it co-existed with various cults, ancient superstitions and religious beliefs together with lay healer and primitive surgery. Competing with it were various sects. There were the Dogmatists who, following the lead of Plato, who adhered to the idea of disease as an essence and discouraged empirical observation. At the opposite pole of belief were the sceptical Empiricists who even took exception to the Hippocratic school's custom of explaining disease in terms of the humoral model.

The dominant Hippocratic tradition continued through Aristotle and his disciples and the Alexandrian school, subsequently spreading to reach imperial Rome and its eastern and western divisions through Galen who acted as the main conduit into medieval thought (Lyons 1987). A tribute to its amazing resilience and adaptability to cultural difference was that its humoral theory of illness survived the Dark Ages and the Renaissance in one form or another to remain the standard explanation of disease and basis for treatment of the practitioner of physic, until its final capitulation to scientific medicine in the West during the latter part of the 19th century. Rome added little to Greek medicine. Furthermore, Asclepiades, the Greek physician who introduced Greek medicine to Rome, was an atomist who did not accept the humoral theory, favoring another rationalistic theory related to the tone of particles in the body (Rhodes 1985).

The giant figure of the period was, however, Galen who saw himself as completing the work of Hippocrates (Porter 1997). He codified medical knowledge and published extensively, although his anatomical knowledge was mostly guesswork and speculation. His great achievement was to reject other sects, and to promulgate Hippocratic rational medicine and to provide the critical link between Hippocratic medicine and Surgery. Surgery was an ancient craft possessed by all cultures in history which made steady progress with experience and development of technology, and was valued especially for its wartime applications. Apart from treppaning (trephining the skull) which may or may not have been performed for medical reasons, surgery obviously could not penetrate the body cavities before the modern era. It is noteworthy that hospitals other than for military personnel did not exist in the Classical world.

Mediaeval Medicine

The survival of the Hippocratic tradition through the Dark Ages was ultimately attributable to the ability of medicine to adapt to cultural difference and to a concurrence of favourable influences (Temkin 1991). The Romans respected the culture of ancient Greece,

Christian doctrines were compatible with the needs of a Roman society living in fear and given to superstition, and the conversion of the Emperor Constantine ensured a Christian Empire. In both Eastern and Western Empire, the traditional Hippocratic paradigm was compatible with the religious beliefs of Judaism, Christianity and Islam, with concern for the individual and with the healing mission of religion.

So, in the West, Hippocratic medicine was nurtured by religion during the early mediaeval lapse of society to the more primitive lifestyle of feudalism. Altruistic medical care and the Pythagorean concept of the honourable man was subsumed by the Samaritan function of doctors or monks or with religious training who cared for a generally god-fearing and respectful population under the umbrella of the church. The hospice offered a crude form of social welfare for the indigent and the traveller. The ethos of medicine was dominated by the Christian construction of disease as punishment for sin but with stress on compassion, care and the worth of the individual. This construction was compatible with the humanist values of the Greek philosophers. The result of this graft was a kind of Christian humanism. Plato and Aristotle, given a Christian interpretation and with varying emphasis placed on the works of each at different times, were central to scholastic philosophy and their influence was preserved by the Church through the mediaeval period. The doctor was either trained in holy orders or closely associated with a monastery which also developed into a hospice caring for the derelict and poor (Temkin 1991). The physician thereby gained prestige as being close to God and someone to be obeyed (Katz 1984).

During the later mediaeval period, death eventually came to be seen as a natural phenomenon rather than the result of an evil agent. The idea of disease communication was becoming established, and there was great fear in the face of epidemic disease. There was also a resurgence in religious attribution of illness with increased interest in faith healing and in seeking the advocacy of Saints during the dark ages (Petrucelli 1978). There was also an attitude of fatalism in the face of disease seen often as punishment for sin or of possession by the Devil. Failure of treatment could be seen as the need to submit to God's will. Hence the role of the doctor, secular or monastic, remained restricted.

An important event of the late mediaeval period was a shift of learning from monastery to university in the late middle ages (Porter 1997). Although the churches controlled the early universities, monastic medicine declined rapidly after their establishment. Formal medical education according to the traditional model and with little clerical control began at Salerno in Italy, a medical school in a city which was the site of a famous spa where there had been a mix of Latin, Greek and Islamic influences, and which became the chief school in the Holy Roman Empire. Universities were subsequently established at Montpellier, Bologna, Paris and many others towards the end of the mediaeval period. After the latter part of the thirteenth century, these remained under church control with theology taking precedence over natural science according to the relationship interpreted by Aquinas.

Doctors were educated with theologian and lawyer in the scholastic tradition (Jacob 1987). This classical training produced an elite polymath of high social rank with much theoretical knowledge but little practical experience, a doctor who prescribed but rarely actually treated patients. The university trained scholastic doctor catered to the privileged, still competing with lay healer and the quack. A continuing doctor-patient relationship was rare, and the bulk of the population had little contact with doctors. For them there was self-help, care in the home, resort to religion or use of the teeth puller, or to folk healer or quack offering herbal remedies and magic, the services of a midwife, with resort to a barber surgeon if absolutely necessary. Physik, the precursor of modern internal medicine, remained a contemplative and supportive activity, and surgery a separate craft of lower status since the Greek bias against manual intervention had continued. Craftsmen were organizing into guilds according to similarity of tools and materials. Doctors also became involved in professional guilds to protect their interests. Physicians were grouped with apothecaries and artists, and surgeons with barbers (Jacob 1987).

Philological Enquiry

Throughout this period, clinical methods remained crude and uncritical and there was no effective treatment in internal medicine. Indeed there had been little progress in medical knowledge. Intellectual inquiry was in the scholastic spirit largely philological, that is, based on discovering what the ancients had thought; with the notable exception of the radical Paracelsus (vide infra), there was neither original thought nor empirical observation. The physician adopted a contemplative approach, essentially content to make a diagnosis in the limited sense of establishing an ontological disease category, to attempt prognosis, and to counsel. Advice included instruction on diet, providing prescriptions, and offering moral support. Medicines ranged from simple folk remedies to the complex medical formulations made up by apothecaries on their own initiative or on the physician's prescription. Therapy was more impressive for the number of ingredients in the prescription or its effectiveness in creating physiological disturbance than for its therapeutic effectiveness.

Physicians had made few therapeutic advances and had little specific to offer apart from mercury for syphilis, often administered in excessive and fatal doses, Cinchona bark (Quinine) for malaria but used indiscriminately for fever, and digitalis for the dropsy. The rationalist humoral theory remained subservient to observation and scarcely articulated with the empirical treatment. The Hippocratic custom of empirical observation with collection of case studies was still in abeyance, and with the exception of the brief return to empirical observation by Paracelsus and by Sydenham, would remain so until the beginning of the modern era in France in the 19th century.

It has to be remembered that medical treatments were, in general, no more rational than the nostrums and superstitious beliefs of the wise or cunning people, the folk healers who continued to meet most of the medical needs of the common folk of the time. In the centuries after the Renaissance, the classical theory of humours was redefined to promote vigorous even heroic treatment. Perhaps it was just as well that medicine did not then articulate with the bulk of patient care as it does today! The more enlightened physicians during the Enlightenment period believed that much disease could be left to nature. Clearly, in days gone by, both doctor and patient must have attributed cure to the doctor's ministrations even when it represented the placebo effect or 'vis mediatrix naturae,' the healing power of nature. Failure on the other hand could be attributed to intrinsically incurable disease, to bad luck or to God's Will rather than to the doctor's incompetence.

Folk-practices rather than doctor or priest helped most people meet death with dignity. Francis Bacon had seen the task of the physician as to attempt to prolong life, although this was disputed, even considered blasphemous by some. The doctor's role was to officiate at the event of natural death, doing no more than assisting nature, providing support for patient and family and exhibiting prognostic skills. Hence what the physician provided was humanistic support and comfort, the illusion of some control over illness for those with serious illness which undoubtedly brought with it reassurance and often the placebo effect. The physician represented a conduit to the public of much prized drugs but the apothecary increasingly took on this role on the evolutionary pathway to becoming the modern general practitioner. The surgeon generally did useful work but was accorded much lower status than the physician. The range of surgery was limited to wounds, fractures, dislocations, amputations, and the opening of abscesses and fistulas, conditions not easily ignored, at least not for long.

The Emerging Welfare State

Various institutions were founded by the Church to cater for the sick, the aged, the destitute, for foundlings and orphans. The transfer of control of medieval hospitals and infirmaries to municipalities in the 12th and 13th centuries could be seen as the first step in the direction of Plato's vision of a utopian state, the modern version of which was the welfare state which took responsibility for the health of its citizens. This shift of responsibility for hospitals to secular control in mediaeval Europe was also the first move towards the university teaching hospital on which the new disease paradigm would be built (vide infra). The achievements of the Romans in public health engineering are well known but even this was lost during the middle ages. However, the idea of contagion was developing (vide infra), as was that of the regulation of training of doctors and the organization of medical care.

Like a chameleon, Hippocratic medicine had merged with a background of Christian culture. Although the continuous development of the classical paradigm of medicine and the ultimate shift to scientific medicine occurred in the West, Islamics, Jews, Persians, Christians in the East - the 'Arabists' - did in fact make significant contributions. Disease was similarly seen as punishment for sin with compassion seen as both proper and holy. Concepts of disease were Galenic, diagnosis was based on observation and emphasized examination of urine. However, formal medicine catered to the needs of the wealthy. There were some outstanding physicians who were capable of good clinical description and pragmatic treatment. The role of women was confined to midwifery. Hospitals were well developed but public health was rudimentary.

Paracelsus - Reading the Future

Often there are thinkers who long anticipate the changes of a paradigm to come, but whose fate is usually to be ignored or persecuted. Such was the lot of Paracelsus, Theophrastus Bombastus of Hohenheim, 16th century physician and alchemist, a radical described as the Luther of medicine who offered a glimmer of intellectual and therapeutic hope by his dissent from the Hippocratic orthodoxy (Feder, 1991). Paracelsus rejected the details of humoral theory but retained the key holistic view of unity of body and spirit and of human microcosm in relation to the macrocosm of nature - organicist rationalist theory. However, an important departure was his belief that disease was usually attributable to an external agent, hence amenable to specific treatment as opposed to the holistic idea of restoration of humoral balance. In the course of his itinerant practice, he sought knowledge of illness from those he knew had the empirical experience of it - from peasants, women, travelers and magicians.

Paracelsus' insistence on empirical observation of clinical phenomena was an important return to Hippocrates. During his chequered career in the early sixteenth century, he attacked the rich and the academic scholastic doctor, and publicly burned the works of Galen and Avicenna in front of the university. Since Aquinas had linked the beginnings of science to religion and Aristotle's influence had increased, alchemy and experimentation was practised. Perhaps training in chemistry related to alchemy allowed Paracelsus to respect the empirical, and to perceive disease as an entity which could have a specific treatment. In fact, he is credited with the idea of treating syphilis with mercury and with the basic principle of homeopathy, of treating like with like. How radical Paracelsus' thinking was can be gauged from the fact that as late as the 17th century, Thomas Sydenham was criticized in Germany for promoting the idea of a specific treatment of disease.

Post-Renaissance Pre-Scientific Period

There were two revolutions after the Renaissance. The first during the 15th and 16th centuries was a revival of classical humanist learning. The second was the emergence of science and statistics during the 17th century. These were the two challenges which were ultimately to transform the traditional paradigm of medicine into its modern form which merged these two influences at the time of the French Revolution. The first challenge was for the Hippocratic paradigm to adapt to the resurgence of the humanist spirit and interest in classical Greek scholarship. This it did by dint of a classical refurbishment with the establishment of the Royal College of Physicians charter designed to reaffirm the traditional Hippocratic paradigm with its Pythagorean ethics. Thus centuries before making the transition to the image of the applied scientist of the modern paradigm, the practitioner of physik had been recast in the mould of classical scholar, of the Latined man!

The second challenge was not so easily dealt with. The seed of scientific thinking sown by the Renaissance exerted a direct influence on doctors and generated scientific biological and medical research which gradually influenced medical thinking. The durable Hippocratic humoral model of illness eventually exhibited the innumerable ad hoc modifications characteristic of a paradigm becoming unstable. There were numerous vain rationalistic attempts to develop clinically useful classifications of the signs of illness in the absence of a valid theoretical explanation, and a spate of speculative theory such as iatrophysics and iatrochemistry which often reflected the influence of the root metaphor of mechanism epitomized by Newtonian physics and analytical chemistry.

Upward Mobility and the Renaissance Man

With the Renaissance in Italy had come the opportunity to be what we now call socially 'upwardly mobile,' to become a gentleman as opposed to being born one (Jacob 1987). This was possible because the new cult of the individual had been merged with the code of chivalry of the nobility. The status of gentleman did not, however, come easily, and was only finally achieved in the second half of the nineteenth century. The doctor with a classical education aspired to be just such a Renaissance Man, given to the contemplative life and possessed of certain attributes as a gentleman. Thus he should be enterprising, loyal, munificent, charming with proportional (not undue) modesty, nonchalance and to exhibit the skills of the gifted amateur who did not seek applause. The 'Practice of Physic was reserved only to those persons that be profound, sad and discreet, groundedly learned and deeply studdied' (Jacob 1987). Such physicians belonged to an international fraternity, the 'Republica Litteraria of Latined Scholars.' For the post-renaissance physician, style as well as substance was the order of the day with emphasis on bedside manner, impeccable manners, and fashionable dress was also de rigeur. The doctor would enter by the front door not by the tradesman's entrance.

The Gentleman Physician

Long before the impact of science, medicine had reaffirmed its commitment to the Hippocratic tradition and style of medicine and at the same time bolstered its status in society. Thomas Linacre, trained at the famous medical school at Padua, was also formally educated in classical philology there. As a classical scholar he was well equipped to translate the work of Galen from Greek into Latin. On his return to England, he served as physician to Henry the VIII upon whom he prevailed to establish the Royal College of Physicians of London, with rights of examination and licensure, in 1518 (Jacob 1987). Ostensibly aimed at raising medical standards and combating quackery, it also had the effect of creating an elite coterie of practitioners of physik who would be sharply distinguished from surgeons and the dispensers of medicine known as apothecaries.

This early manifestation of what would become professionalism bears an interesting resemblance to the concerns over quackery which restored medicine's fortunes when under attack after the French revolution. It is also reminiscent of the reform of medical education early in this century which formally acknowledged the importance of science in medicine and established the profession as the dominant force in health care.

The Royal College of Physicians of London was established with Linacre as foundation president, and with a constitution in close accord with the Oath of Opollo and with the traditions of Greek medicine. Thus were accommodated the interests of these elite university trained Latined men who operated as consultants and counsellors to the aristocracy. They laid the foundations of the 'medical dominance' with which many thinkers since have taken issue, forming an influential group in conjunction with the cloth and the law since their advice might be sought concerning matters of state. Their training, in keeping with classical education in general, was based on the assumption that reading the litterae humaniores produced a humanist in the sense of a refined and cultured gentleman. Professional training by apprenticeship could subsequently be undertaken to acquire specific skills.

Apprenticeship was, on the other hand, the sole mode of education of the surgeon and apothecary. Membership of the College, their associations and their influential contacts distinguished physik sharply from the crafts of the barber surgeon and of the apothecary, the family doctor of the future, who had no classical education. Ultimately, however, both would ride the coat-tails of the College of Physicians to Royal status and greater professional recognition. All three became united by the modern concept of the profession, and profited greatly from the rapid rise in status which followed with medicine's identification with the rapidly rising star of science during the 19th century.

Thus long before scientific medicine took hold, the ancient paradigm was reaffirmed and formalized with a renewed commitment to the role of Pythogorean gentleman, bound by the Oath of Apollo to ethical and altruistic behavior, but with authoritarian overtones. Physicians, at least, had attained a position of power and social influence by virtue of the commitment to the humanities as a gentleman with a classical education. The influences were such therefore that the modern doctor would remain authoritarian, a parent figure commanding trust, respect and obedience, working in a brotherhood of doctors committed to the education of the next generation. The essential characteristics of clinical ethics would continue to adhere to Hippocratic principles, including the confidentiality of information, an altruistic stance free of the taint of materialism, and the assumption of identity of interest between doctor and patient. Training by apprenticeship continues to ensure that these attitudes and beliefs are thoroughly internalized by a process of role-modelling, mentorship and socialization, as part of the tacit knowledge of the traditional medical paradigm. Breeches of these principles, even today, tend to create a feeling of unease in doctors without them necessarily being aware of its origin.

The post-Renaissance university trained doctor continued to cater to the rich, then still only offering an empirically learned ability to prognosticate, support and render reassurance to the ill and frightened, and comfort to the dying and family. Like his forebears, the doctor's ministrations had to rely on impressive appearance or some striking physiological effect, impressing the patient and perhaps eliciting a placebo effect or buying time for natural cure. Poynter put it graphically: 'there are few reasons for believing that the actual treatment of the patient, judged from its efficacy, was any better in nineteenth-century Britain than it was in second-century Rome, when Galen was bringing together all the leading ideas of his leading predecessors of the preceding five centuries, from Hippocrates on, into one coherent system.' (Poynter 1973).

An extensive pharmacopoeia was invoked to fill prescriptions comprising long lists of drugs with arcane Latin names or distinctive taste and smell which would boost their placebo effect. Others were used to induce puking or diarrhoea; along with cupping, blood letting and sweating, treatments were based on the ancient principle of plethora and eliminating peccant humours. During all of this time, methods of clinical examination had changed almost not at all. The history was simply an account of the illness and of personal habits. Examination was, as in ancient times, simply general inspection, examination of the tongue, pulse and urine. The procedure was uninformed by anatomical or pathological knowledge hence by any understanding of the link between abnormality of a specific organ and clinical symptoms. It is now hard to conceive that this basic connection, now so obvious to the greenest of medical students, was not part of the disease paradigm.

There were rules of etiquette and of demeanour designed to impress, to conceal ignorance, to bolster hope and to maximize the chance of placebo effect. Included was an injunction to act quickly and boldly which was in keeping with an era of aggressive pharmacological intervention. Patients did not appear to be complaining of the need for more information or of lack of participation in decision-making, any more than doctors considered straying from their traditional code of silence and control. Most of the populace, of course, never saw a doctor. Before the late 19th century, around the time when scientific medicine became the consensus position in the profession, the great majority of people helped themselves, were assisted by their family, by a feudal mistress or by a lay healer of some kind.

That is to say, the threshold for seeking the assistance of a doctor was necessarily high. For one thing there was the cost but there were also other considerations that medicine in general was held in quite low esteem. When doctors did become more readily available, it was men rather than women and children who sought medical attention. There was also a sturdy lay tradition of self-help with the assistance of books such as Wesley's or Buchan's guides for the lay person or recourse to the bone-setter, tooth puller, wise man or of the midwife.

In Britain and on the continent of Europe, physicians had achieved social respectability, a good income, powerful links to the other great professions and to the influential, without the benefit of a scientific basis, with treatment which was of little consequence except that some was potentially harmful. Medicine had achieved all of this while resisting corporatisation, and in opposition to the laissez-faire principles of classical economics! Small wonder then that medicine is seen as the exemplar of the socially and politically successful profession. The row was somewhat harder to hoe in the United States where the profession lacked a home grown aristocratic tradition and competed in a culture with a tradition of self-reliance (Starr 1982). During this long rather sterile period in medicine, surgery was not linked to science and its progress was blocked pending the discovery of anaesthesia and antisepsis which would allow penetration into the body cavities with an acceptable rate of success. Nevertheless, anatomical knowledge relevant to surgery advanced rapidly through the work of Pott and of the Hunter brothers in Britain. With this, the surgeons emerged closer to parity of status with the physicians.

Medical Education – Severing the Religious Ties

In Britain, a utilitarian push to disengage medical education from its religious connection at the traditional universities was successful. Just as science engaged industry and became professionalized, so too did medicine develop professional organization and gain status and the protection of the state. The institutions of medicine also reflected the unifying influence of science, competition within the profession reflecting the rising status of surgeon and apothecary, and externally the competition between medicine, lay healer and family care. Science profoundly influenced the shape of the emerging industrial state and its technologies shaped its towns. Public health, initially only in the form of statistics, was developing its social conscience and doctors were involved.

Altogether some 300 years were to elapse between the first stirrings of medical science and the emergence of a new scientific paradigm. Medicine gained its first toe-hold at the end of the Enlightenment in revolutionary France. During this long hiatus, a great deal of progress in the natural and biological sciences had nevertheless laid the foundations for the basic medical sciences to come. Knowledge of human biology, and to a lesser extent of pathology, accelerated from the 16th century onwards but initially had remarkably little specific impact on clinical medicine. Nor was anatomical advance closely linked to surgical progress. However there was beginning to appear evidence of instability of the belief system of medicine, a sign of competition between the old classical beliefs and the new ideas and findings of the emerging scientific medicine, engaged in mortal combat prior to the impending shift of paradigm when the political space was created by the French Revolution. This was the 'paradigmatic instability' of Thomas Kuhn, preceding the shift.

Sydenham – Taxonomics and a Glimpse into the Future

An interesting island in a sea of ignorance and speculation was the work of Thomas Sydenham. The first and most fundamental requirement was for accurate description of the pictures or patterns of illness, the mechanism of which any theory must then endeavour to explain. Hippocrates had begun this crucial task of mapping the clinical scene. Long afterwards, Thomas Sydenham, 17th century admirer of Bacon, friend of the utilitarian John Locke and of empiricist scientist Robert Boyle, a man referred to as the English Hippocrates, had insisted that 'pathological phenomena should be described with the same accuracy that a painter observes in painting a portrait' (Faber 1930). Sydenham was a brilliant clinical observer – 'Anatomy, botany, nonsense. No, young man, go to the bedside; there alone can you learn disease.'(Jacob 1987). He left us accurate empirical descriptions of the patterns of signs characteristic of gout, smallpox and other infectious diseases, of syphilis and of St. Vitus' Dance (a manifestation of acute rheumatic fever).

Although he still clung to the Galenic orthodoxy, Sydenham was opposed to speculation about disease mechanism, and strongly opposed to those who constructed fanciful speculative systems to explain disease which his friend Locke described as 'castles in the air' (Faber 1930). Nevertheless, like Paracelsus before him, he foresaw the possibility of a specific cure for disease. Unfortunately, this revival of scepticism and empirical observation was short-lived since it was followed by degeneration into meaningless and largely useless classifications of symptoms - useless because of the lack of a coherent basic understanding of the basic nature of disease. An observational science based on taxonomy did, however, develop in imitation of botanical classification, a medicine of species dormant until rediscovered for medicine by Feinstein (1967). Since these rationalistic and speculative classifications, based on shuffling the clinical signs of disease, were developed with little empirical content, they had no hope of forging a useful theory of disease.

Medical Science Emerging

One sign of the early inroads made by science was the scepticism of the anatomist Vesalius. Just as Copernicus was dislocating mankind by proposing a heliocentric universe, Vesalius' empirical anatomical observations were challenging the Galenic version of the classical medical paradigm. So too did the empirical studies of William Harvey, pioneer physiologist and contemporary of Francis Bacon, who discovered the circulation of the blood. In the eighteenth century, Morgagni published his 'De Sedibus et Causis Morborum' in which he correlated the morbid anatomical changes findings at autopsy with the clinical details of the patients he dissected. This could have been the beginning of modern medicine were it not for the blinkering effect of the prevailing Traditional paradigm of medicine. So the significance of these results was not evident to those not yet ready to accept the radical new idea that disease was a consequence of damage to internal organs. Similarly too the evidence of Auenbrugger that percussion of the chest could reveal the presence of fluid carried the same implications of internal disease but its significance was similarly not widely appreciated until the work was translated, practiced and promoted by Corvisart, pioneer of clinic-pathological correlation and mentor of Rene Laennec.

The Old Paradigm Falters

Lacking an understanding of underlying cellular structure and function, the science of the 18th century continued to rely solely upon the systematic classification of phenomena based upon evidence of identity and difference – by itself an intellectual dead-end. The discipline of 'taxonomy' was however highly developed in botany, and the classification of Linnaeus has become the basis of modern biological taxonomy. Thus there was a long period, extending through 17th and 18th centuries which was characterized by a profusion of elaborate rationalistic classifications and speculative theories (Jewson 1974), often intermingled with causal notions derived from Newtonian mechanics. It appears that clinicians still hungered for some satisfactory method of classification of the patterns of illness symptoms and signs to structure and explain their clinical observations. This explains the popularity of the classification of Boissier de Sauvages who published his definitive work 'Nosologia Methodica Sistens Morborum Classes Genera et Species' in 1763 not long before the major impact of science on clinical medicine. Following the suggestion of Sydenham, he applied Botanical principles to disease classification, as did his admirer the great botanist Linnaeus. However, in the grand classification of Sauvages, almost every symptom constituted a disease. His system was simplified by Cullen's modification which referred to 'pathognomonic' symptoms and symptom complexes, the first step towards the recognition of an empirical clinical pattern of findings.

The last of these great classifiers of illness was Pinel, a great French physician and humanitarian whose detailed classification applied anatomic criteria to break diseases down into species, orders and families. His misfortune was to practise in Paris just before the establishment of the famous clinical school which would render his scheme obsolete. This classificatory work was a dead end. What emerged however had been arbitrary and unsatisfactory. These systems were fumbling attempts to generate a new nosology in the absence of sufficient understanding of the nature of disease. Nevertheless Pinel left an important legacy – the idea that a single disease could manifest itself as different patterns of clinical findings. It was this insight which was elaborated by Bichat who became aware of the existence of individual tissues.

This proclivity for classification is understandable since clinical diagnosis rests chiefly on the recognition and categorisation of illness patterns. However, at the turn of the 18th century, the philosophy of mechanism was strong in science, as a powerful response to the spectacular achievements of Newtonian science by now linked firmly to mathematics. All of this was going on in England during the intellectual ferment which was building up in association with the discoveries of the heyday of the amateur laboratory scientist in the natural sciences and of the Royal Society. This meant that there was also a drive to find a causal explanation underlying the patterns of symptoms and signs. Before the time of Sydenham and afterwards, there were attempts to develop broad systems to explain disease in terms of body chemistry - iatrochemistry, or in terms of physics - iatrophysics or iatromechanics. Theoretical systems of medicine based on the same basic Hippocratic conceptual foundations were modified under the influence of Newton. These theories attributed disease to a disturbance of solid body structures rather than simply to humoral imbalance (Jewson 1974). A specific example was the system of Cullen who developed iatrochemistry into a notion of explanation of disease in terms of body 'tone' (Saffron 1987).

This was a return to the ancient doctrine of atomism, to the root metaphor of mechanism, to the clockwork model which explained disease by reduction to simple mechanical cause and effect which would dominate the new biomedical paradigm. But these early transitional models of disease were doomed to failure since they were not yet based on sound biological knowledge. Yet like the small premonitory tremors which precede a major earthquake, these were evidence of a senescent paradigm no longer adequately satisfying the physician's need to understand human illness.

A New Version of 'Evidence' - Another Break with the Past

Another important development for a scientific basis for clinical medicine was the notion of evidence for generating and testing an hypothesis, and the application of statistical analysis. During the 17th century, the scholastic concept of a 'sign' as a portent of things to come, of the course of illness, began to give way to the idea of collecting evidence from observation (Hacking 1975). At the same time, the meaning of 'probability' shifted from the support of respected authority to likelihood in the light of external evidence which could be supported by mathematical calculation. The analogy between pictures of illness, comprising symptoms and signs, and the combinations of elements to form chemical compounds or of letters to form words was recognized in France (Foucault 1976). Furthermore, it was recognised that all such conjunctions of symptoms and signs could be analysed by the mathematics of combinatorial probability.

Medical theory and practice changed quite dramatically during the 19th century in Western European societies. During the latter part of the 18th century, there was the culmination of a period of transition similar to what we are experiencing today. Just before the key developments of the teaching hospital and medical laboratory which brought the modern paradigm to dominance, a large variety of theories had by now become grafted onto the humoral balance theory to generate 'a chaotic diversity of schools of thought' (Jewson 1976) – a sign of a paradigm shift to come. Private practitioners competed for the patronage of the affluent patient, striving to offer an acceptable explanation for the client's illness of the, preferably based on a distinctive theory, preferably with an aura of the scientific which then justified active, impressive, even heroic therapy. Nevertheless the clinical approach remained holistic, as it had always been since Hippocrates; illness involved the whole person and its genesis included the emotional and the spiritual dimensions. Will this attribute survive the inroads of scientific evaluation? The emphasis was still on the clinical pattern of signs of illness garnered mainly from the patient's account and from a perfunctory, superficially and theoretically uninformed physical examination. The individual doctor's perceived social skills and moral integrity were important ingredients for professional success in addition to his reputation for competence. There was still almost no effective treatment and speculation still centred on finding a single all-encompassing cure for illness.

Conclusion

Thus the major elements of the classical medical paradigm were forged over thousands of years from those of ancient Greek medicine. Modern medicine is only as old as the democratic nation state. The focus on the individual, on clinical judgement, respect for authority, the gentlemanly demeanor, the authoritorian stance, the lack of communication with patients were all features of this ancient paradigm. So too were the reliance on clinical pictures of illness and upon clinical experience for diagnosis of illness, and a system of specifically clinical ethics. Our detailed account of this early paradigm is justified by the fact that it has been incorporated into the modern scientific one which followed, bringing with it essential features of clinical practice so closely adapted to practice that they are unlikely ever to change.

Unfortunately the remnants of the old paradigm known as the 'art of medicine' have come into some conflict. This cut both ways. Thus the old paradigm has shown some resistance to the inroads of science; on the other hand, science has sometimes resulted in naive oversimplification of clinical phenomena. There have also been clashes with an emergent desire for patient autonomy and communication, and the expectation of clinical autonomy has proved incompatible with the fiscal political pressures on modern government. Signs of a further shift of paradigm were evident during the 18th century, and the major shift occurred early in the 19th century. This is the subject of the next chapter.

References

Faber K. F., Nosography. the evolution of medicine in modern times. Paul B Hoeber, New York, 1930, p. 7.

Faber K. F., Nosography. the evolution of medicine in modern times. Paul B Hoeber, New York, 1930, p. 17.

Feder G., Paradigm lost: a celebration of Paracelsus on his quincentenary. *Lancet* 338:803-5; 1991

Foucault M., The Birth of the Clinic. Tavistock, Bristol, 1976. p. 120.

Hacking I., The Emergence of Probability. Cambridge University Press, Cambridge, 1975, p. 39-48.

Jacob J. M., Doctors and Rules: A sociology of professional values. Routledge, London, 1987. p. 89.

Jacob J. M., Doctors and Rules: A sociology of professional values. Routledge, London, 1987. p. 95.

Jacob J. M., Doctors and Rules: A sociology of professional values. Routledge, London, 1987. p. 117.

Jacob J. M., Doctors and Rules: A sociology of professional values. Routledge, London, 1987. p. 93.

Jacob J. M., Doctors and Rules: A sociology of professional values. Routledge, London, 1987, p. 33.

Jewson N., The disappearance of the sick man from medical cosmology, 1770-1870. Sociology 10: 225-44; 1976.

Jewson N., Medical knowledge and the patronage system in 18th century England. *Sociology:* 8:369-85; 1974.

Katz J., The Silent World of Doctors and Patients. Free Press, New York, 1984. pp. 7-8.

Louras N. K., First Steps in the Darkness. In: The Origins of Medicine in Greece. Tsakonas P Ed. Christos Christou, Athens, 1968.

Lyons A. S., Hippocrates. In: Lyons A S and Petrucelli R J II. Harry N Abrams, New York. 1987. pp. 214.

Lyons A. S., Hippocrates. In: Lyons A S and Petrucelli R J II. Harry N Abrams, New York. 1987. pp. 219.

Lyons A. S., Medicine in Hippocratic Times. In: Lyons A S and Petrucelli R J II. Harry N Abrams, New York. 1987. pp. 186.

Lyons A. S., Medicine in Hippocratic Times. In: Lyons AS and Petrucelli RJ II. Harry N Abrams, New York. 1987. pp. 196.

Macnaughton J., The humanities in medical education: context, outcomes and structures. *Medical humanities.* 26: 23-30; 2000.

Marinatos S. M., The Medical and Human Genius of Hippocrates. In: The Origins of Medicine in Greece. Tsakonas P Ed. Christos Christou, Athens, 1968.

Petrucelli R. J. II., The Rise of Christianity. In Lyons A S and Petrucelli R J II. Harry N Abrams, New York, 1987, pp. 265-278.

Porter R., The Greatest Benefit to Mankind: A medical history of humanity from antiquity to the present. Harper Collins. London. 1997.

Porter R., The Greatest Benefit to Mankind: A medical history of humanity from antiquity to the present. Harper Collins. London. 1997, p. 57.

Porter R., The Greatest Benefit to Mankind: A medical history of humanity from antiquity to the present. Harper Collins. London. 1997. p. 61.

Porter R., The Greatest Benefit to Mankind: A medical history of humanity from antiquity to the present. Harper Collins. London. 1997. p. 59.

Porter R., The Greatest Benefit to Mankind: A medical history of humanity from antiquity to the present. Harper Collins. London. 1997. pp. 73-7.

Porter R., The Greatest Benefit to Mankind: A medical history of humanity from antiquity to the present. Harper Collins, London, 1997. pp. 113-8.

Poynter N., Medicine and Man. Pelican, *Harmondsworth*, 1973. p. 27.

Rhodes., An Outline History of Medicine. *Butterworths*, London, 1985.

Saffron M., The eighteenth century. In: Lyons AS and Petrucelli RJ II. Harry N Abrams, New York. 1987. P467.

Starr P., The Social Transformation of American Medicine. the rise of a sovereign profession and the making of a vast industry. *Basic Books,* 1982.

Temkin O., Hippocrates in a world of Pagans and Christians. Johns Hopkins University Press, Baltimore, 1991.

Temkin O., Hippocrates in a world of Pagans and Christians. Johns Hopkins University Press. Baltimore, 1991, p. 164.

Chapter 6

The Shift of Paradigm
to Modern Medicine

The Forces for Change

In the 18th century, science as the font of invention and technology drove industrialization which, in turn, provoked radical politics. The social application of science, the so-called Enlightenment Project which epitomized the aspirations of empiricist philosophers, aspects of the Romantic reaction against it, together with the dedication of revolutionaries to democratic principles, can be seen as the political motive forces responsible for radical changes in medical institutions and practice following the French Revolution. Political revolution in France spawned a new political order with radical restructuring of public health and clinical medicine. During the second half of the 19th century, beginning in Germany then spreading centrifugally through the Western world, there was a move towards reform of universities. There was, as we noted in the last chapter, refinement of research procedures, first in the humanities involving the humanistic interpretive paradigm, then in the natural and biological sciences involving the analytical scientific paradigm. The key event in France, where modern medicine was conceived, was the establishment of the university teaching hospital which nurtured the new scientific paradigm in which illness was simply the outward manifestation of dysfunction of bodily organs which could culminate in death.

The ancient humoral model of illness, nearly 2500 years old, was swept aside during the early nineteenth century paradigm shift. The role of science in precipitating the shift was direct in the sense that it cracked the code of illness causality by disciplined correlation of clinical illness with autopsy evidence of organ pathology. Its impact was also indirect in that it was commitment to science which provoked a political attack on the institutions of the old paradigm in France. The organization of clinical medicine was radically changed, so that the teaching hospital thereafter became the flagship of scientific progress. The patterns of illness, interpreted first empirically in terms of the new mathematics of probability, were then explained in terms of disease mechanism. This, in turn, cried out for identification of a cause and possible treatment of that cause.

Hence the way was now clear for development of the specific treatment of disease which had been previously anticipated by but a few medical seers. At the birth of the modern paradigm, there was even an appreciation of the need for the scientific evaluation of clinical care; however, this insight did not survive so that it had to be rediscovered after the Second World War. The adverse consequences of rapid industrialization and urbanization drew doctors and social activists into the public health debate. The movement was revolutionary in France and Germany, and there were strong evolutionary pressures in Britain. Such pressures were more scientifically driven and politically muted in the USA.

The Crack in the Dyke Widens

The traditional holistic view of illness might well have survived in a more sophisticated form. After all, better understanding of the homeostatic balance mechanisms of the body and their disturbance by disease, and the link of illness to poor social conditions were really only more sophisticated versions of the Hippocratic attribution of disease to imbalance within the body and between body and external environment. However, any possibility of a refurbished holistic model of disease was thwarted by the strong movement from organicism and holism to mechanism and atomism. This reflected both the acceptance of the worldview of the analytical tradition of classical science with its spectacular vindication by germ theory, and the ultimate success of the anti-bacterial vaccine and 'magic' bullet in conquering the infectious illness, the scourge of mankind. The complex interplay of biological disturbance, psychological reaction and social context of illness had therefore been reduced to a simple chain of cause and effect.

The root-metaphor of mechanism appeared to have prevailed over that of organicism in the paradigm of modern medicine. However, the stage had already been set for a counter-revolution. Slowly it became clear that the technological fix so successful for infectious disease would not be repeated for chronic illness and cancer, for mental illness and the anxieties of living brought to the doctor; nor would scientific medicine abolish disease in the community according to early naive hopes based on the early successes of science in the positivist analytical tradition. We now consider in more detail these events which moulded the paradigm of modern medicine and which have ultimately lead to its current crisis of confidence.

In Kuhnian terms, the gradual progress of clinical medicine since the shift after the French revolution, the gradual extension of knowledge and its application to diagnosis and treatment, was the activity of 'normal science' with consolidation of gains and gradual evolution of new methods of diagnosis and treatment. Barely 100 years further on again, we are in the throes of re-evaluating this dramatic impact of science and, I believe, are set for another shift of paradigm. The events in France and Germany are therefore of particular importance to us. The controversies of the nineteenth century represent the birth pains of scientific medicine and the beginnings of the strong interaction between the ancient clinical traditions and the ideology of the new science. To fully understand this paradigmatic conflict is important for analysing current problems. For these reasons we discuss this period in detail.

The Modern Scientific Paradigm - Birth and Infancy

In the last chapter we discussed the first great watershed in medical history, the original paradigm shift which established a rational conception of disease. The second, more than 2000 years later, saw the substitution of this rationalistic humoral theory of disease by a scientific model. It took 300 years for post-Renaissance science which was evolving from natural philosophy to precipitate this paradigm shift which established biomedical science and its concepts of disease. Once it had started, at the end of the Enlightenment period early in the 19th century, the shift from the traditional Hippocratic paradigm to the scientific model was relatively quick, taking place over about thirty years. However, the remainder of the century would pass before this change percolated through to achieve consensus in the medical community, or to have a major impact on medical treatment. It is a sobering thought that the practitioner of internal medicine, heir to the traditions of the ancient physik, had little to offer apart from the placebo effect until well into the 20th century, barely a full life-time ago.

Such a fundamental restructuring of medical thinking did not occur all at once. We can identify stages or resting places on the road to the new scientific model of illness model. We have already mentioned the first which was related to the better understanding of the mathematics of probability in 18th century France - the recognition that the variable patterns of illness represented a statistical distribution around a typical one characteristic of a particular disease. The other two occurred in the first and second halves of the 19th century respectively. The second was to see that the disease was a mechanical derangement of the body which could result in death. The third was to attribute the infectious illnesses to an external agent in the form of bacteria. All of this thinking depended on observation of patients and of the course of illness in hospital, and on relating clinical illness to autopsy findings. The existence of such hospitals was itself the result of new medical institutions established in a climate of seething political revolution. The trust in science for purposes of social engineering was part of the great Enlightenment Project initiated by Bacon and by British and French empiricists. We now trace this fascinating development in more detail.

The first step towards the modern understanding of the relationship between illness and disease of the body was the move away from the mediaeval notion of disease as a Platonic essence, a definable but abstract disturbance of the whole body. Such 'diseases' were simply patterns of signs manifest by ill people such as had been first described by the Hippocratic school and revived by Thomas Sydenham. These clusters of signs were the species of disease categorized by the hierarchical classifications of the Enlightenment nosologists. Characteristic of concepts from a different paradigm, it is hard for us now to imagine how disease could be thought of as not located in any particular region of the body. In fact a Hippocratic disease could move about from one organ to another. Similarly alien to us now is that disease was not seen as a process evolving over time, rather the changing clinical signs were interpreted as one disease replacing another. There was no basis for its further explanation beyond invoking the operation of morbid forces related to disturbed humoral balance. To identify a disease 'essence' it was necessary first to abstract it from those variable features which were seen as complications related to individual patient constitution and context.

The next stage of understanding was the first evidence of real scientific thinking and undoubtedly related to the pioneering work in mathematical statistics in France around that time. An analogy was drawn between the aggregation of symptoms to form disease patterns and the combination of the elements as atoms to form molecules. The variety of disease patterns could then be explained by operation of the rules of combination postulated by Pascal (Foucault 1976). The fundamental clinical concept which emerged was of a typical disease picture around which was distributed a range of allowable variations which overlapped with the patterns of other diseases. This huge range of potential variation is consistent with the clinical truism that no two patients ever present an identical disease picture. This was a crucial observation since the different patterns of presentation of the same disease is the basis of modern choice of treatment in the individual patient.

The genius of French clinicians, the first evidence of clinical science, was therefore to apply statistical thinking to explain clinical observations more parsimoniously and usefully, rather than dismissing disease variations as 'complications' or as a constantly changing disease entity. We return to the importance of probability in medicine after we consider the circumstances and impact of the next and crucial insight necessary en route to the modern paradigm. This was to invoke the root metaphor of mechanism, the core of the analytical paradigm, to organize these patterns according to a cause-and-effect explanatory model of disease. A necessary first step was to recognize that illness was the result of disease afflicting the individual organs of the body. The idea is implicit in Vesalius' and Morgagni's earlier autopsy work but it was most convincingly established by Bichat, who extended the ideas of Pinel by demonstrating the existence of the different kinds of body tissues which constitute the organs, and their proneness to specific kinds of pathological derangement.

Surgeons must have been aware of the localized nature of diseases they treated such as abscesses and bladder stone but their contribution was limited by their inability to access most internal organs. Such was the blinkering effect of the traditional paradigm. This vital connection was that made by Xavier Bichat, physician to Napoleon, anatomist and physiologist at the Hotel Dieu at Lyon. By comparing his clinical observations to postmortem findings, he recognized that tissues reacted in characteristic fashion to disease, in particular to inflammation. Hence he was the first to interpret disease as a dysfunction of body organs, and to link the process of illness with the outcome of death. When he died at the age of 31 years, Bichat had established the basic concept that 'it is the body itself that has become ill,' and in so doing, shifted the clinician's 'gaze' from the more obvious surface signs of illness to the anatomical context of the deep organs accessible to autopsy, and later to the palpating hand and listening ear (Foucault 1976). Bichat's legacy was the French tradition of clinicopathological correlation whereby changes in organs at autopsy were compared with clinical findings, the diseased organ with the healthy, one disease with another. This was the basis of his great work 'Anatomie Generale' first published in 1801 (Foucault, 1976).

The Key to Disease Understanding – Clinicopathological Research

Corvisart, Bichat's successor at the Hotel Dieu, carried the torch for this new tradition, cultivating the art of physical examination (Faber 1930). He also revived Auenbrugger's work on percussion first published 50 years earlier by translating it. Corvisart also influenced Laennec, his famous pupil at the Hopital de le Charite in Paris, whose stethoscope added auscultation as another dimension to the clinical armamentarium. Even more important was his emphasis on meticulous clinical examination and its correlation with disease at autopsy. For example, Laennec's studies of tuberculosis, the most serious chronic disease of the time, established the important principle that a single disease not only had a characteristic pattern of abnormalities but could have multiple clinical manifestations. French physicians subsequently identified a number of specific disease patterns in this way, including diphtheria, typhoid, general paralysis of the insane, gastric ulcer, mitral regurgitation (valve leak) and rheumatic endocarditis (valve inflammation) (Faber 1930).

The New Gaze - Seeing Inside the Body

Foucault's metaphor of 'the gaze' for the new biomedical paradigm which emerged in the French Clinic was a deliberate double entendre intended to convey both the idea of looking beyond the surface of the body, examining the deep organs. But it was as well the sense of a general perspective or vision - the realization that disease was in fact a physical bodily abnormality located in body organs (Foucault, 1976). Undoubtedly, this realization is related to a pervasive medical obsession with methods to see inside the body; after all 'seeing is believing.' Just as surgeons have always had the reputation of taking the opportunity to operate whenever it presented, physicians set about examination of internal organs with similar zeal. Physicians have also taken any opportunity they had see inside the body with a 'scope or to record the activity of an organ which emitted some kind of signal. With the constant pressure of the development of ingenious instruments for looking at the inside of the body came diagnostic tools designed to gain access to the organs of the body interior in the living person not just the cadaver. The first, a major stimulus for the new science of clinicopathological correlation was the discovery of the simple yet effective stethoscope. This created the first window into the interior of the body.

Hippocrates had been aware of abnormal sounds in the abdomen in disease - the succussion splash in pyloric stenosis which causes obstruction to stomach emptying. William Harvey was also aware of sounds heard in the chest. Pioneer British laboratory scientist, Robert Hooke, showed remarkable prescience about the way in which diagnostic information would be obtained by auscultation: 'it may be possible to discover the Motion of Internal Parts of Bodies, whether Animal, Vegetable, or Mineral, by the sound they make,' based on his own auscultation of the heart, lung and joints (Reiser 1978). Laennec, however, designed an instrument to capitalize on this information, then proceeded to provide a masterly account of its powers of diagnosis. Although the stethoscope relates to hearing, the skilled auscultator of the heart does construct a detailed mental picture of the anatomy of the heart. Laennec was therefore able to use the stethoscope to detect signs, and to correlate them with autopsy findings to detect as the pathological footprints of disease which corresponded to clinical illness. As a result of the stethoscope's unsurpassed combination of accuracy, diagnostic relevance and portability it remained unsurpassed as a clinical tool.

The Floodgates Open

Impressive applications of science to medical practice involved new diagnostic technologies, beginning with the stethoscope and X-ray, which provided both a source of excitement with the expanded prospects for diagnosis, and also some scepticism in the face of misapplication and discovery of limitations and error (Reiser 1978). The stethoscope has been a great survivor, worthy of the honour of being the badge of the practising physician, providing a glimpse of living physiology which, for its accuracy and diagnostic relevance has remained unsurpassed as a portable clinical instrument. Even more importantly, the success of auscultation conveyed the important message that it was possible to tune in to body signals for purposes of diagnosis. The doctors' compulsion to probe the body interior was further crowned by early success with regard to the eye (opthalmoscope), throat (laryngoscope), ear (auriscope), stomach (gastroscope), bowel (sigmoidoscope), bladder (cystoscope), cervix uteri (speculum), and abdominal cavity (laparoscope) (Reiser 1978). Since then various scopes have been designed for passage into just about every other accessible organ, bodily orifice and cavity to allow direct viewing and sampling of tissues for microscopy.

Physicians not only learnt to recognize disease as signals from abnormal images from the body interior but also as abnormal signals which bore the signature of disease - for recording of heart sounds (phonocardiography), for recording its electrical signals (electrocardiogram), electrical brain signals (electroencephalogram) or muscle signals (electromyogram), and even those from the tiny conducting system of the heart (His bundle recording). This process of discovery has continued unabated, extending to therapeutic intervention. Recently, major and quite delicate surgery, such as removal of the gallbladder, has been performed by an abdominal 'keyhole' (laparoscopic) method. It has even proved possible to view the interior of a coronary artery and to obtain local ultrasonic images. The kind of device which has done most to satisfy this drive to see the cause of disease has been the indirect imaging of the internal organs as shadows, what is now known as 'organ imaging.'

Far and away the first, and still the most versatile organ imaging device has been the use of X-rays, discovered by Roentgen in 1895 and immediately applied to medical diagnosis. Here was the promise of an Aladdin's Lamp for diagnosis, the epitome of Foucault's medical gaze, a direct way home likely to render less direct methods of examination superfluous, a test which quickly caught the imagination of doctor, patient and public alike (Reiser 1978). These advances were gratefully accepted by most physicians but there were, nevertheless, some dissenting voices (Reiser 1978). Despite the obvious utility of stethoscope and X-ray, some physicians have had legitimate concerns about the way diagnostic modalities were used with regard to subjectivity and inaccuracy, and use for social rather than medical purposes (Reiser 1978). Even today, there are serious problems related to the range of normal, false positive diagnosis, harm from doubtful sounds or images which are a potent source of anxiety and iatrogenic illness.

Pathological Interpretation - The 'Glue' of Clinical Interpretation

A less obvious but no less important advance was the gradual incorporation of knowledge of pathological anatomy and physiology and into the traditional clinical interview and examination, now competing with impressive diagnostic tests. The biomedical model of illness developed in the name of scientific medicine has obviously contributed greatly to the clinical examination of patients by providing information on the structure and function of internal organs. The modern clinician only rarely indulges in extensive explicit reasoning in terms of disease mechanism unless confronted by a particularly difficult diagnosis or when writing a report or explaining to students. However, this knowledge forms an indispensable subconscious reservoir of tacit knowledge which underpins all clinical thinking; it also aids the fine-tuning of knowledge applicable to groups to fit the unique diagnostic pattern and treatment needs of the individual patient. Biomedical knowledge allows the clinician to conceptualize the mechanism of patients' complaints, to explain the signs of illness in terms of changes in the deep organs when the problem is organic disease, to plan treatment and to anticipate the effects. Pathological knowledge is a kind of glue which holds the clinical picture and disease manifestations together.

As scientific thinking permeated clinical discussion of disease, the feeling that there should be some external causal agent which explained the patterns of illness must have grown stronger. Having applied the science of taxonomy and combined it with statistical thinking, the missing piece at last fell into place. The superficial model of illness as a pattern of pieces of clinical evidence was virtually swept aside by a deep mechanical cause-and-effect scientific model of illness as a manifestation of the irritation of the tissues of body organs (Foucault 1976). There was increasing recognition of the localisation of disease in body organs, more specifically involving specific tissues, lead to the idea of illness as a bodily affliction which could culminate in death, not as a separate abstract entity.

Identifying One Cause of Illness – At Last!

The way was then open to identifying a specific cause of disease which came not long afterwards in the form of bacterial infection. Robert Koch got the credit for enunciating 'germ theory' and won the 1905 Nobel Prize. Bretonneau of the Paris school had earlier argued for diseases like diphtheria being specific entities, speculating about the 'quid divinum' responsible for them (Faber 1930). In fact, there had already been something of an overswing. The disease model which came to be seen as co-extensive with illness, that is to say the disease was the illness. The drama of the emergence of scientific medicine notwithstanding, the superficial model comprising clinical pictures remains the raw data of practice, as postulated much later by Feinstein (1967). It is tunnel vision to ignore the fact it is the clinical pattern or picture, tied to knowledge of prognosis and to treatment, which is even more important today to underpin decisions concerning the deployment of the formidable arsenal of scientific intervention spawned by biomedical science in the 20th century.

In effect, the new disease paradigm provided an interpretive grid which allowed the clinician to interpret the signs and symptoms of disease, and later abnormal diagnostic tests and responses to specific treatments, in terms of scientific understanding of the body interior and disease mechanism. This was tantamount to having learned a new 'language' which allowed the experienced clinician to read the patient's symptoms and signs elicited from inside the body (Foucault 1976) and to interpret this pattern in terms of disease. If postmodern doctors could similarly understand the languages of the social sciences and humanities, as well as they do that of biomedicine, they could read the whole person in social and cultural context! This will be the aim of the new clinic in the 21st century. Clinical medicine is an organ of society. Its characteristics must, in the longer term, match those of society. Major change cannot be expected in its institutions and practice without a concomitant social change. Hence before we consider further accomplishments in establishing the mechanism of disease, the new germ theory, we digress to consider the social and political background to this momentous change.

The Social Context of the Paradigm Shift

In France, in the first half of the 19th century, it was the birth of the teaching hospital system which nurtured the new paradigm in its formative years. The beginning of the scientific paradigm was indeed catalyzed by a sea change in social thinking which provoked radical change in medical institutions following the political disruption of the French Revolution. It required a conjunction of social and cultural revolution in France with scientific progress in disease understanding to provoke the shift of belief which led to the final overthrow of a rationalist system of medical knowledge which had lasted for thousands of years. The social and political changes which impacted on medicine and the church were related to the idea of a 'social physics' part of the Enlightenment Project which involved the application of science to the critique and reform of societal institutions. This was the ideal of the French philosophes and British empiricists. Contributing factors in France included fear of epidemic illness and the need to control rampant quackery.

Hence the transformation of health care was almost a side-show to the massive social transmogrification which accompanied the crumbling of feudalism and its replacement by the liberal democratic state and its market economy. Important aspects of the historical context in France were the objectives of health care reform, particularly that involving the poor (Foucault 1976). For example, the conservative university Faculte de Medicin, with its scholastic orientation still committed to the Galenic model of disease, was replaced by the Societe Royale de Medicin ideologically linked to science. Hospitals, medical guilds and the faculty were to be abolished. Scientifically trained doctors would replace the clergy as a secular source of counsel about illness. In response to the problem of quacks, doctors were to be licensed according to knowledge, both theoretical and practical, as well as moral worth but without the need for explicit governmental regulation. The doctor was therefore to be the one who would set the standards of good health. However, doctors would ultimately be unnecessary with the return to health of a good society. They thought that the cost of health would therefore fall. There is a striking similarity to the trap into which modern health administrators fell in this century – 'the finite need model' of health care delivery.

Should Patients Be Treated at Home?

Since disease was thought to exhibit a more natural form at home, this is where health care should be undertaken. However, this proved impractical because of the sheer number of poor and the economic implications (Foucault 1976). The compromise struck was to establish the charity hospital to take care of the poor. As it happened, this provided the ideal environment for the clinical research, the clinicopathological correlation which would in turn benefit the rich as well. What was generated in this serendipitous way was a feed-back loop, a hermeneutic circle, whereby empirical signs of illness were interpreted according to the footprints of disease found in the body after death according to the new disease model based on pathological anatomy. In this way, the knowledge edifice of new biomedical model of illness was built up and applied as an additional instrument of diagnosis, complementing the empirical recognition of the clinical patterns of illness. The paradigm of science had joined that of traditional medicine in the new medical paradigm.

Early Paradigmatic Controversy

The establishment of a new paradigm may involve advance and retreat before a final consensus position is established. So it was for the new medical paradigm. The Romantic idealist movement in Germany held to holism in reaction to the advance of classical science and of its root-metaphor of mechanism. Hence there was a functionalist school in Germany and in France took a more holistic perspective on the nature of disease which stressed abnormal organ physiology, with disease as the consequence of the disequilibrium consequent on disturbed organ function (Faber 1930). The French view of disease was attacked as 'ontological' since disease was portrayed as a 'thing' rather than a process.

The German functionalist view represented the emergence of pathological physiology as opposed to pathological anatomy, the emphasis of the French clinico-pathological correlation. This was the trend followed in Germany by the famous German physiologist and anatomist Johannes Muller, Professor at the University of Bonn. He undertook an extraordinary range of studies in physiology and anatomy, as well as establishing a reputation as a fine teacher of students, one of whom was Rudolf Virchow. Under his reign and under Virchow, German medicine flourished but with 'extremely narrow and limited views concerning clinical medicine' (Faber 1930). They stoutly resisted the notion of typical clinical pictures and of individual diseases with a specific cause; these were seen as incompatible with the functional view of disease as disturbed physiology generating an infinite array of clinical manifestations. Ultimately these would be seen as complementary views.

In this sometimes strident debate, the French physician Broussais was a seminal though paradoxical figure. He was an ardent advocate of the 'physiological medicine,' the most popular medical doctrine in Paris at the time, hence he prescribed blood-letting and fasting according to the old paradigm. Yet he accepted Bichat's localization of disease in the tissues of organs, indeed claimed that this applied to all diseases including fevers and mental disease when little may be found at autopsy. Thus his creed was: 'seek in physiology the characteristic feature of diseases, and by skillful analysis disentangle the often confused cries of the sick organs' (Foucault 1976). In this he was on the side of the German functionalists and a bitter opponent of Laennec and of the Paris school. In particular, he strongly objected to disease being labelled as a 'thing,' a stance which he rejected as ontological, the reification of disease as a Platonic abstraction. Rather he emphasized the infinity of physiological responses to disease, hence of clinical patterns of illness, in keeping with the clinical heuristic that no two patients ever present an identical clinical picture.

The Other Science - Still-Birth of the Empirical Statistical Approach

By the end of the 19th century, science was at the core of the Enlightenment project and had at last impacted powerfully on clinical medicine. At the time, quantitative sociology had emerged as the major tool of social research in response to advances in mathematical statistics, pioneering social research spearheaded by Laplace, Poisson and Quetelet. There was an explosion of statistics which were being extensively applied in the analysis of social problems by the infant welfare state in Europe (Hacking 1990). The eminent Laplace had even targeted medicine as a fruitful area of application of statistics. Inevitably the idea did spread to medicine. One would be forgiven therefore for assuming that the impact of science allied with statistics would have extended beyond forging a new model of disease. Surely science would be exploited as a means of bringing the rigour of the laboratory to the bedside. But it did not work out that way.

A new discipline of epidemiology arose in the mid-19th century which brought scientific statistical refinement to public health research. It was via epidemiology that empirical science entered the thinking of clinical practice in the mid-20th century, and which is now flourishing as 'clinical epidemiology' and 'evidence-based medicine'. There had, however, been a false start in Paris much earlier. Pierre-Charles-Alexandre Louis, one of the pioneers of the clinical research of the Paris school did conceive the notion that scientific and statistical concepts could be applied to confront and to quantify the inherent uncertainties of clinical practice. He even put into practice the more radical idea of scientifically evaluating the effectiveness of treatments. He applied sceptical scientific reasoning to the techniques of clinical care with the aim of minimising observational error, long an obsession of natural scientists and of astronomers and a prime application for the new statistics. History-taking required care to avoid the serious bias which could be introduced by using direct questions which might influence a patient's responses.

Louis stressed the importance of scientific objectivity in interpreting clinical observations, specifically emphasizing the importance of quantitative expression of data. He also introduced a kind of structured interview – a check list of questions about symptoms. Like Feinstein much later, Louis applied his science to clinical methods with proper respect for the art. Thus he recognised the importance of eliciting the patient's own opinion of illness, previously the cornerstone of a consultation but subsequently neglected by clinicians whose attention was focussed on the more objective but generally less germane investigation results in the name of scientific objectivity. He also retained the clinical outlook. While he is widely quoted as saying that 'it is indispensable to count,' he also stressed the need to pay attention to individual 'distinguishing factors of age, sex and patient history,' noting that 'it is not sufficient to count' (Louis, quoted in Matthews 1995). As a dedicated dissector, Louis also applied his 'methode numerique' to the new clinical research using quantitation when documenting the relative frequency of individual clinical manifestations, their severity, duration and progress. In fact, the contribution for which Louis is best remembered is his evaluation of blood-letting, one of the most popular treatments of the Hippocratic tradition (Matthews 1995, see Faber 1930). He proposed the evaluation of treatment through comparative studies of two populations selected 'indiscriminately' with only one being subjected to the intervention (Louis, 1836). Louis used his numerical method to demonstrate the ineffectiveness of blood letting, one of the most popular treatments of the Hippocratic tradition. Bretonneau of the Paris school had convincingly argued for diseases like diphtheria being specific entities, speculating about the 'quid divinum' responsible for them (Faber 1930).

A False Start to Evaluation

Louis' work was a clear anticipation of modern moves to make clinical practice more scientific in the spirit of clinical epidemiology. Although therapeutic nihilism was rife, scientific skepticism vis a vis clinical methods did not take root in the nineteenth century and the numerical method failed to gain lasting support. The question is why this was so. An obvious explanation lies in the threat posed to traditional clinical skill which sustained the authority of the medical profession. Louis' demonstration of the ineffectiveness of bloodletting for typhoid fever damaged the reputation of his enemy Broussais, and threw into question an extremely popular practice. The very idea of putting medical treatment to the empirical test directly challenged the doctor's clinical authority and this, in turn, undermined that patient trust in the doctor which was believed to be a crucial element in the success of treatment (Katz, 1984). It could also be argued that the new democratic states had a stake in supporting scientific medicine but there were as yet no effective and expensive treatment which would tax their budgets.

Although Louis' interest was simply about scientific thinking and the appropriate use of numbers, not statistical theory or analysis, his 'methode numerique' did become a focus of some concern. At issue were the value and propriety of using data from groups for the treatment of individual patients, the role of clinical judgement, and the value of probability as a concept for clinical diagnosis based upon the manipulation of clinical patterns or pictures. The controversy was played out in two debates conducted in Paris in the late 1830s (Matthews 1995). These raised issues related to the application of statistics in clinical medicine which still echo in current controversy surrounding health services research and evidence-based medicine.

Changes in Clinical Thinking – Evidence Redefined

At this point it is worth taking stock of the depth of the change in thinking which had so far influenced clinical medicine by the mid-19th century when the new disease model had become widely accepted. The most fundamental was not the idea of controlled collection of data in the laboratory which underpinned biomedical science. It was the very notion of collecting evidence to support a belief about which there was uncertainty. The scholastic tradition prized 'scientia,' the Aristotelian idea of certain knowledge of the true nature or essence of things obtained deductively by syllogistic reasoning and mathematical calculation. Such knowledge was the province of physics and astronomy, the 'high sciences.' Medicine was, along with alchemy and mineralogy, a 'low science' (Hacking 1990). Its knowledge was uncertain, 'opinio,' derived from interpretation of signs. Initially the 'probability' of a sign was the extent of support from acknowledged authorities as we have stated. Later signs were read from nature, as Paracelsus and Sydenham had done in medicine, and as Francis Bacon recommended in his call for empirical research.

After the mid-17th century such empirical data began to be interpreted according to a new idea of probability based upon the frequency of observation of signs in nature. Eventually the patterns of disease, their prognosis and best treatment would be seen in terms of probability and controlled studies. As in the case of Newtonian mechanics, probability was the bridge required between deterministic mechanical cause-and-effect and the uncertainty of outcome in a complex dynamic system. As an interesting diversion, we should note the role of 'uncertainty' in the evolution of scientific thinking, responsible for the intellectual revolution from cause and effect, via systems theory and thinking to postmodern complexity theory which is currently finding its place in clinical research.

The Aristotelian concept of disease was as an essence, an ideal type. Science replaced this with two concepts. The first was a mechanical model based upon causality. The other was a variety of patterns representing the unique interaction between provoking agent and individual person, distributed as combinatorial probabilities. The latter is an early explanation of the clinician's view of illness as patterns of clinical pictures. Clinicians rely on these patterns and their frequency in making diagnoses, and on the opinion of acknowledged experts with long experience. They tend to assess the effectiveness of treatment according to their own experience and that of professional consensus, as they have always done, and now rely on what would be expected from the biomedical disease mechanism. I agree that empirical statistical science in the accessible form of epidemiological thinking can improve clinical judgement by evaluating effectiveness as Louis initially proposed. Hence many different kinds of evidence contribute to clinical judgement, a fact of life not readily accepted by proponents of evidence-based medicine. Controversy is stirred when one is accorded a privileged status as we will see in Chapter 13. Most clinicians simply cannot accept this.

Another reason that clinicians did not pursue statistical thinking was the rapid and exciting advance of biomedical science and its clinical applications in the first half of the 19th century. The idea of a specific cause of disease hence specific treatment had been anticipated by seers such as Paracelsus, Robert Boyle and Thomas Sydenham but was not in keeping with the traditional paradigm which saw the specificity of illness as a manifestation of humoral imbalance, with specific features related to individual constitution and environmental influence. Following the breakthrough in the Paris school, there was a kind of paradigmatic interregnum during which there was rapid progress in diagnostic testing without much prospect of treatment. As a reaffirmation in scientific garb of the primacy of diagnosis in the traditional paradigm, it is relevant to the modern doctor's tendency still see diagnosis as an end in itself rather than as a staging post on the way to specific treatment.

Surely There Must Be Some Cause?

Nonetheless, there was mounting concern, a veritable obsession with the cause of disease and its implications for treatment. The concept that any effect is the result of some cause is, of course, deeply rooted in commonsense. It was also one of Kant's intrinsic basic categories used for our interpretation of external world events. Moreover simple cause and effect is the basic assumption of the mechanistic reductionist model which had came to ascendancy with the scientific revolution following the Renaissance. The cosmos was widely seen as the result of linear interaction between variables according to the analogy of colliding billiard balls, a concept based on the atomistic theory of the Greeks and deeply rooted in the thinking of such men as Descartes, Newton and Laplace. Descartes proposed that the body was a machine but carefully excluded the workings of the mind. La Mettrie (1747), French physician and philosopher, was not so coy. In his 'L'homme Machine,' he proposed the highly materialistic view that psychic phenomena were also related to organic changes in the brain and nervous system, an idea which caused considerable outcry at the time. Broussais, an erratic genius, opponent of the Paris school spoke of 'irritation' of tissues, explicitly introducing the notion of a specific disease cause in his ('The Examination of Medical Doctrines' 1816, Foucault 1976). The pathological changes found in organs and tissues at autopsy surely begged for a causal explanation.

Infection and Contagion

The idea of a transmissible agent as a cause of contagious disease has ancient roots. Varo had suggested the idea in ancient times. Fracastoro explicitly postulated disease transmission by minute particles, 'animalicules.' Antonio van Loewenhoek had seen bacteria through his microscope but did not associate them with infection. This kind of thinking was outside the traditional paradigm and had not been generally accepted before the 19th century. Daviaine (Reiser 1978) demonstrated that anthrax micro-organisms caused disease in sheep; Bassi demonstrated that bacteria caused muscardine, a fatal disease of silk worms. Nevertheless, the idea remained contentious. The problems posed by viral diseases muddied the waters, as did the earlier problem of the absence of localized disease in some cases of fever. Alternative theories of transmission were non-bacterial infectious particles and miasma emanating from filth.

This debate and the rather fruitless and confused argument over ontology and the nature of disease was cut short by the identification of bacteria as the cause of the most important diseases of the time, the endemic and epidemic infections. The establishment of germ theory put into place the last piece of the disease mechanism of the new paradigm. The impasse was resolved when Pasteur convincingly linked organic putrefaction with bacteria (Dubos 1960), and by the success of Lister's application of these findings by using disinfection to reduce surgical infection. Koch clinched matters with his work on anthrax and his meticulous demonstration of the mycobacterium as the cause of tuberculosis based on a specific set of scientific postulates.

Here too we have examples of those 'paradigm prophets' who are before their time. Of these the most famous was Semmelweiss who correctly identified a transmissible agent as the cause of puerperal fever in 1847; indeed he was able to successfully institute preventive measures (Porter 1997). However, the medical establishment, including the great Virchow, rejected his findings. The corollary is that the old ideas die hard, often along with their most rabid, fervid, and influential adherents! Germ theory was a further radical departure from the orthodoxy of the traditional disease paradigm of medicine. It is therefore not at all surprising that Louis Pasteur encountered strong resistance when he attempted to convince the French Academy of Sciences of his theory.

However the evidence for germ theory was too strong to be resisted for long. Its impact on clinical medicine and on public health was profound. The claim of the functionalists that disease was not a real entity, merely patterns of physiological disturbance, was finally vanquished. As so often happens, there was an overswing. The experience, dating back through Sydenham to Hippocrates, which related individual constitution and environmental conditions to disease, was swept aside by the dramatic demonstration of invading bacteria as the single cause of disease. This idea also resonated with Darwin's theory which emphasized competition between species, in this case between germ and man (Dubos 1960). Thus infectious disease so obviously supported the mechanistic root-metaphor of the analytical tradition that it dealt the final blow to the organic holism which had guided traditional clinical care under the ancient paradigm!

Holism Vanquished – But for How Long?

To paraphrase an old aphorism, 'it's a good wind that blows nobody ill.' Put in another way, with the sharp turn towards mechanism in the interpretation of illness, the baby soon went out with the bath water. The balance of humors model of illness might have been a fanciful theory but its emphasis on holism was entirely realistic in medicine. On the other hand, the apparently simple nature of the causation of infectious disease was seriously misleading as a general guide to the nature of illness. In particular, the great importance of psychological factors and of the healing milieu, of social problems and of economic and environmental conditions and factors in illness, became all too easy to overlook.

In the second half of the 19th century, germ theory provided a somewhat misleading though compelling exemplar of a simple cause of disease which came to dominate thinking, raising as it did the possibility of the 'magic bullet' cure. However, acute infection provided a quite misleading model for chronic disease such as coronary heart disease, cancer, cirrhosis of the liver and mental illness. The irony is that although infectious disease can be explained largely in terms of a single specific agent, its real complexity and the importance of environmental context was evident to Pasteur and others in light of the great difficulty they encountered when culturing bacteria in the laboratory. This complexity became evident later when the importance in infection of host and environmental variables were recognized, and much later when the problem of drug resistance emerged.

The Rise of Laboratory Science

The spectacular success of scientific medicine in the analytical tradition was to have serious distorting effects on clinical practice and on public health (Chapter 7). Early evidence of this was the extent of rise of laboratory medicine in Germany then in the United States, as graduates went to study there. A highly attractive alternative to science based upon clinical observation was soon offered by the laboratory science which was developing rapidly in Germany, overshadowing clinical medicine (Faber 1930). In hospital settings doctors focused on the body and its organs, and medical research became increasingly detached from whole patients and their social context. Scepticism about science gave way to the belief that laboratory science would transform medicine. There would, in the future, be less need for an art of medicine, a 'future belongs to science' point of view. To define the disturbance of bodily physiology - the key to diagnosis was the task of the medical laboratory.

Doctors as 'Medical Scientists'?

Laboratory science generally flourished in Germany in the second half of the nineteenth century. Laboratories were established in conjunction with clinics, pathological physiology and anatomy became separated from clinical medicine, and doctors as medical scientists from their patients. Clinical observation based on the traditional holistic view of organicism was de-emphasized and considered subordinate to the reductionist mechanistic view of laboratory science. New German journals demanded greater emphasis on laboratory science in medicine, promoting explanation over description, the laboratory result over the clinical observation. Clinical thinking was distorted by inordinate efforts to explain clinical phenomena in physiological terms. The great French physiologist Claude Bernard also overestimated the importance of the basic sciences to clinical medicine when he said 'Medicine, rich with facts acquired in the hospital setting, can now leave it to go into the laboratory. In taking the form of experimental medicine, it becomes pure science.' (Faber 1930).

The Textbooks Mirror the Paradigm

Contrary to what one might imagine, it is the medical textbook which tells us most about the modern paradigm of medicine. The essence of a professional paradigm is that it comprises a shared profile of beliefs. How then are these beliefs manifest? One of these concerns its epistemology, the way in which it shapes the body of professional knowledge upon which it calls, determining both its content and mode of how it is classified. The medical text therefore holds a mirror up to the paradigm. The nature and the arrangement of medical knowledge must reflect the composition of the nature and the arrangement of the medical paradigm. A subset of these medical beliefs is the clinical paradigm. The modern clinical paradigm is, we have proposed, consists chiefly of a biomedical component (the science of medicine), traditional techniques and related knowledge (the art of medicine) co-existing in an uneasy equilibrium. The textbooks from which students learn their clinical science and their craft are, at the same time, both a reflection of the structure of the prevailing clinical paradigm and a powerful mechanism contributing to its reproduction, to its transmission to the next generation of doctors.

The failure of these texts to respond to change with the time must exert a conservative influence on students and on their clinical tutors. Our objective in mounting a critique of these texts is not in any way to denigrate them since they clearly meet perceived educational needs. Our objective is to use them to examine unstated paradigmatic assumptions. The texts we have chosen are those recommended for students at the University of Melbourne. The same texts are in widespread use in the United Kingdom, United States and other Western countries. Examination of the content of medical textbooks does, however, provide a concrete embodiment of the characteristics of the current modern paradigm. The point to note is that 35 years of development of the rational scientific approach to methods of clinical examination, and of evaluation of evidence and interpretation of information in the medical literature, has almost entirely slipped through the cracks between the text book of medicine and the text book of clinical examination.

The Textbook of Medicine

Professional knowledge, including that of medicine can be conveniently divided into the data base of theory and empirical observation related to illness, its detection, classification and treatment on the one hand, and the methods or techniques used to obtain, process and apply information in the course of patient evaluation and treatment on the other - the technology of the clinical process as it were. The data base consists of two major components, the scientific and the clinical. The scientific component is a body of information comprising chiefly biomedical science, including pathological anatomy and physiology related to disease mechanism, and characteristics of diagnostic and therapeutic technologies. The clinical component is the description and classification of clinical patterns of illness related to prognosis and choice of treatment. These two components are brought together, and as far as is possible related to one another in the textbook of medicine.

The standard textbook of medicine covers the bulk of the curriculum of the undergraduate or postgraduate student in internal medicine. The units of discussion in the standard textbook of medicine, which we take entirely for granted in keeping with the idea of tacit acceptance of a paradigm, are moulded by the structure of the knowledge base hence reflect that of the paradigm. A brief description of the disease entity, rather than any attempt at a formal definition is followed by a discussion of mechanism, description of the typical or modal pattern of clinical features, of the commonly observed variations, and of diseases which resemble it, and an account of prognosis and treatment options. We could refer to these units as the illness patterns of the paradigm. As discussed earlier, these provide templates for recognition and classification of illness in the individual patient, guides to its clinical behaviour untreated and its response to treatment. These encapsulations of illness in the form of interconnected facts are, of course, an indispensable means of communication between clinicians. Products of the modern paradigm, their construction faithfully reflects the way that clinical knowledge has been structured since the rise of the teaching hospital in France early in the eighteenth century introduced clinicopathological correlation, clinical conjecture checked against autopsy findings.

Thus the texts quote the biomedical fact, say the proportion of patients with lung cancer who have haemoptysis (blood in the sputum); this autopsy observation is of limited interest to the clinician who would be better served by the empirical clinical observation of what proportion of people with blood in the sputum, the clinical observation, have lung cancer, since this knowledge can be directly applied to making the diagnosis. The clinician faced with the problem of making a disease diagnosis for a specific patient has totally different perspective. The clinical problem is that we have in front of us a particular patient with a specific pattern of clinical findings. Confronted by a patient with headache, the doctor's immediate need is to be able to generate a short list of likely causes in any particular practice environment, say in primary care or in a neurology clinic. All that is to hand initially is the presenting complaint, a letter of referral, patient's age, sex and general characteristics. There may be no physical signs. The physician can scarcely seek help since there is, as yet, no diagnosis to look up!

'The Epidemiological Slant'

It was this very contradiction, this focus on interpreting clinical findings at autopsy in lieu of documenting the natural history of illness and response to therapeutic intervention which Feinstein exposed in his 'Clinical Judgment.' This kind of epidemiological information is still scarce for it requires detailed scientific study of prognosis and treatment which, as we have seen, began only in the 1960s, at the beginning of the postmodern era when Feinstein and later others developed the new discipline of clinical epidemiology to correct just this deficiency. So far clinical epidemiology has not progressed further than a cameo appearance in the textbook of medicine. It has certainly not reshaped the way that knowledge is presented to clinician and student.

A partial response to this problem has been the evolution of a different kind of medical text book which has evolved dedicated to the problem of differential diagnosis. In this kind of text, information is framed according to how the patient presents clinically addressing the question of which disease is most likely to explain these findings (Harvey and Bordley 1955). The standard text books of medicine give only brief descriptions related to the technique of clinical examination. It has been the custom for students to learn these at the bedside and from the text books of clinical examination. Unfortunately, as we will see, none of these text books incorporates the scientific critique of clinical method which is the stuff of 'clinical epidemiology' which has fallen between the stools. In chapter 15, we discuss the daunting task facing the 'reflective practitioner' whom we see as coordinating trainees, graduates and staff of the Centre for the Study of Clinical Practice, reflective physicians all conducting 'clinical practice research' of which clinical epidemiology is a key ingredient. Then the problem will be to get the information into the textbooks!

The Importance of Functional Symptoms

Most symptoms in the community, and those of the peripheral zone, are either minor and of unknown or speculative cause, psychosomatic or in combination. Hence their differentiation from the manifestations of organic disease is the first and most crucial step in diagnosis. To fail here can make a fit person into an invalid or, less commonly, can result in the dismissal of symptoms of early perhaps treatable disease. Given that symptoms are so common in the community and that their distinction from the organic is of such crucial import, one might expect that those which most aided the differentiation of the functional illness from the organic would be accorded the highest priority in these texts, and that the distinctive patterns of functional illness would also. Nothing could be further from the truth. Even the characteristics of the extremely common and important symptoms which can spuriously suggest serious or life-threatening heart or lung disease, such as functional shortness of breath, chest pain and palpitations, are given scant attention. So strong is the pull of the biomedical component of the clinical paradigm, the emphasis on organic disease, that the functional symptoms, the patterns of psychosomatic illness, which are so hard to explain under this mechanistic paradigm, are given short shrift.

In particular, little attention is devoted to understanding the psychosocial influences which impinge on the decisions of doctor and patient in seeking and cooperating with care and in providing it respectively. Clearly these textbooks are oriented towards the Central Zone of clinical care, the teaching hospital reflecting the focus of medical education and research on the hospital in-patient (vide infra). What is important is that under the conditions of practice in the Peripheral Zone, the ambulant patient in general practice, the functional symptom and reassurance dominate reality. In the practice of primary care medicine and in internal medicine, it is not all that easy for most doctors to do a lot of good in their professional life time. It is, however, distressingly easy to do harm by diagnosing disease when none is present, by ordering a test which delivers a doubtful result when the test was not really necessary, or by intervening inappropriately because of misinterpretation on the basis of a functional symptom believed to be organic. Symptoms associated with neurosis in the absence of demonstrable organic disease, functional symptoms, form a large proportion of all presenting complaints in all areas of clinical practice. Hence their accurate recognition is crucial to the avoidance of much fruitless worry, expensive investigations and wasted resources in terms of clinicians' time and hospital beds.

Functional Illness as 'Background Noise'

The textbook of medicine can be seen as largely representing a repository of knowledge necessary for practice in the Central Zone of medical care with emphasis on the positive identification of disease. Students are not encouraged, on the other hand to make a positive diagnosis of functional illness from the clinical pattern of the symptoms and from the associated psychological manifestations and social circumstances. Rather functional illness, unexplained symptoms, psychological response and problems of living were seen as 'background noise' rather than as very common and central to the understanding of illness. The tendency encouraged by modern medicine and reflected in the text book is the tendency to regard symptoms as evidence of organic disease until proven otherwise. Relevant input from behavioural science, from sociology and anthropology comprise only a small fraction of the content of the textbook of medicine. Not only that, in some cases the textbook has gone backwards; short, limited but useful sections on functional symptoms have disappeared between editions. The student could certainly be forgiven for drawing the implicit conclusion that the patient's symptoms are attributable to organic disease until proven otherwise, often by extensive investigation, and that reassurance is simply a matter of telling the patient that the exclusion of organic disease has been successfully accomplished.

Common functional symptoms such as tension headache, atypical chest pain, air-hunger described as 'breathlessness,' early morning fatigue and insomnia are discussed in the standard text books. However, the descriptions are scattered among the differential diagnoses of various organic illnesses when they are not given the emphasis which their diagnostic and therapeutic importance warrants. Thus the tension headache may mimic cerebral tumour, the breathlessness described as 'air hunger' heart or lung disease, the chest pain - angina in a patient with an asymptomatic coronary stenosis leading to inappropriate angioplasty, dizziness - disseminated sclerosis, and abdominal pain - biliary colic in a patient with asymptomatic gallstones leading to ultrasonic lithotripsy or cholecystectomy. Yet in each case, careful interrogation often reveals features highly suggestive of a psychological origin not typical of the organic symptoms and the holistic pattern of psychological and psychosomatic response, and the social circumstance may allow a positive diagnosis.

Heart Murmurs and All That

An important inhabitant of the Peripheral Zone has, in fact, sometimes been invited inadvertently into the system by the medical profession. Apart from community screening, this is most often the result of a query raised by a doctor in the course of a routine physical examination. The prime physical sign which is discovered by doctors is the heart murmur, so that such a query can be used as an exemplar. Murmurs suggest either a valve problem, hole in the heart or are 'innocent,' simply a thickened valve as a normal accompaniment of aging or rapid blood flow in a high proportion of children and pregnant women, and, most significantly, in the anxious! By far the majority are innocent. Given the frequency with which such doubts are raised, the number of specialist referrals requested and number of tests ordered for clarification, and given the potentially serious consequences of misdiagnosis, even of raising the query which invariably causes anxiety, the accurate clinical recognition of the innocent heart murmur is a matter of great concern.

Yet it is difficult to find in medical texts clear statements to the effect that murmurs are commonly encountered in normal people. This is all the more distressing since it may adversely affect the lives of the family of a child who has been queried, of a pregnant woman, of a job candidate or insurance applicant whose future may be compromised. Like functional symptoms, the innocent murmur can be classified and distinguished from organic heart diseased on positive grounds by its character as well as by the absence of other evidence of heart disease. However, such an invaluable classification of innocent murmurs is not presented in standard textbooks, is not systematically taught to medical students, is not well known even to specialist physicians. Cardiologists learn to recognize innocent murmurs from their own experience but often do not make any attempt to classify them.

Typically, medical students get a thoroughly skewed experience. They may examine their own heart (and sometimes find a murmur!) and that of a few of their colleagues; they do not usually examine a large number of normal children, anxious people or pregnant women. On the other hand, in a university teaching hospital with an open heart surgical unit, 'interesting cases' with serious heart disease are not hard to find; teaching on such patients is not hard to justify since students are regularly confronted by such patients in their examinations. Evidence is in support of this is the problem which can be created. Given the potential damage which can arise from failure of a doctor with this instrument around his or her neck to clearly understand the range of normal findings causing misinterpretation of heart murmurs, it is hardly surprising that there is a clinical aphorism which says that 'the good cardiologist is a little bit deaf.' Alternatively, no student should be let loose on patients until he or she has demonstrated an accurate and comprehensive grip on the normal range of heart sounds.

The strong biomedical emphasis on organic disease can be seen from analysis of the contents of textbooks according to the number of pages devoted to the above topics. Moreover, this balance has changed little between the 1950s and the present time. The pathogenesis, clinical description and treatment of disease comprised, on average, 97% of the contents in the 1950's, 96% for recent editions. Chapters or sections related to psychology or psychiatry constituted 0.6% of the earlier texts, 2.5% recently. A mere 0.3% of space in the 1950's was devoted to material that could be classified as population health or social science. These topics and the new science of clinical technique (clinical epidemiology) now accounts for 2.4%. The recent additions also included specific topics such as the general approach to the practice and art of medicine, problems of aging, medical ethics, epidemiology and preventive medicine, clinical epidemiology and decision analysis, economic costs, personal health, human growth and development, public responsibility of physicians, terminal care and, in one of these texts, concerns and fears of the patient in hospital and sports medicine. The very fact that these topics have been included points to recognition that these texts do aim to cover the ground occupied by internal medicine.

Textbook of Clinical Examination

While information on disease is presented to students in the lecture hall, in the clinicopathological conference and in text books of medicine, clinical technique is taught almost exclusively at the bedside. In this situation, we note a strong tendency for clinicians to continue to teach what they were themselves taught. The student's guide to the techniques of patient evaluation is the text book of clinical examination, used as a complement to bedside teaching, the traditional method of transmitting the craft which has continued uninterrupted since Hippocrates. Hence the text book of clinical examination directs its attention towards teaching the skills associated with the clinical interview and the physical examination which are the basic methods used to collect clinical data from patients.

A rather startling observation in the scientific era is that the text book of clinical examination has also changed little since the last century, exhibiting an archaic emphasis on description of the typical, even of the gross abnormality, with little evidence of a sceptical attitude, of awareness of the need for critical evaluation of the accuracy and reliability of clinical information whether from the examination of the patient, from diagnostic tests or from the medical literature. Classifications include lists of symptoms and signs which show little discrimination of what aspect of diagnosis they address such as disease severity or aetiology. There has been some intrusion of biomedical science as a means of explaining symptoms and signs in terms of pathological physiology. In short there is a lack of any scientific spirit.

The text books in physical examination currently recommended for students at the University of Melbourne are of relatively recent origin. Hence we have compared their content with two which were recommended in the mid-1950's which have editions dating back to 1897 (Hutchinson and Hunter) and 1936 (Chamberlain). Eponymous nomenclature persists and obsolete concepts and signs clutter the text, propagated from one book to the other and from one edition to the next. The vital distinction between normal and abnormal which is so often the key task in the peripheral zone of care is not stressed. Missing is any awareness of attempts over 50 years to refine and improve of clinical techniques of diagnosis and management, to minimize diagnostic error by measuring the accuracy of tests highlighting the threats to their reliability, to critically assess the effectiveness of treatment and the reliability of the medical literature, to relate clinical symptoms and signs to prognosis and choice of treatment. A series in the Journal of the American Medical Association in 2001 represented an attempt to do this in the case of some physical signs, as did Joshua et al. (2005), McGee (2005) and Simel (2008). However symptoms and most physical signs still remain unevaluated.

What is lacking, in fact is the territory of modern clinical epidemiology. This is, of course, the consequence of the failure of P-C-A Louis' and of Jules Gavarret's attempts to introduce a scientific spirit into the clinical enterprise in the early days of scientific medicine, and the subsequent divorce of epidemiology from clinical medicine was to deprive it of the opportunity to develop methods of harvesting and analyzing clinical observations in a systematic way. Only traditional views of the nature of diagnosis, the applied science chimaera, are ever presented. No attempt has been made to incorporate the insights of cognitive science into how clinicians actually make a diagnosis. Some clinicians confess to the fact that it is difficult to discontinue some routine aspect of the physical examination even when long experience has shown it to be worthless. Thus the chest wall was routinely tapped (percussed) in a futile attempt to determine the heart size long after Sir Thomas Lewis (1946) had pronounced the sign to be worthless!

What Influences the Patient's and Doctor's Puzzling Decisions?

Even less in evidence is any appreciation of the need for and availability of information on why and when patients seek medical help, whether and why they are or are not satisfied with clinical consultations, comply with treatment recommendations or are reassured by exclusion of serious disease, or why doctors make the decisions they do. As a result of this profound lack of interest in matters psychological and social, the standard social history taking taught to students is a pathetic brief stereotyped ritual with regard to marital status and habits especially smoking and alcohol consumption. Nor is there much discussion of the great difficulties which can confront communication between doctor and patient beyond advice to 'establish rapport and understanding' to attend to body language and to note that proper interpretation yields only to practice (Talley and O'Connor 2009). Instead attention is focused on disease diagnosis. Conspicuously absent is any attempt to encourage the interpretation of symptoms in the light of the multitude of influences relevant to the reason for and success of the consultation. The fruits of research into the doctor-patient relationship important to interpreting patient complaints, and handling them without unnecessary, potentially damaging and costly investigations, are not incorporated. All of these relate to an emerging patient-centred or humanistic care.

The need for the doctor to be aware of the way the patient experiences illness and seeks to attach meaning to it, the extent of lay consultation and the need to develop a more patient-centred style of consultation are subjects never addressed. These texts appear to inhabit some kind of a time warp, presenting a nineteenth century view of the medical consultation which is seriously out of touch with the task of the doctor, especially in the peripheral zone of practice. This is a serious problem since the risk of diagnostic error and of failure to appreciate crucial psychological and social complexities are greatly magnified when doctors work, as most do, in the Peripheral Zone of clinical care (mainly primary care).

Rarely is any attempt made to distinguish symptoms and signs which contribute to disease diagnosis from those which provide additional necessary for management, that is necessary detail on its cause, severity and progression, complications and likely response to treatment. For example, clinical signs of a leaking aortic valve (aortic regurgitation) include a murmur resulting from leakage of blood past the incompetent valve leaflets, and evidence of the severity of the leak; the latter includes highly reliable evidence in the form of the blood pressure and size of the overloaded heart chamber (left ventricle). These vital pieces of evidence are grouped with a wide variety of other physical signs which frequently carry an eponymous name honouring one of the greats of the last century - Corrigan's sign and pulse, De Roziez's murmur, pistol-short femorals, de Musset's sign - wobbling of the ear lobes in severe regurgitation, none of which has any specific value in clinical assessment!

Nowhere is there information indicating how accurate these signs are in which clinical context, nor are errors related to patient idiosyncracy or environmental conditions. It is well known that jaundice may be missed if the patient is examined in artificial light. The measurement of jugular venous pressure, a vital sign of heart failure, can usually be elicited easily by the expert under good conditions, with difficulty in the obese or collapsed patient, and, since an erroneous estimate may be seriously misleading, it is frequently best ignored or left to the specialist rather than guessed at by the less expert. Similarly, the distinction between the organic and functional symptom is one of the most important responsibilities in clinical practice since it is such an integral feature of medical practice in the Peripheral Zone. Information on this distinction is scattered through the text books of medicine. Stress on this vital distinction might be expected to be picked up by the text books of clinical examination but it is not. Information is scanty or absent in the case of functional breathlessness, chest pain and fatigue, for example, some of the most important symptoms proffered by patients under stress.

The Medical Literature

Long ago, Feinstein et al. (1967) drew attention to the shift which had occurred in medical research. By analyzing the content of the American Spring Meetings, they were able to demonstrate a progressive shift to basic science away from the immediate concerns of the clinician and bedside medicine. Brief inspection of the contents of current journals will readily confirm that biomedical science is still the focus. There are relatively few reports of clinical cases. Discussion of clinical symptoms and signs is uncommon, even more so is information on their accuracy. There has been some increase in health services research, the great bulk of which is study of drug efficacy using randomized trials.

Conclusion

We have considered the paradigm shift which accompanied the shift of medical paradigm from the classical to the modern. It represented a delayed event following the enlightenment. The social epoch of the arrival of modern medicine bears a close resemblance to present conditions, a period of paradigmatic instability, part of which is a pressure on medicine to adjust its mandate with an emerging postmodern society just as it was obliged to do in Revolutionary France. The conditions are rather different and obviously so will be the specific solutions.

It is ironic that the last shift heralded an increase in the commitment of the medical paradigm to science - this time around, an important component will to reaffirm its need for the humanities and due recognition of the place of the social sciences. Just as we could discern the shape of the modern paradigm, so too will the shape of the new one be eventually manifest in the composition of the postmodern paradigm, and similarly reflected in the structure of medical textbooks. I hope that a combination of evolving university reforms, the training of reflective physicians, programs of clinical practice research, and the establishment of centres for the study of clinical practice (chapter 15) will soon provide concrete proof of our intention to go with the flow of the new paradigm.

References

Armstrong D., Political anatomy of the Body. Cambridge University Press, Cambridge, 1983.

Chamberlain E. N., Symptoms and signs in clinical medicine. An introduction to medical diagnosis. 1st edition. 1936.

Dubos R., Mirage of Health. Allen and Unwin, London, 1960.

Feinstein A. R., Koss N., Austin J. H. M., The changing emphasis in clinical research. I Topics under investigation. An analysis of the submitted abstracts and selected programs at the annual 'Atlantic City Meetings' during 1953.

Faber K. F., Nosography. the evolution of medicine in modern times. Paul B Hoeber, New York, 1930.

Flexner A., The Flexner Report on Medical Education in the United States and Canada. Bulletin Number Four. A Report to the Carnegie Foundation for the Advancement of Teaching. New York, 1910.

Foucault M., The Birth of the Clinic. Tavistock, Bristol, 1976. P190.

Freidson E., Medical Work in America: essays on health care. Yale University Press, New Haven, 1989, p. 77.

Hacking I., The Taming of Chance. Cambridge University Press. Cambridge, 1990, p. 39.

Harvey A McG., Bordley A., Differential diagnosis: the interpretation of clinical evidence. WB Saunders, Philadelphia. 1955.

Hunter D., Bomford R. R., Hutchinson's clinical methods. 13th edition (1st edition 1897).

Illich I., Limits to Medicine - Medical Nemesis: The Expropriation of Health, London, Calder and Boyars, 1974, p. 152-3.

Katz J., The Silent World of Doctors and Patients. Free Press, New York, 1984. pp. 5, 6.

Katz J., The Silent World of Doctors and Patients. Free Press, New York, 1984. p. 191.

Lewis T., Diseases of the heart. 1946.

Louis P. C-A., Researches on the Effects of Bloodletting on Some inflammatory Diseases, and on the Influence of Tartarized Antimony and Vesication in Pneumonitis. Milliard Gray and Co, Boston, 1836.

Matthews J. R., Louis, quoted in Quantification and the Quest for Medical Certainty. Princeton University Press, Princeton, 1995.

Simel D. L., Rennie D., Keitz S. A., eds. The Rational Clinical Examination. McGraw-Hill, New York, 2009.

Odegaard C., Dear Doctor: a personal letter to a physician. The Henry J Kaiser Foundation, Menlo Park, 1986.

Odegaard C., Dear Doctor: a personal letter to a physician. The Henry J Kaiser Foundation, Menlo Park, 1986 p. 49.

Porter R., The Greatest Benefit to Mankind: a medical history of humanity from antiquity to the present. Harper Collins. London. 1997, p. 396.

Reiser S. J., Medicine and the Reign of Technology. Cambridge University Press. New York, 1978, p. 23.

Shorter E., Doctors and Their Patients: a social history. Simon and Schuster, New Jersey, 1991.

Simel D. L., Evidence-based physical diagnosis. Evidence-based Med. 6:167, 2001.

Starr P., The Social Transformation of American Medicine. the rise of a sovereign profession and the making of a vast industry. Basic Books, 1982.

Talley N., O'Connor S., Clinical examination. Elsevier Health. 6th edition, 2009.

Chapter 7

Paradigms Close to Medicine - Public Health, the Social Sciences and Medical Ethics

The Threat to Cooperative Effort Posed by Paradigmatic Conflict

We have now examined the evolution of the paradigm of medicine which exerts such a dominant influence on every doctor's thinking. Under the influence of the globalising impact of information technology, health systems are becoming more closely integrated. This means that doctors and the disciplines with a stake in implementing and studying health care policy and delivery are obliged to work together. Such a cooperative venture augurs well for efficiency in the long run. The fly in the ointment again, however, is paradigmatic difference. In particular, there are fundamental differences in orientation towards individual and the community, and differences in allegiance of research methods to the analytical scientific and humanistic interpretive paradigms respectively. We examine these differences in this chapter as they relate to public health, medicine's sister discipline, to the social sciences, often a vocal critic of medicine, and to the humanities, particularly ethics. These differences are important because they threaten the cooperative effort required for the generation of policy, and for the implementation and study of health care.

Paradigmatic Commitments of the Players

The paradigms of public health and of the social sciences were conceived at the time of the Enlightenment and Industrial Revolutions, after the French and American Revolutions. The paradigm of public health and that of economics adopted the perspective of the community rather than that of the individual. That of sociology adopts the perspective of both individual and community. The interests of anthropology, with a more circumscribed interest in health services than the others, has been focused on the individual. The paradigms of public health and of economics are strongly committed to the scientific quantitative paradigm of inquiry, anthropology to the interpretive qualitative, while psychology and sociology have commitments to both. Although the discipline has much to offer, the involvement of anthropology in cooperative 'health services research' have been limited and we will not discuss the discipline further. Sociology and economics are more closely engaged with clinical medicine which nevertheless still holds them at arm's length. Sociology has provided much of the ammunition used for the public criticism of medicine. Economics to most doctors conjures up the vision of 'bean counting' and of 'big brother,' of inappropriate pressures to contain costs against the interests of patients.

Public Health

Major paradigmatic differences, bones of contention, between public health and clinical medicine have been historically the relative extent of the contributions of social improvements to improved health of the community, and currently the role of public health, fostered by governments, in the evaluation of clinical care and cost containment. The paradigm of modern public health grew out of the early recognition of the importance of statistics to the state, and in response to the social and health problems thrown up by industrialisation, mainly in the 18th and 19th centuries. It does not therefore have the deep roots of the traditional medical paradigm which stretches back to antiquity. Public health has its primary allegiance to the quantitative analytical paradigm through epidemiology.

Improved Community Health – Who Should Get the Credit?

Doctors were involved early in the activities of public health. However, following the dramatic surge of understanding which came with the scientific model of disease mechanism, clinical medicine concentrated on pursuing the single curative intervention, the 'magic bullet'. This 'conquest of disease' achieved such dramatic results that this kind of intervention got the credit for improvements in the health of the community since the middle of the last century. In retrospect, this rejection of the real complexity of illness was a serious overswing. The complexity of even bacterial infection and the importance of host factors under natural circumstances was effectively concealed by the highly controlled conditions of a laboratory, a fact known to the pioneers including Pasteur. The objective of carefully controlled laboratory conditions was to eliminate such factors in order to allow bacterial growth in vitro (Dubos 1960). German workers in the 19th century had challenged the narrow view of the microorganism as the 'cause' of disease, recognising the importance of biological context and host constitution.

Microbiologist Renee Dubos reactivated the debate started by Virchow about the relative importance of environmental conditions versus medical care (Dubos 1960). This he did in a scholarly way by taking a broad view of the relationship between humankind and the environment. Hippocrates was aware of the importance of public health measures and this was also of prime concern of the Roman Empire. However the mechanical concept of bacteria and disease as a problem of simple cause-and-effect, and the casting of the problem into the

Darwinian mould of battle between organism and mankind more readily captured the public imagination. Dubos perceived the dangers of this reductionist view. As a microbiologist, he was keenly aware of the role of his own discipline in producing such tunnel vision.

The Enlightenment view was that scientific progress could deliver mankind from the burden of disease but it was the sanitary revolution, not laboratory science, which was responsible for most health gains in the 19th century (Dubos 1960). What Dubos did was to promote a holistic view of man, society and environment as a single ecological system. Seen in this light, the real complexity of disease, especially of chronic illness, became clear. So too did the limited role of curative medicine and the basic medical sciences in ameliorating the health of the community at large, however important they might be to the survival and well-being of the individual in modern society. Pragmatism and enlightened self-interest rather than revolutionary zeal was the basis for a successful sanitary revolution. Cleaning up the cities together with the rising standard of living and improved nutrition resulted in a major health impact. Laboratory science improved understanding of disease so that therapeutic advances subsequently completed the conquest and got most of the credit. All in all, Dubos saw the new biomedical model of illness which placed such stress on a mechanical conception of illness as an understandable but temporary aberration from the holistic one inherited from classical Greece (Dubos 1960).

Thomas McKeown (1979) more specifically examined the major determinants of the decline in the death rate in England in the nineteenth century. Was it a reduced death rate contingent on better medical care, the conventional wisdom of the day, or was it a rising birth rate related to economic growth and industrialization? McKeown marshalled impressive evidence, given the problems of past record keeping, which led him to the conclusion that the influences were first some improvements in agriculture leading to better nutrition and resistance to infection, improved hygiene, and also contraception. The contribution of medical treatment was smaller and came later, becoming evident during the second quarter of the 19th century. The impact of biomedical advances, even on infectious diseases, seen from the community perspective, was less than had been previously appreciated. Responding to earlier criticism, McKeown does document as far as is possible, the reduction in morbidity and suffering for which medicine can reasonably claim credit.

Medicine as a Social Science

At a time when there was intense debate over the role of social conditions in predisposing to disease, both clinical medicine and public health can be seen to have placed a narrow emphasis on the prevention of bacterial infection as 'the cause.' The idea that the wider environment was related to disease dates back to Hippocrates; it was certainly emphasized by Thomas Sydenham in the 17th century, and appears to have been intuitively accepted by physicians. The connection between industrialization, occupation, poverty and ill-health was known to social thinkers and to physicians in the early decades of the 19th century at the very time that scientific medicine was establishing itself. So too was the belief that science should address such problems.

However, it is the German doctor Rudolf Virchow who is remembered as the physician who proclaimed in 1847 that 'medicine is intrinsically and essentially a social science'

(Rosen 1993). Virchow's claims followed his investigation of an outbreak of typhus which convinced him that social conditions of living, economic and political conditions were the primary causative factors in epidemic disease. He saw an analogy between the sickness in the body and the social malaise (Rosen 1993). Virchow also proclaimed the view that doctors must be involved in public health. These radical views he published in his newspaper 'Medicinische Reform' until it was closed down following the revolution of 1848. He was briefly suspended from his academic post by the government but remained politically active. The irony is that he was also a pioneer of biomedical science, especially important for his characterization of disease as due to cellular abnormality.

Biomedical science made counter claims. A contemporary of Virchow, Emil von Behring, founder of immunology and inventor of the diphtheria vaccine, while conceding Virchow's point, nevertheless saw the study of bacteriology as the way to go, rather than the pursuit of social policy. His thinking, of course, reflected the position of the rising star of biomedical science in Germany at that time which subsequently spread to become the dominant paradigm of medicine in the western world. In the heated debates in Britain and on the Continent, an important issue was the relative contribution of miasma related to filth, a public health concern, and of bacterial infection, a medical matter. More correctly, the debate concerned 'exciting' and 'predisposing'causes (Hamlin 1992). The idea of 'predisposing' causes had potential class and political overtones; for one thing it could be implied that 'structural improvements provided in wealthy areas (e.g., drainage) also be provided to the poor.' The overwhelming victory of germ theory and microbiology effectively suppressed this debate; the great 'bug hunt' was on (White 1991).

Social Class – Not Part of the Main Game

Since that time, both clinical medicine and public health have been criticised for ignoring the ecological perspective and accused of paying insufficient attention to the importance of social class. The traditional public health movement has been seen as not doing enough to spotlight the social and environmental causes of illness, so that this emerged as one of the planks of the New Public Health platform. Certainly the clinician's training in the Central Zone, an academic centre currently leads to a lack of a community perspective. Where doctors draw the line with regard to their responsibilities is a difficult question, involving the ideology of medicine and the paradigm of the modern clinician. Some doctors would simply see politics as none of their concern or would support the status quo politically. Others might see the problem as a public health issue outside the sphere of influence of the clinician. Still others would see the need to avoid a counterproductive backlash which might follow overt political action; this would entail supporting selected less controversial issues like childhood poverty or provision of adequate housing as part of the 'treatment of symptoms and end-stages of social failure,' since to go further is to enter 'the central arena of politics' (Morris 1957).

In any case, the fact is that the profession of medicine eschews the politics of health, and the profession as a whole has gained an unfortunate reputation for self-interest rather than of concern for the wider community. This is a far cry from the political activism which Virchow felt was their duty. Yet, as Dubos predicted, doctors can no longer remain aloof from the politics of cost-containment and allocation of health resources (Dubos 1960). Surely they must take a position individually or as a profession if a system of rationing threatens restriction on the basis of class, as was the case in Oregon, U.S.A. (McBride 1990). The medical profession should be seen to be a responsible advocate of the public interest and a professional prod to the conscience of the state. To follow Virchow is to risk the wroth of government and conservative forces and perhaps to court his fate in this regard. To promote specific issues and to engage in winnable skirmishes might be analogous to the successful pragmatic pressure which led to large gains in 19th century public health in Britain as opposed to the unsuccessful revolutionary movements in France and Germany.

The Evaluation of Clinical Practice

In the ancient and mediaeval worlds, there was no concept of scientific evaluation of medical care in the paradigm of ancient Hippocratic Traditional Medicine. Then indeed, there was no system of delivery to evaluate! In the modern world, a number of disciplines have emerged to meet that need. The next chapter examines the roots of these, and their relationship with clinical medicine and the state which has by no means always been harmonious. We saw that there was downside to the impact of science on clinical practice and education. There two kinds of science relevant to medicine. To date, we have considered the effects of the burgeoning biomedical science with which we are all familiar. Serious paradigm clashes have, however, marred the practice and scientific evaluation of medicine – in this case the science can be identified as the 'empirical, statistical, analytical and reductionist science' with which most of us are not familiar rather than the 'biomedical science' which has revolutionised medicine as part of society. The pernicious effects of disciplinary bias and blinkering can be readily seen. This has been most apparent for the new disciplines of 'clinical epidemiology' and its derivative, 'evidence-based medicine.' Hence we will examine their claims and practice in more detail in Chapter.

Another important criticism has been that clinical medicine, until recently, has been unwilling to devote itself to the critical examination of its own treatment interventions. As a result, public health has been prominent in this area - to a considerable extent by default. (clin epi andquantitation) One might have thought that the scientific attitude which transformed clinical thinking early in the 19th century would similarly have led to a skeptical attitude towards treatment and to its critical evaluation. And so it did. In an atmosphere in which statistical thinking was a powerful political and social instrument, indeed, right at the starting point of scientific medicine in Paris, statistical comparison was used to evaluate treatment scientifically. Thus the effectiveness of medical care first became the subject of formal inquiry with Charles-Pierre-Alexandre Louis' 'Methode Numerique' but his brilliant idea fell on barren soil, despite the fact that early French clinicians had been exposed to mathematics and statistical thinking. This initiative lay dormant until the mid 19th century and beyond.

Louis was much criticized by his colleagues and his initiative lapsed. We could speculate that it did so because doctors are, by and large, pragmatists given little to reflection about the way they work and the assumptions they make. Any tendency to do so might also be inhibited by the fact much clinical work is performed at an intuitive level and using rules of thumb

(Ch.13), a mode of operating which might seem 'unscientific.' Or we could suspect from their reaction that clinicians were threatened by exposure of the uncertainties of practice, their reliance on the placebo effect and their threadbare therapeutic armamentarium of specific treatment. A little later, their attention was diverted by the promise of magic bullets, the new scientific therapies promised by microbiology soon afterwards. Another possibility is that diagnosis and the traditions of patient care, largely transmitted as an oral culture and learned by apprenticeship, are conservative and resistant to rapid penetration by the new scientific paradigm. Finally, we could argue evaluation of what meagre therapy was available was not a pressing issue at that time nor was it of concern to government at the time. The net result was that it was public health and epidemiology not clinical medicine which cultivated a strong interest in statistics and quantitative research methods.

Science by the Back Door

Whatever may have been the explanation, this was a false start for empirical science in clinical practice. Science had been embraced as providing solutions concerning what should be done but did not successfully challenge traditional beliefs about how that diagnosis and treatment should be implemented. It was epidemiology, the population biomedical science and sister of the basic clinical sciences, and her bedfellow, biostatistics which played such an important role as the vehicle for the re-introduction of empirical statistical science into the medical paradigm, and for the initiation of the philosophy of evidence-based medicine. In Britain, not long after the Second World War, Morris (1957) introduced the idea of applying epidemiological methods to the study of health services and the randomised trial was first used to assess the effectiveness of a drug. Cochrane later castigated the medical profession for failure to study its own performance, advocating the systematic use of such trials to evaluate health interventions (Cochrane 1971). Cochrane's timely clarion call has since been answered slowly in the form of health services research and related disciplines such as quality assurance, technology assessment, effectiveness and health outcomes research (Chapter 12).

Although doctors had pioneered clinical audit (Codman 1914), and have been active in quality assurance under medical control, the initiative for formal assessment of technology has clearly come from outside, as public health enterprises backed up by moves by government for establish accountability of the medical profession. Thus, although clinical audit was introduced early in the century as a means of checking the outcomes of interventions, it was more than a century after Louis before a science of clinical management re-emerged through Alvan Feinstein in the 1960s. This movement has only recently caught on as clinical epidemiology and evidence-based medicine. The criticism is not so much that medicine has resisted evaluation rather that it has not led the movement.

Essentially, the emphasis on biomedical science decontextualized the clinical process. An open-minded view of the cause of illness would have acknowledged the truth of the claims of both clinical medicine with regard to specific aetiology, and of social medicine with regard to the social and environmental context of illness. Their roles were complementary not in competition at all, and both had been shown to be important to the health of the community. Similarly, clinical experience is essential to evaluating the effects of treatment in individual patients. On the other hand, epidemiological methods can also yield important information concerning the choice of treatment in the individual. Unfortunately clinical medicine and public health went their separate ways during the two centuries past. In the United States, separate schools of public health were set-up under the auspices of the Rockefeller Foundation. In White's (1991) view, this was a retrograde step for public health, creating a 'schism' which became an impediment to recruitment of good physicians and which fostered a narrow intellectual focus on disease aetiology and mechanism rather than extension of epidemiological skills into what came to be known as 'Health Services Research.'

At the same time, germ theory distracted academic clinical medicine which became specialised, withdrawing into its academic centres and losing its community perspective, its point of contact with primary care practice and with public health issues. Clinicians have lost touch with the importance of social factors in the genesis of illness, have lost balance in appreciating the relative prevalences of various diseases in the community, on the common presentations of illness in general practice, and of the limitations of the biomedical model in this setting, of the difficulty in modifying behaviour and of promoting health in an unfavourable social context of deprivation and poverty. It could also be argued that clinical medicine's single-minded obsession with disease mechanism could have been muted by closer contact with epidemiology with a tradition of empiricism and statistical methods which could have exposed problems much earlier by the evaluation of clinical care. Rapprochement is still possible, however. Following a report of the Institute of Medicine which is critical of public health in the United States, the American Medical Association published a report which promoted closer interaction between public health and practising physicians, with an editorial in the Journal of the American Medical Association under the title of '(r)eductionist biology and population medicine - strange bed fellows or a marriage made in heaven?' (Bulger 1990).

Sociology

The social sciences, particularly sociology, have been marginalised in public health and play almost no part in medical practice, are almost entirely excluded from the conventional medical school curriculum and are rarely part of clinical research. The importance of the patient's social environment was stressed by Henderson in the U.S. in the 1930s. Even earlier, one of the 'holistic elite' physicians, Cabot in the 1920s had recognised the importance of attending to these issues but believed that this was a task for the social worker. The paradigm of sociology has also come into conflict with that of clinical medicine. So much so that that sociology therefore has a reputation for 'doctor bashing.' We see the justification if not the justice of the clinician's mistrust of sociology when we see the extent to which sociological research has provided the ammunition for critics demanding political action, and for trenchant critics such as Ivan Illich!

The interests of sociology look outwards to the community, toward studies at the societal or 'macro' level, as well as inwards towards the individual and group behavior or 'micro' level. Thus, in medicine, sociology has contributed much to understanding of health care both at the level of the impact of social factors on health and their political determinants, and the delivery of health services to the community including study of the role of the medical profession. It has contributed rather less to our understanding of the interaction of patients and doctors in medical encounters, although it has access to the qualitative investigational tools required for the task. Its statistical skills have contributed most in community studies. Its qualitative methods, especially those involving interview of the clinical players, patients, doctors and others, have a great deal to offer for those 'reflective physicians' engaged in 'clinical practice research' in the future (Chapter 15).

The Need for the Field Study
with Qualitative Analysis

Denied much access to the clinical scene, the analyses of sociology been almost entirely academic and theoretical, based to only a small extent on empirical studies where its focus has been on the most vulnerable – in ambulant care. Despite this theoretical orientation and concentration of inquiry, the impact of sociology has been profound, sparking, as we have seen, criticisms and demands for reform. Medical sociology began in the 1930's but achieved maturity in the 1960's with a subsequent move to change the name to 'sociology of health' to reflect a broader perspective. Sociology, on the other hand, in its 'micro' form, has a vital concern in dissecting out the complex motivations and reactions of the players in clinical transactions, and the complex interplay of technical, social and cultural influences on their decision-making. In particular, sociology attends to the perspective of the patient. After all it is the patient, often assisted by a coterie of advisors, who makes the fundamental decision of whether or not to become a patient in the first place, and whether or not to accept reassurance or treatment. Such detail can only be delivered by field studies applying qualitative analysis.

Such illness behaviour cannot be interpreted except in the context of a patients personal attributes, past experience and social milieu. The sociological perspective has also revealed the patient to be active as a diagnostician with a network of lay consultants, striving to understand the illness and its meaning in terms of likely outcome and available treatment. Indeed woe betide any healer who fails to satisfy in this area since the penalty is likely to be an unsuccessful outcome in the sense of failure to reassure in the absence of serious illness, of failure to relieve symptoms or to achieve patient cooperation with treatment, and ultimately failure to satisfy patient and kin. Sociology has therefore, much to offer as part of clinical practice research, working side by with physicians, especially in multidisciplinary studies as 'continuous clinical practice research' (Chapter 15).

Sociology, Parsons and the Patient-Doctor System

The link between the individual encounter between doctor and patient, and the community interest was clearly laid out in Talcott Parsons' classical analysis which was based on the model of doctor, patient and society as a social system in equilibrium (Parsons 1951). Parson's sick role model's emphasis on equilibrium in the doctor-patient relationship was challenged. First it was branded as conservative by its adherence to the view held by the medical profession - that the interests of doctors and their patients are entirely complementary. Thus it was argued that patients and doctors occupy separate worlds of experience, and Parsons was accused of bias towards the perspective of the medical profession (Freidson 1989). The symbolic interactionist movement objected that reality is socially constructed. Thus doctors and patients negotiate their positions, largely unconsciously, and may bargain. The doctor is in a dominant position, and the use of professional definitions may result in disease labelling, a criticism most strongly voiced by anti-psychiatry movement.

These attitudes reflected seeing the patient as the underdog, a victim of 'medicalisation.' Deviance in the sick role model was regarded as a construction of the dominant elite. This was also the contention of the socialist left and Marxist who saw the social role of medicine of gatekeeper to the sick role as amounting to some kind of conspiracy between the profession, the state and the corporate sector to prevent depletion of the work force by minor illness. Doctors can be complicit with the state in subtle ways of which they are quite unaware. Under this conflict model, much illness is seen as the result of stress and alienation of workers which are a direct consequence of the mode of production of the capitalist system and of its consumerist ethic. C.W. Mills (1959) called for a 'sociological imagination' to see how personal troubles related to social issues.

These can be unintentionally reinforced when doctors, through the use of language and control of the consultation agenda, emphasise personal issues in the face of social stress related to poverty, unemployment or lack of welfare support. Thus '(d)octors' messages of ideology and social control arise within sincere, but usually uncritical, attempts to help people to cope with contextual problems.' (Waitzkin 1991). In all of this, medicine is then seen as an agent acting to cover up the politically sensitive connection between failure of redistribution of income and ill-health by transmogrifying a social problem into a technical one which can be solved by its experts, in this case the doctor (Habermas 1976). In addition, health is treated as a commodity like any other in a free enterprise system, so that patients from lower classes in general and minority groups in particular have been subjected to discriminatory and oppressive management, particularly in the U.S.A..

As we have seen in our earlier discussion of public health, the state has also been seen as systematically ignoring the contribution of social, economic and environmental factors to illness in the community. Even in the pluralist health systems such as those of Canada and Australia there is inequality in the standard of health care offered to rich and poor, manifest as a 'two-tiered' health system in which the affluent have ready access to private practice. 'Technological fixes' in the form of community screening programs as a means of disease prevention, and behavioural modification as a means of health promotion can be used as substitutes for increased spending on social problems such as housing, work place reform and social support systems which are so much less tractable, but which might be more effective in improvement of community health. In this way, governments can avoid political conflict of interest, and actions which do not sit well with the requirements of economic rationalism. Medicine has been seen as failing to raise its collective voice to point out the importance of the relation of illness and premature death to poverty and low social class, and the importance of economic and environmental factors in its genesis.

The Nature of the Power Struggle

The thrust of the medicalisation debate as proposed by Marxist and political liberals has implied conspiracy by medicine in collusion with the state, hence the need for 'demedicalisation.' This has been applauded or recommended by the most radical of the social critics. However, the waters have been muddied by the influential writings of Michel Foucault. His interpretation is much more subtle interpretation of power which does not lend itself to conspiracy and such naked deployment. As components of a cultural discourse, doctors and patients are powerfully constrained by paradigm, a tacit network of beliefs and attitudes shaped by their socialisation as members of a community, and in the case of the doctor, by medical training as well.

For Foucault (1980), power is not simply repressive, it is the energy which drives change in society. Such power is 'capillary' in the sense that it is pervasive invisible and largely self imposed social discipline. It can also be effectively opposed as what a doctor might see as 'peripheral resistance.' Hence the relationship between public and medical profession, between doctor and patient is dynamic in a constant state of negotiation and renegotiation. This process of give and take can be observed in medical encounters, mainly in the form of unconscious response and manoeuvring. Noncompliance, failure of the doctor to reassure the worried well, and failure of medicine to convince patients of the need to present early with serious symptoms are all surface manifestations of this struggle. Lay knowledge and perceptions may be subjugated knowledge but patients are neither passive nor ineffective in their dealings with doctors.

In all of this medicine is then seen as an agent acting to cover up the politically sensitive matters such as the connection between failure of redistribution of income and ill-health by transmogrifying a social problem into a scientific one which can be solved by experts, in this case the doctor. This is an extension of Weber's concern over the rationalisation of society following the renaissance. He saw society as likely to be imprisoned in an 'iron cage of bureaucracy' administered according an 'instrumental rationality' narrowly focused on means rather than broad social ends. Critical theory, as represented by Habermas (1983), criticises the use of the scientific expert to force technical solutions on what are really social and political issues, and of the dishonest communication required to publicly maintain this deception and inhibit genuine public debate.

In the late premodern era, just before the scientific revolution in medicine, doctors were in intense competition with each other and with a wide variety of lay healers (Jewson 1976). In an atmosphere such as this, especially in the case of the social elite who were medicine's main customers, it was obvious that the successful practitioner had to prescribe according to the patient's individual requirements. The patient's views were therefore to be carefully considered. This catering to patients' needs was eroded by the standard prescriptions of scientific medicine and the doctor surely knew best where science was concerned. The basic ingredients for 'consultation failure' are therefore the 'patient decentred' interview with lack of the level of communication needed to resolve doubt, to resolve misunderstandings, to persuade the patient regarding the accuracy of diagnosis, of prognosis and of the need for the treatment chosen.

Medical dominance does not, however, have to be seen as a conspiracy. Another reasonable interpretation is that the structure of society determines the kind of mandate given to healers, and specifically to medicine. Hence medicine as one of society's technologies is largely shaped according to society's needs and in turn makes its contribution to shaping society. Like other professions, medicine can be manipulated to support the interests of the more powerful in society. The practitioner of physik, the university trained doctor, together with the legal profession and the clergy in the past has long enjoyed the confidence of the aristocratic class, frequently acting in an advisory capacity. This political influence has persisted although somewhat eroded by rising costs and public dissatisfaction with medicine which have tended to spoil this cosy relationship. Nevertheless, the profession still enjoys a large measure of autonomy, is left to regulate itself to a considerable extent, and is still well placed to exert a strong influence on the structure of health institutions and on health care policy.

In any case, medicalization may be replaced by health promotion which is scarcely liberating. This activity tends to emphasise the individual risk factors, ignore the powerful constraints of culture and class on behaviour to discount the complex and as yet unexplained connection between class and health, unable to see the wood for the trees. This has been condemned as victim blaming and also as collusive with the state. The cultural relativist viewpoint of Foucault's thinking, as applied to concealed medical surveillance of the community by Armstrong (1983), has medicine, epidemiology and sociology accused of colluding with government in mounting surveillance over the health of the community as part of the 'dispensary gaze.' Public health and sociology can be seen to have colluded with the state through population surveys and research which has led to an epidemiological definition of normality in terms of a statistical index, or absence of demonstrable risk factors for illness. The net effect has been the two-edged one of expanding community medicine to provide services for school children, population screening, community care of mental illness, expansion of paediatrics and geriatrics as a result of locating disease in the community as a 'clinical ice-berg' (Last 1963), as well as providing testimony to the magnitude of the problem of the trivial illness in general practice. Thus the activities of public health and clinical care have been expanded further by the act of surveillance itself.

Health Economics

The paradigm of economics is such that the thrust of this profession is more clearly at the societal or community level than is the case for that of sociology. Health economics has only a limited contribution to make to the day to day processes of clinical care of patients. Governments have called upon economists to assist in difficult decisions of allocation of resources involved in managing the economy since the 1930s, and health economics has burgeoned internationally since the economic downturn of the 1970s. The major topics of their studies have been the organization of health care, consideration of the determinants of health, of value for money, including attempts to evaluate the impact of medical care on community health, and implications for allocation of resources taking account of opportunity cost. Also important has been consideration of the atypical nature of the health market leading to the concept of 'market failure.'

Economists have to take an active interest in the determinants of the decisions of individuals, of doctors, patients, administrators and politicians, since collectively these determine the expenditure on health care and its distribution. They rely on simple models of human behaviour as the basis of decision-making - 'homo economicus'. The decision model was assumed to be entirely rational, and specifically to be an entirely to the complete exclusion of important emotional influences (vide infra). These models are quintessentially modern in their assumption of rationality, deeply imbued in neoclassical economics which is a product of the Enlightenment. This conservative approach was reinforced early in the 19th century, and further reinforced by Marshall in Britain early in the 20th. However the importance of the paradigm of economics to us is that it is an important part of the top-down scrutiny of clinical care on behalf of health bureaucracies and government.

Patient decision-making, according to the economic doctrine of Maximisation of Expected Utility, is cast as an entirely rational affair with emotions playing no part other than to introduce error (Chapter 14). The gap in knowledge between patients and their doctors makes it difficult for patients to make independent decisions as consumers. The 'invisible hand' concept cannot apply when the consumer cannot be sufficiently informed to allow personal judgement to operate as a regulator of demand. Moreover, the patient is too dependent on the good will and technical skill of the doctor for the latter to be regarded as a disinterested supplier. In addition, the conflict of interest between the consumer and the financial provider is seen as a 'moral hazard' which can encourage excessive expenditure. The ubiquitous regional variation in medical decision-making, of intense interest to health services researchers, has been interpreted as the product of uncertainty, of custom and of over-servicing. The reality is far more complex in light of the multiplicity of interacting influences involved for even the most routine decisions in practice. Both clinician and patient have to interact as they both consider technical 'facts,' including risks, under the influence of a host of personal, social and cultural factors which, as we shall see, are not problems normally discussed in a medical school's curriculum.

Social Sciences and the Quantitative Analytical Paradigm

All of the disciplines with a stake in health care, most of all economics, have paradigms imbued with the analytical quantitative intellectual paradigm. Yet medicine, for all of its protestations about being an applied science, goes about its daily business of evaluating patients blissfully unaware that the clinical techniques it is predominantly employing - interpretive qualitative methods - belong to a 'foreign' paradigm! Obviously, these disciplines must compromise because clinical practice criticism and research must call upon the skills and methods of both intellectual paradigms. The sooner those in both camps accept this as given, the sooner will clinical research into the clinical process itself make progress!

In particular it must be appreciated that qualitative research methods, especially the interpretation of interview data, are essential for success. The charge should be led by medical education forging a postmodern paradigm. In all humility, we have claimed to have put to the test a centre for the study of clinical practice designed to complement university efforts to introduce social sciences and humanities into teaching and research, and to foster closer interdisciplinary cooperation in teaching and research. Such a centre would train the 'reflective physicians,' which we will describe, to supervise clinical practice research, and organize a comprehensive repository of research skills at the host hospital. Of particular importance is that clinicians should be appropriately represented in such research and evaluation.

Empirical studies of clinical decision-making in the field, almost entirely lacking in the literature, should therefore be a high priority for research. Economists criticise doctors for adopting a narrow view of clinical practice which does not take account of cost and the community perspective, implying that their decisions would be more rational if informed by economic concepts. Economists are vexed by the problem that the physician is the major determinant of health care expenditure but expects and enjoys a large measure of autonomy. The question is how responsibility for spreading benefits over the community at large can be balanced against the physicians' obligation to represent the needs of the individual patient. This also involves basic paradigmatic conflict. Clinicians are also suspected of capitalising on 'supplier induced demand' whereby the affluent class of patients may be overserviced. There are also economists who, while acknowledging the gains of the past, are convinced that more medical care cannot be expected to bring about much more improvement on community health. Some even contend that more medical care might be counterproductive!

Fuch's Diagnosis

During the 1970s when cutbacks in welfare spending in the U.S. became a priority, Fuchs, an economist member of the United States' Institute of Medicine published 'Who Shall Live? Health, Economics, and Social Change' (1974). This provides a convenient summary of an economist's view of health services. Fuchs was modest in his claims and flagged his understanding of the limitations of economics when confronted by the complexity of the health system. The basic problems of health care he identified as excessive cost, limited access and unsatisfactory levels of health. Pointing to the loose connection currently between health and health care, he argued that '(in) the developed countries the marginal contribution to medical care to life expectancy is very small' (Fuchs 1974, p144). He identified the physician, the 'Captain of the Team,' as the major determinant of costs, astutely locating increased medical discretion in the face of uncertainty as a potential contributor to excessive intervention and cost. He also understood that the organization of medicine cannot be considered independently of a culture it serves, and insisted that remuneration arrangements must be seen in their social and political context. In his recommended general approach to reform, he came close to the concept of continuous quality improvement which was later developed in Japanese business, imported to the United States and extended to the case of quality assurance in medical care.

Given the interest in reform of medical education at the time, Fuchs supported the need to pay more attention to selection of students and to paying attention to the 'incentives and constraints' of medical practice. Fuchs also foresaw the rise of the generalist disciplines of primary care and general internal medicine, as opposed to training ever more specialists. Among Fuchs' practical recommendations were universal comprehensive insurance, decentralization of health care delivery, payment to physicians by capitation, competition between health plans, and relaxation of licensing restrictions. He advocated the use of 'physician extenders' working under the supervision of physicians, saw that hospital costs could be reduced by eliminating unnecessary admissions and reducing bed stay, as well as by reducing the number of beds - all measures which have become central planks in cost-containment policy. He also targeted inappropriate use of drugs and insufficient post-marketing surveillance. In a somewhat more provocative conclusion, Fuchs suggests, no doubt with tongue in cheek that 'it might be better to redistribute income and allow the poor to decide which additional goods and services they want to buy.' (Fuchs 1974). He concedes that it would be more practical, however, to redistribute services!

A feature of the New Public Health was the recognition of social policy as an important determinant of community health, a competitor with medical expenditure in this regard. This perspective is reflected in a later review from an economist's perspective (Evans and Stoddart 1990). Their systems model is based on the Lalonde 'health field framework' which conceptualizes 'well-being' as the end-product of a complex interaction of prosperity, health and function. This is determined, in turn by individual biological and behavioural response to social and physical environment, modulated by genetic endowment, diminished by disease and favourably influenced by health care. By framing the problems of health in this way, it is possible to develop a more rational approach to health policy, aiming to optimize health without the current bias towards the primacy of medical care, even of health care.

Seen from this perspective, allocation of finance to public housing might well be accorded higher priority than a community screening program of doubtful efficacy, and social support services might gain resources ahead of a new medical technology. Evans and Stoddart also made the astute observation that the perception of a crisis in the cost of health care is common to all countries despite the fact that the proportion of national income involved varies substantially. This they interpret to mean that the perception of crisis means the occurrence of conflict concerning health care expenditure when any attempt is made to place limits on it, a political concern unrelated to any consideration of community health (Evans and Stoddart 1990).

Medicine parted company with its traditional base in the humanities when it embraced science. The result is that there is a highly scientific basis for technological intervention, a well developed science of medicine, but no correspondingly humanistically refined art of medicine which has drawn academically on the knowledge base of the social sciences and humanities. Recent developments in health care can only be properly understood in historical context. Several areas of philosophy relating to ethics, knowledge and modelling of health processes have a direct bearing on current problems. It has also been strongly argued that better doctors are produced by a curriculum which includes the humanities, especially literature pertinent to the human experience in medicine, and the moral dilemmas which it throws up. It could also be argued that doctors, and especially medical students, would benefit from more medical history teaching, if only to allow reflection upon the impact of science and how recent this has been. We will not go into the debate over the place of history literature in the medical curriculum. We will discuss only ethics, that branch of philosophy which is unavoidable in the modern era.

Ethics

Not so long ago, medical ethics was the province of the individual doctor confronted by a particular clinical problem, and the professional societies concerned with codes of conduct. The ethics concerned had not changed in its essentials since Hippocrates. It was not a field for the professional philosopher. We argue that academics whose primary interest is in clinical care, clinical scholars, cannot avoid an encounter with some basic philosophical concepts. While few other health workers will take much of an interest in the more abstract reaches of philosophy, none can avoid encounters with ethics. The Hippocratic ethics which has evolved with the traditional discourse of clinical medicine have simply not proved equal to the challenges of modern medical practice and research. Doubts about heroic measures for the low birth weight or severely deformed infant, the problems of in-vitro fertilisation, of euthanasia, of abortion on demand, of the futility of intensive care for some of the terminally ill, the moral dilemmas of clinical trials, the intrusion of surveys on privacy and questions of conflicts of interest could obviously not have been anticipated. Important ethical issues, apart from those arising from medical practice include the question of distribution of scarce resources, and the related problem of possible rationing of expensive technologies, problems of distributive justice.

The paradigm of medical ethics has evolved as all paradigms do. The two basic philosophies are deontological and consequentialist ethics. The first deals with the intrinsic good or evil of an act or series of actions. The second relies on the consequences to decide whether an action is moral or not. Even the paradigm of medical ethics has been influenced by the positivist turn in the societal way of thinking. In clinical practice, the first challenge to the traditional Hippocratic ethics came from analytical philosophy, in the United States during the 1960s. This has an analytical flavor about it. As a result, there has been a backlash against the proliferation of consultants and committees, and objections to what has been called the 'engineering model' of ethics in which set rules are applied to solve complex problems, applying the mantra of respect for autonomy, justice, beneficence, and non-malificence without due regard, at times, to all of the circumstances of the particular case.

More recently there has been more attention paid to the interpretation in the individual case with full attention to the specific context, essentially taking an approach analogous to the clinical case-study, an application of casuistry similar to case law, using the general rules only as guidelines. Similarly, in research ethics, there is a move to take account of the precise circumstances of research rather than rely on abstract principles. The objective is to seek the free consensus interpretation of a group of disinterested people, including patient representatives, in a clinical care or research ethics committee. However, this is not as easy as it sounds since institutions involved in research and biomedical researchers are perceived to have too much influence - another example of the links between knowledge and power. Research ethics has also been extended to take account of the interests of those on whom research is conducted, and an ethical obligation to publish and to disseminate results.

It is important to note that an aspect of clinical thinking, important to continuous learning, is the process known as 'reflection.' It is a form of conscious rumination about cases. This should be seen as an ethical matter as well as an educational requirement (Sanders 2009). To reflect upon experience is morally essential for professionals. An excellent coverage of matters pertaining to ethics and the law has been provided by Breen et al. (2010).

Behavioural Science

A phenomenon which is behind much of the conflict within the health system during the current transitional period is the increased contribution of the human and social sciences to the debate on health. Psychology is a special case since Freudian psychology formed the foundation of medical psychiatry, and has had a strong influence on the interpretation of the medical history. For much of this century, the basic concepts have also tacitly underpinned clinical thinking about psychosomatic illness and about functional illness in general. Psychology is now well established in the medical curriculum. However, the relationship of psychology with scientific medicine has been an uneasy one because of doubts about the scientific status of clinical psychology and psychiatry which date back to the pioneering reforms of the medical curriculum early in this century.

One of the major contributions of behavioural science and 'micro' sociology has been to emphasise the individuality hence the variety of patient decisions, and the multitude of influences which impinge on them, and more recently to emphasize the role of the emotions. After all it is the patient, often assisted by a coterie of family advisors, who makes the fundamental decision of whether or not to become a patient in the first place, and illness behaviour cannot be interpreted except through an understanding of the context of a patient's unique tapestry of personal attributes, family and social milieu, cultural context, and past experience, including past history of medical encounters. The sociological perspective has the patient as an active agent, striving to make sense of the illness and its meaning in terms of likely outcome and available treatment. They too will decide whether or not to take the treatment recommended or accept the advice that none is needed, or they may decide to defect to an alternative practitioner.

Conclusion

The delivery of health care is primarily the responsibility of clinicians and public health practitioners. The research into clinical care, upon which informed reform must depend, also involves sociologist, economist and ethicist. For each of these disciplines, every interdisciplinary discussion, every choice of research design, in fact every judgement and decision, is influenced by powerful paradigmatic forces. These commitments are largely at an unconscious level, so that misunderstanding is rife, disagreement frequent and acrimony often the outcome.

Some of the practical effects of these problems we have illustrated in this chapter. For our purposes, the most important implications of paradigmatic conflict between medicine and other disciplines have been manifest in the evaluation of health care. So far, clinical doctors have played only a minor part in this evaluation but are becoming more involved. The paradigmatic tensions are therefore likely to get worse before they get better.

References

Armstrong D., Political anatomy of the Body. Cambridge University Press, Cambridge, 1983.

Breen K. J., Cordner S. M., Pluekhahn V. D., Thomson C. J. H., Good Medical Practice. Professionalism, ethics and the law. Cambridge, 2010.

Bulger R. J., Reductionist biology and population medicine - strange bed fellows or a marriage made in heaven? *JAMA*; 264:508-9; 1990.

Cochrane A. L., Effectiveness and Efficiency: Random reflections on health services. Nuffield Provincial Trust. London, 1972.

Codman E. A., The Product of the hospital. *Surgery, Gynecology and Obstetrics* 18:491-6; 1914.

Dubos R., Mirage of Health. Allen and Unwin, London, 1960.

Dubos R., Mirage of Health. Allen and Unwin, London, 1960. p. 125.

Evans R. G., Stoddart G.,. Producing health, consuming health care. *Soc Sci Med* 31:1347-63; 1990.

Foucault M., Power/Knowledge: Selected interviews and other writings 1972-1977. Gordon C ed. The Harvester Press, Sussex, 1980.

Freidson E., Medical Work in America: essays on health care. Yale University Press, New Haven, 1989, p. 77.

Fuchs V., Who Shall Live? Health, Economics, and Social Choice. Basic Books, New York, 1974, p. 144.

Fuchs V., Who Shall Live? Health, Economics, and Social Choice. Basic Books, New York, 1974.

Fuchs. V., Who Shall Live? Health, Economics, and Social Choice. Basic Books, New York, 1974, p. 149.

Habermas J., Legitimation Crisis. Polity press, Cambridge, 1976.

Hamlin C., Predisposing causes and public health in early nineteenth-century medical thought. *Soc His Med;* 50: 43-70; 1992.

Illich I., Limits to Medicine - Medical Nemesis: The expropriation of health, London, Calder and Boyars, 1974, p. 152-3.

Jewson N., The disappearance of the sick man from medical cosmology, 1770-1870. *Sociology* 10:225-44; 1976.

Last J., 'Completing the clinical picture' in general practice. *Lancet:* II: 28-31;1963.

McBride G., Rationing health care in Oregon. *BMJ* 301:355-6;1990.

McKeown T., The Role of Medicine: Dream, Mirage or Nemesis? Basil Blackwell, Oxford, 1979.

Mills C. W., The Sociological Imagination. Oxford University Press, Oxford, 1959.

Morris J. N., Uses of Epidemiology. Williams and Wilkins, Baltimore, 1957.

Morris J. N., Social inequalities in health: ten years and little further on. *Lancet* 336:491-3;1990 Nuffield Hospitals Trust, London, 1971.

Parsons, T., The Social System. Routledge and Keegan Paul, London, 1951.

Porter R., The Greatest Benefit to Mankind: a medical history of humanity from antiquity to the present. Harper Collins. London. 1997, p. 396.

Porter T. M., Trust in Numbers: The Pursuit of Objectivity in Science and Public Life. Princeton University Press, Princeton, 1995.

Rosen G., A History of Public Health. The Johns Hopkins University Press, Baltimore, 1993.

Sanders J., The use of refection in medical education. *Medical Teacher* 31: 685-695, 2009.

Waitzkin H., The Politics of Medical Encounters. How patients and doctors deal with social problems. Yale University Press, New Haven, 1991, p. 8.

White K., Healing the Schism: epidemiology, medicine, and the public's health. *Springer-Verlag,* New York, 1991.

Chapter 8

Paradigmatic Conflict in the Peripheral Zone – The Case of Alternative Medicine

Complementary medicine has been defined according the Institute of Medicine thus: 'Complementary and alternative medicine (CAM) is a broad domain of resources that encompasses health systems, modalities, and practices, and their accompanying theories and beliefs other than those intrinsic to the dominant health system of a particular society or culture in a given historical period. CAM includes such resources perceived by their users as associated with positive health outcomes..' They also pointed out that '(B)oundaries within the CAM domain or between CAM domain and the domain of the dominant system are not always sharp or fixed.

There are several cogent reasons for our reflective physicians to be well versed in the evaluation of complementary medicine. The first is that our centre's concerns paradigmatic frictions impacting on medicine of which CAM provides a valuable exemplar. Discussion of alternative medicine highlights and brings this notion of conflict between paradigms to a concrete focus, including the issues of paradigmatic power and subjugated paradigm, and it certainly constitutes a conflict for many patients in the 'Peripheral Zone' of ambulant care where the paradigms of allopathic medicine, complementary medicine and the lay paradigms are potentially all in conflict. We discuss the meaning of the term 'Peripheral Zone' fully in the next chapter. By contrast with hospital care, the 'Central Zone' of clinical care, this is in primary care practice where functional illness and somatization are so common, and where the art of medicine and the placebo effect are most in evidence.

The second reason is for teaching purposes related to the evaluation research expertise sought by reflective doctors working in the centre for the study of clinical practice. The third is that the case of complementary medicine is an area where the centre can meet the evaluation needs of government. As we have noted, perhaps the most important effect might be to oblige medicine to attend to the commonly quoted neglect of supportive care for patients, thus they might get the best of both worlds. We will next outline what the scope of the reflective physician's knowledge in this area should be.

The use of Traditional Chinese Medicine as my example of alternative medicine is because the Centre for the Study of Clinical Practice at St. Vincent's subjected it to evaluation on behalf of the Victorian Government, including conducting an analysis of their trials. I also saw it in action, and discussed procedures with local practitioners during a visit to China. That the social and scientific issues are similar for other forms of complementary medicine is confirmed by analyzing the contributions and problems under an umbrella term such as 'CAM' – complementary and alternative medicine. Western and complementary medicine do occupy different worlds in the sense of being different cultural products with different worldviews and classifications of knowledge or epistemologies, based upon a different paradigm of health care. The evidence suggests that the use of alternative medicine is on the rise. This has been thoroughly discussed by Coulter and Willis (2004). The most popular forms are chiropractic, acupuncture, homeopathy, herbal therapy and mind-body techniques. Since 75% in the U.S. have had resort to alternative medicine, and 30% of patients with cancer worldwide in the past year, to reject it out of hand would be tantamount to trivializing more than 50,000 years of history, or ignoring an elephant in the living room!

It has been shown to save money for the government but can it cure people? It is tensions between these component paradigms of medicine, public health, complementary medicine and the lay culture which is at the root of the current debate. A substantial proportion of the community who object to medical dominance of the consultation or with the outcome, decide to undertake more of their own treatment and to vote with their feet by invoking the assistance of complementary medicine. This cannot be solely a matter of ignorance since many who seek it are highly educated people. While, in some instances, patients may be desperate when medical interventions have failed, others have found that patient-centred, individualised treatment and supportive care is often better delivered by the practitioner of complementary medicine. This, of course, is an indictment of modern scientific medicine and neglect of the art. It is obviously important to understand why people choose a form of health care which is mostly without scientific foundation.

The historical break with superstition and religion in health in the West came with Hippocratic medicine in Ancient Greece, the great survivor which underpinned medicine until around 1800 when science had such a dramatic impact (Chapter 5). The classical Hippocratic paradigm was strongly reminiscent of that of Traditional Chinese Medicine, and of many other kinds of complementary medicine, with its holistic model of disease as humoral imbalance, an emphasis on empirical observation and collective experience, strong focus on the supportive care of the individual, on symptom relief, and undoubtedly in most cases for both paradigms, reliance on natural healing and the placebo effect. The paradigm of modern scientific medicine which arrived in the early 1800s was based upon vastly different beliefs from its Chinese and other alternative counterpart. The rise in the use of complementary medicine in the West could be seen as an attempt by the community to regain supportive clinical care. Moreover, current trends indicate that it may yet bear fruit by some form of merger with allopathic medicine such as 'integrative medicine' (The Royal Australian College of General Practitioners 2011).

The mood of evaluation accompanying economic rationalism has inevitably caught up with complementary medicine. Governments are about listening to community concerns but also about cost-containment. There is a widespread move towards recognition of complementary medicine. In China, at least, this was seen as a cost-effective way to provide care in the Peripheral Zone where functional symptoms and minor illness predominate. Western governments have looked to epidemiology and biostatistics to provide the tools for evaluation of health interventions with a strong emphasis on the randomised trial and cost-effectiveness analysis. Cynics, or at least the more skeptical among us, have seen the emphasis on scientific evaluation of medicine as a technological fix for political problems, and quantitative methods, sometimes as a tool for control of a profession whose judgement they see as tainted by vested interest. A paradigm being what it is, we would expect that both the aura of science and political interest would have the medical profession supporting the use of the randomised trial to evaluate complementary medicine such as traditional Chinese medicine. But is this right and is this possible? To the extent that the claim of complementary medicine is satisfaction of the individual, then this must be the logical end-point.

The application of modern analytical reductionist methods to the evaluation of a holistic approach to treatment is logically problematic, both as an exercise in scientific research and as a claim to representing an evaluation of the practice of complementary medicine. Ambulatory clinical care, in particular, calls for a supportive role which modern Western medicine stands accused of neglecting. This is most of what devotees of alternative medicine see it as providing. Unhappily, when science bestowed great benefits on patients and much status on doctors, it did so by distorting its view of care to a considerable extent. A desire to gain credibility in the eyes of Western science by placing inappropriate emphasis on the analytical quantitative approach to testing traditional herbal remedies using the clinical trial could have a distorting effect on the ethos and practice of complementary medicine, taking it too down a path of excessive reductionism. Indeed the challenge of alternative medicine has been that complementary medicine has acted as a lightning rod for discontent with modern medicine, and one of its contributions could be a rejuvenation of medicine's commitment to supportive, contextually sensitive care.

Science and the Placebo Effect

Ambulant medical care means general practice and hospital outpatients where medical specialists work. In both settings we see the clash between the art and science of medicine, and between scientific medicine and the lay paradigm of illness. The disease model of the scientific medical paradigm is often inappropriately applied - a serious problem in ambulant care. Doctors we have seen, trained under the Flexnerian curriculum in acute hospitals, especially specialists in the outpatient departments, tend to think in terms of organic disease and to be sometimes inappropriately swayed by a technological imperative. Thus the holistic idea of 'functional illness' is part of a subjugated paradigm. Such illness may be seen as seen as trivial. It is rarely discussed, seldom taught, now almost synonymous with neurosis (Jewson 1976). This narrow view of illness creates difficulties by impairing the mainstays of supportive care, disowning the 'placebo effect,' the direct impact of caring, the positive effect of the healer, and often ignoring the personal and social context of illness. The residue of the old Western tradition, 19th century clinical traditions nurtured in Britain with the accent on knowing your patient and social context, good supportive care, and prudent intervention are in full retreat in the face of U.S. trained specialists in particular (Jewson 1976).

These changes have occurred just when the population is most in need of these traditional skills, and ironically, the very success of scientific medicine has been a major reason. Thus an expansion of ambulant medical care reflects an increase in medical consultations associated with an historic decline in self-help, family care, and use of the lay healer. Patients have been drawn to the medical consultation by the successes of science, assisted by subsidisation of cost by health insurance. Many feel that complementary medicine has something to offer - but it is a subjugated paradigm like the art of medicine. Uncertainty also creates space for the social construction of illness. The scientific bent of the medical discourse is troubled by holistic illness with unclear mechanism, a concept which evolved in France as 'functional illness' of which there was no evidence at autopsy. Diagnosed by a process of exclusion following investigation, the 'living autopsy,' it is rarely discussed as such or taught in medicine, and journals use oblique terms like 'undifferentiated illness.' In any case, symptom complexes with a focus on a single organ but without a clear biomedical explanation tend to be subsumed under a presumptive biomedical mechanism. A classical case has been chronic fatigue syndrome, sometime biomedicalised as 'myalgic encephalitis,' and a prominent inhabitant of the Peripheral Zone of medical care.

What Are the Outcomes of All of This Dissonance Between Paradigms?

The Peripheral Zone of clinical care, which will discuss further in Chapter 10, comprises mainly primary care, that is general practice. An important effect of the clash of paradigms, especially in the large Peripheral Zone is an epidemiological risk whereby investigation for organic disease of low prevalence runs a high statistical risk of harmful false positive or doubtful test results. There is also a lack of awareness of personal motivations; at the same time, pervasive social factors lead to misattribution of functional symptoms hence failure to spot the role of problems of living, anxiety and depression. Both can lead to ill-advised interventions.

The risk of choice of inappropriate treatment is further increased because uncertainty associated with lack of clear diagnosis and treatment creates a discretional space into which diagnostic error can creep. In addition to the technical issues related to intervention which are often not controversial, there intrude on judgement a vast number of interacting influences such as the doctor's age and personal philosophy, medical specialty and attitudes to science, clinical experience and training, vested interests and perceived legal threat, peer or administrative pressure, as well as the patient's attributes, attitudes and beliefs and those of the family and referring doctor, all under the influence of cultural issues. Although the patient is often unaware of diagnostic errors, even inappropriate treatments, patients reject dominance of the consultation process by a scientific technical preoccupation. This is unfortunate for both parties but the story does not end there. Clearly related to lack of patient satisfaction are noncompliance, and failure to accept reassurance with patients remaining anxious or vulnerable to further doubts, and, as the doctor sees it, often as defection to alternative medicine because of unhappiness about the outcome or the consultation.

Paradigmatic Tensions in Clinical Practice – The Two Cultures Problem in Evaluation

The mood of evaluation accompanying economic rationalism has inevitably caught up with alternative medicine. Governments are listening to community concerns but are also currently fixated about cost-containment. There is a move towards recognition of complementary medicine, and in China at least, this has been seen as a cost-effective way to provide care in the Peripheral Zone. On the other hand, there is also pressure on government not to finance alternative care - because it is 'unscientific.' Western governments have looked to epidemiology and biostatistics to provide the tools for evaluation of health interventions with a strong emphasis on the randomised trial. This emphasis on science as a technofix and substitution of quantitative methods for political problems, 'trust in numbers,' as a tool for control of a profession whose judgement they see as tainted by vested interest. A paradigm being what it is, we would expect that both the aura of science and political interest would have the medical profession supporting the use of the randomised trial to evaluate complementary medicine. Is this right and is this possible?

Methodological Mismatch

So when it comes to evaluation, the same problem of tension between discourses has emerged as that which is causing conflict within the medical discourse, and between it and complementary medicine. The evaluation process itself is hostile to complementary medicine because of the Two Cultures Problem, the lack of mutual understanding between those trained in science and those grounded in the humanities which Snow highlighted in the 1960s (1964). Science, emphasising control and statistical analysis, sees the randomized controlled trial as the only way to evaluate complementary medicine. A humanistic approach would argue that interview with patients indicates that - surprise, surprise - that those who opt for alternative medicine are generally satisfied with their choice - surely the outcome that matters! Both schools of thought are right. To the extent that the claim of complementary medicine is satisfaction of the individual, then this is the end-point which can and should be measured by interview and survey. The randomised trial which deliberately excludes the placebo effect on which the outcome of alternative therapy may depend, measures outcomes related to imputed mechanism and delivers standardized care when individualised treatment may be more appropriate.

To apply the Western analytical method of the clinical trial to the evaluation of an aspect of Traditional Chinese Medicine exposes a mismatch inherent in the intellectual paradigms of two cultures. Evaluation of a healing practice must first and foremost provide a personal service to an individual consumer by achieving relief of symptoms. If the objective is different, for example to trawl the Chinese pharmacopoeia for new wonder drugs, to tap into a source of pharmacologically effective, standardisable potentially commercial treatments, then randomised trials are appropriate, unavoidable but a daunting undertaking. In addition, if the practitioner of alternative medicine makes claims about cure or specific effects related to palliation, there are issues involved of public health related to safety and effectiveness, and of public interest related to honesty and fair trade. It is quite legitimate then to insist on trials to deliver scientifically acceptable answers. There has been debate over the place of the randomized controlled trial in the armamentarium of health services research, but none concerning their central place in the process of testing drugs for efficacy and toxicity. If the claim is about mechanism, the physiological laboratory has its skills to offer.

To point to the limitations of trials is not, therefore, intended to denigrate a worthwhile and necessary scientific enterprise. It is simply a statement that the application of modern analytical reductionist methods to the evaluation of a holistic approach to treatment is usually inappropriate, both as an exercise in scientific research and as a claim to representing an evaluation of the practice of Traditional Chinese Medicine. Ambulatory clinical care, in particular, calls for a supportive role which modern Western medicine stands accused of neglecting. When science bestowed great benefits on patients and much status on doctors, it did so by distorting its view of care to a considerable extent. A desire to gain credibility in the eyes of Western science by placing emphasis on the analytical quantitative approach to testing traditional herbal remedies using the clinical trial could have a distorting effect on the ethos and practice of Traditional Chinese Medicine, which has a holistic orientation.

Nevertheless, once the decision has been made to embark upon trials, they must be of high quality if clear answers are to be obtained. Lessons learned by bitter experience in the West about the need to be paranoid about all potential sources of bias should be heeded. In particular, double blinding, when feasible, is absolutely essential. My review of trials of Traditional Chinese Medicine revealed that very few rigorous trials had been conducted. In fact, indirect evidence indicated that many were not, in fact truly randomized. In fact, the Chinese symbols used for allocation into treatment and control groups, 'sui ji' had been translated 'as they come,' presumably meaning patients unselected in a broad sense but not randomly allocated to treatment and control groups.

The Rigour of the Randomized Controlled Trial - The Issue of Validity

The modern RCT has an exceptionally rigorous structure - but no more rigorous than it needs to be in order to yield valid and credible results in the face of chance events and the pervasive susceptibility to bias to which all human agents are prone. Its current form has been cast in the crucible of constant criticism, moulded by the pressures of claim and counter claim over trial results. What has emerged above all else has been the frailty of the human experimenter in avoiding unconscious bias, in a setting where there seems to offer an almost unlimited opportunity for error. A preoccupation with those biases related to patient response and experimental observation is simply a legacy of the many mistakes recognized in past trials. The credibility of the result of a clinical trial in the scientific community therefore depends on the quality of the design features which purport to adjust for chance occurrences, to avoid known experimental biases, and to exclude both the natural process of recovery from illness, and the effects of healer, of intervention, and context of care as contributors to clinical improvement. The study is ultimately credible to the extent that these unwanted effects can be seen to have been effectively excluded. In addition the clinician consumers of research results have another important concern - they must know the degree to which the results can reasonably be generalized to the treatment of their own patients. To allow this is also a requirement of good trial design.

The Challenge to the Randomized Trial – Locating the Active Agent

Before mounting a trial or when interpreting the result for scientific or commercial purposes, it is usually important that a putative active agent be identified. In a herbal concoction, there are multiple ingredients, and the composition is not uniform from the point of view of the character of each ingredient and the formula for each patient. Each ingredient has multiple constituents which can interact with each other in a reinforcing or inhibitory way, according to the factorial mathematics of combinatorial probability. The potential therapeutic or toxic effects which could arise from innumerable such interactions are a scientific nightmare for the evaluator. The problems confronting a scientific, reductionist approach to controlling this degree of complexity are formidable indeed.

These nuances of study design represent an evolutionary response to an environment of constant professional criticism and the public demand for proof of effectiveness and assurance of safety of drugs in general. Indeed, the rise of clinical epidemiology and of 'evidence-based medicine' can be seen as responses to this demand. However, at present, only relatively few centres in the West can meet the exacting standards required for validity. By the same token, if the practitioners of Traditional Chinese Medicine claim therapeutic effectiveness in terms of disease mechanism rather than a placebo response, and they should put these claims to the test of a trial, then such trials will inevitably be subjected to same critical scrutiny to which Western trials are subjected. Their credibility in this area will therefore stand or fall by these standards of Western technical rationality and science.

Outcome

The outcome of a trial is usually judged by an impact on a single variable, generally on group morbidity or mortality. To evaluate a symptomatic response is difficult and to allow for patient priorities even harder. This poses a problem if a herbal treatment is claimed to be tailored for the treatment of the individual. The requirement that treatment must be individualised could be met using a methodological device known as the N-of-1 trial design. A medication is administered to an individual patient in a randomized way, using clinical symptoms to test response (Guyatt et al. 1986). We applied, as a compromise, less stringent check list for the rigour of trials of Traditional Chinese Medicine. Major problems were lack of randomisation and blinding, keystones of a valid study design. Blinding of trial participants is necessary to prevent unconscious bias. The reason for this apparently paranoid approach is that the most conscientious of observers have been deceived by their own biases, patients have sometimes gone to extreme lengths to break the randomisation code, and unblinding has occurred by the most subtle of mechanisms. However, blinding was rarely mentioned for the alternative treatment even for subjective clinical outcome measures.

The other major problem was that although 'randomization' was specified in many studies, the numbers in the treatment and control groups strongly suggest that, in many if not most cases, this did not mean allocation to treatment group by lot, that is according to the operation of chance alone. As we have seen, randomisation was rendered by the word 'sui ji' in the text which was translated by the Chinese reviewer as 'randomized.' In no case, however, was a method of random allocation actually described. There is no reason at all to suggest that patients were allocated to groups in a deliberately biased way. Rather, patients were 'taken as they came' or 'according to opportunity' - for example, allocation of alternate patients - which can be subject to bias. This does not automatically invalidate their results but it does substantially increase the risk of bias. And there were other problems. Statistical analysis was rudimentary. Negative trial results were very uncommon in my review which raises the spectre of publication bias. It is also worth noting that I applied a much more stringent set of criteria for trials conducted in the West.

Western and Alternative Medicine in the Postmodern World

In the future, I suspect that it will be a case of 'render to Caesar the things that are Caesar's and to God the things that are God's.' Not negotiable to our current way of thinking are free patient choice, with the proviso that it is optimally informed, that is with protection against toxic products, deception and fraud. With a great deal of hard work, it will gradually become apparent to all which treatments work predominantly through some specific effect like a Western drug, or through the placebo effect like most of the treatments of Traditional Chinese Medicine, and to what extent the placebo effect itself represents is an impact on identifiable physiological processes or simply some kind of halo effect on the feelings of the ill. 'Although heterogeneous, the many CAM treatments, include individualizing the treatment, treating the whole person, promoting self-care and self-healing, and recognizing the spiritual nature of each individual.' (White House Commission on Complementary and Alternative Medicine Policy 2002). It would be unfortunate if allopathic and alternative continued on a collision course, and if any chance of mutually advantageous rapprochement were to be lost.

Conclusion

What complementary medicine has certainly done is to act as conduit for discontent with an excessively technically oriented medicine, reminding us that thousands, of years of empirical human experience should not be arrogantly dismissed. What we hope, of course, is that postmodern medicine will come in from the cold, as it were, to become a syncretic product of rejuvenated contextual supportive care, such as is provided by alternative medicine but refined by the benefits of science, social science and the humanities. This could be achieved by some form of 'integrative medicine' which is practised by some orthodox as well as by alternative practitioners. Should this trend become stronger, alternative medicine in such a form could provide just the kind of therapy that many patients are seeking for the problematic Peripheral Zone of medical care, in the form of holistic and contextual care as a supplement to orthodox allopathic medicine.

References

Bensoussan A., Myers S. P., Towards a Safer Choice: the practice of traditional Chinese medicine in Australia. Faculty of Health, University of Western Sydney Macarthur, 1996.

Board of health promotion and disease prevention of the Institute of Medicine (2005), Complementary and Alternative Medicine in the United States. National Academies Press.

Conrad L. I., Neve M., Nutton V., Porter R., Wear A. Eds., The Western Medical Tradition 800 BC to 1800 AD. Cambridge University Press, Cambridge, 1995.

Coulter I. D., Willis E. M., The rise and rise of alternative medicine. *Med J Aust* 180; 587-89; 2004.

Foucault M., The Birth of the Clinic: an archaeology of medical perception. Tavistock, London, 1976.

Guba E. G., Lincoln Y. S., Fourth Generation Evaluation. Newbury Park Sage, 1989, p. 35.

Gutting G, Michel Foucault's Archaeology of Scientific Reason. Cambridge University Press, Cambridge.

Guyatt G., Sackett D., Taylor W., Chang J., Roberts R. Pugsley S.,Determining optimal therapy - randomised trials in individual patents. *New Eng J Med* 314: 889-92:1986.

Haynes B., Can it work? Does it work? Is it worth it?: the testing of health care interventions is evolving. *BMJ:* 319: 652-3;1999.

Jewson N., The disappearance of the sick man from medical cosmology, 1770-1870. *Sociology* 10:225-44; 1976.

Kuhn T., The Structure of Scientific Revolutions. University of Chicago Press, Chicago, 1970.

Lindblom C. E., The science of muddling through. *Public Administration Review* 19:79-88. 1968.

McDonald I. G., Information technology as a challenge to evaluation: a blessing in disguise? Telehealth International (in press).

Porter T. M., Trust in Numbers: The pursuit of objectivity in science and public life. Princeton University Press, Princeton, 1995.

Rittel H., Systems analysis of the 'first and second generations.' In Laconte P, Gibson, J, Rapoport A eds. Human Energy Factors in Urban Planning. NATO Advanced Study institutes Series D. Behavioural and Social Sciences No. 12, Martinus Nijhoff, The Hague, 1982, 35-63.

The Royal Australian College of General Practitioners., Curriculum for Australian General Practice 2011 Integrative medicine. The RACGP Curriculum for Australian General Practice 2011.

Snow C., The Two Cultures and A Second Look: an expanded version of the two cultures and the scientific revolution. Cambridge University Press, 1964.

White House Commission on Complementary and Alternative Medicine Policy., Final Report, 2002.

Chapter 9

Clinical Inefficiency

We devote this chapter to the basic problem of clinical inefficiency, a major contributor to the fire which has generated the pall of smoke over medicine in the latter part of the 20th century and beginning of the 21st. We emphasise how faulty clinical decisions can both impair the quality and inflate the cost of clinical care. These are problems which primarily afflict the science of medicine by influencing decisions about technological intervention. Recourse to empirical scientific and statistical thinking accessed mainly through epidemiology already offers hope of major improvements in clinical decision-making in this area. The social component, the traditional doctor-patient relationship, comprises communication with the objective of achieving mutual understanding of the illness, counsel, and the supportive or Samaritan offerings of empathy and sympathy. In practice, these two components tend to interact with each other. There are many points in the diagnostic process where things can go wrong, where mistakes and misjudgements can lead to error and misunderstanding, iatrogenic harm and dissatisfaction, inefficient management and unwarranted expense.

Definition

We therefore define 'clinical inefficiency' as clinical error or inappropriate diagnostic or therapeutic intervention which increases the risk of patient harm or of reduced treatment benefit. Clinical inefficiency, comprising physician errors, inappropriate intervention and adverse events, is also the real culprit in the escalating cost of health care. These matters we consider in this chapter. We define 'consultation failure' as patient dissatisfaction resulting from problems of communication or inadequate supportive care, lack of cooperation with medical management plans, or abandonment of medical care for self help or alternative medicine. Consultation failure we discuss in the next two chapters.

Our conception of clinical inefficiency rests on a basic notion derived from mechanics. The efficiency of an engine is limited by the sum total of the energy losses in the system. Similarly, the limits to the efficiency of a clinical consultation are set by the sum total of errors and misunderstandings at all points of the system. According to our definition, 'clinical inefficiency' is the collective effect of physician error and misjudgement on technological care which is what ultimately sets the upper limit of its quality. Clinical inefficiency obviously interacts with problems of communication and inadequate support defined as consultation failure, the subject of the next chapter. The technical, the personal and the social variables are inseparable in the complex dynamics of the clinical consultation. Many doctors sincerely believe that they work as applied scientists like engineers, bringing scientific knowledge and technical training to bear in an objective manner on the problems of their patients. To some extent this is so, but they are generally unaware of the extent to which non-technical issues intrude. These issues are integral to sound judgement in the individual but are also a potent source of misjudgement and error hence a basis for inefficient practice.

Few patients would be aware of the way in which these non-technical issues affect the planning of their management and quality of their care. Errors which are the consequence of technical mistake or inappropriate personal or social influence will result in errors of diagnosis, prognosis and choice of interventions. Technical uncertainty has, of course, become greater as the complexity of biomedical, technical and scientific knowledge has burgeoned with fragmentation, specialisation and demands for high precision of diagnosis for sophisticated but potentially hazardous therapies. Many sources of error have been identified in the clinical transaction but empirical studies of their actual impact on patient care have been few. Such errors may be demonstrated in various parts of the process of diagnosis or management, or may become evident as suboptimal care processes of care detected by clinical audit, as inappropriate interventions, as unjustifiable variations in clinical care or as adverse events.

Technical Error

Errors may be called cognitive if they involve the physician's basic, largely unconscious, problem-solving activity. They are procedural if they pertain to the specific techniques which have evolved for the of collection and interpretation of clinical information, including the clinical assessment, the ordering, performance and interpretation of diagnostic tests and of acquisition and interpretation of data from the medical literature. Among the least blameworthy of clinical errors pertain to the nature of human reasoning itself. Such cognitive errors abound in everyday life and in professional practice (Kahneman et al. 1982).

Problems with the handling of probability are common and important. For instance, the clinician may place too much weight on evidence which is readily recalled, on diseases recently encountered, and on the significance of evidence already to hand. Clinicians have also been shown to sometimes fail to adjust disease probabilities adequately in the light of new evidence, and to take more notice of data which confirms rather than conflicts with existing beliefs. They may also have a tendency to premature closure, that is to accept a diagnosis while there is still adequate evidence, or fail to consider the possibility that an unusual event was, in fact, a fluke unlikely to be repeated because of the statistical phenomenon of regression to the mean. Misconceptions of chance are common such as the occurrence of a random event by chance may be inflated by failure to appreciate independence of outcomes in say a coin tossing sequence, individuals frequently fail to appreciate the role of sample size when thinking in probability terms, anchoring as when individuals make estimates based upon an initial value and make insufficient adjustments when establishing a final value, individuals tend to seek confirmatory information for what they think is true and fail to search for conflicting evidence. They may fall victim to hindsight bias or have a tendency to overconfidence. Some sources of error may be unconscious and much related to emotional factors, such as disappointment effects, illusion of control, chagrin effects, status quo-bias, and reaction to 'sunk costs.' This kind of behaviour has been elicited for the most part in studies of experts other than doctors and under laboratory conditions, however experience suggests that such problems do occur in medical practice!

Procedural errors involve the process of collection and interpretation of clinical information from the examination and use of diagnostic tests leading up to the planning of management. All methods of gathering and interpreting information are subject to human foible, and diagnosis is no exception. Some are systematic errors, that is, biases; others involve the vagaries of chance. These errors may be the result of inexperience, of lack of specific knowledge, of or working with misleading information. Murphy's law applies. Procedural errors can occur at all stages of diagnosis involving the clinical history, examination and ordering of tests, diagnosis and setting of therapeutic objectives. For example, the clinician may make errors in taking the history, performing the physical examination, obtaining information from the medical literature and interpreting it (Koran and Koran 1975). In the case of a test, errors range through inappropriate selection of the test for the patient's problem, misinterpretation of artefact, interpretation inappropriately biased by clinical knowledge, or a mistaken reading of the test result by the clinician looking after the patient. Errors may interact, one with the other. Thus, in a patient with chest pain, careless history-taking, misinterpretation of an exercise electrocardiogram and failure to detect a social problem might lead to the false diagnosis of angina when anxiety is the correct answer.

The risk of error, being a matter of statistics, increases almost in direct proportion to the number of tests a patient has done. After 20 tests, on the grounds of chance alone, approximately two-thirds of patients who are normal will have returned at least one false positive test result. So a normal person has been defined as someone who hasn't had enough tests yet! Doubtful results also often cause apprehension. For every false test result, there will be many more which are doubtful. The risk of error also depends very much on the context, more specifically on disease prevalence. Breast cancer, however important, is nevertheless an uncommon cause of a lump in the breast. Hence a positive result for a mammogram performed in a community screening program is perhaps ten times more likely to be false than true. Conversely, if an older male has chest pain with clinical features suggesting angina and an exercise stress test is negative, this is likely to be a potentially misleading false negative result. A curious feature of the medical paradigm is that clinicians have only recently shown any interest in clinical errors. This could be seen as a self-protective mechanism.

A clear clash between the art of medicine, the residue of the ancient classical paradigm of medicine, and the modern scientific paradigm is seen in the evidence that clinicians use for their judgements. Traditionally, clinicians have drawn on their personal experience, sometimes from collective experience from working with colleagues, and attending clinical conferences. This experience is interpreted against a background of generally accepted knowledge obtained from meetings, and found in textbooks and reviews in the medical literature which, until recently, comprised mainly case-reports. Clinical experience alone is not enough to ensure sound decisions. A strong case has been made for greater reliance on accessible data from rigorous, clinically appraised studies in the medical literature. This is the basis of evidence-based medicine (Chapter 15).

Further evidence of the clash of art and science is that the accuracy of the most basic of all clinical information, the symptoms and other narrative data obtained from the clinical interview and of clinical signs elicited by the clinical examination of patients, have yet to be comprehensively studied some 200 years after the beginnings of scientific medicine. Louis pointed to the need early in the 19th century, and Feinstein documented the magnitude of the problem in the 1960s – some 150 years later - but to little effect. Different observers may obtain different evidence, interpret it differently or reach different conclusions after they have synthesised the data. Despite the paucity of studies, evidence of serious disagreement between clinicians has been documented with regard to the interpretation of bread-and-butter symptoms, physical signs and results of investigation commonly used for diagnosis (Koran and Koran 1975). Added to all of this uncertainty is the fact that the accuracy of most clinical symptoms and signs have not been evaluated at all, most diagnostic tests have never been adequately assessed, and what information is available on choice of treatment is confined to efficacy data, the effectiveness of intervention under ideal circumstances not including important 'soft data' such as failure of reassurance, and not at all representative of local day-to-day clinical practice. In these instances, the art of medicine has quite inappropriately resisted the legitimate inroads of the science.

Psychosocial Influences

The combined effect of the residual classical paradigm, the clinical art, and of the modern scientific paradigm is to largely conceal the operation of other important psychosocial influences on clinical judgement. Doctors tend to imagine that decisions regarding choice of interventions are made solely on scientific and rational technical grounds. That this is not the case can be seen from a moment's reflection. All clinicians occasionally use a diagnostic test to reassure a dubious patient or to comply with the expectations of a referring doctor. The decision to operate on a patient with obscure and troublesome symptoms may be influenced by family pressure. In addition, there are often emotional influences which may be inappropriate. This is arguably the main reason that doctors are commonly advised not to treat their own families. Governments believe that inducements to overservicing are inherent in fee-for-service reimbursement. These psychosocial factors involve personal beliefs and attitudes of a doctor or of a patient, as well as social and cultural pressures. It is worth noting here that the contribution of these psychosocial factors is amplified by uncertainty which opens a discretional space for doctor and patient. They are therefore of great importance in ambulant care which is such a large part of clinical practice. In Chapter 14, we will take note of the emotions of both doctor and patient which have long been neglected despite rather obvious evidence of their importance since can greatly influence a decision.

A doctor's decisions may be influenced by such basic traits as optimism or pessimism, nihilist or interventionist tendencies, beliefs about and attitudes to patients as people, to medicine, to science or to technology. A doctor may also respond to personal interests such as the need for diagnostic confidence in the face of uncertainty, or such vested interests as personal reputation, financial gain or legal protection. A doctor should be responsive to patient wishes and values, and may be influenced by their personal relationship. Finally we call 'paradigmatic'- any influence which invokes the basic traditions or collective wisdom of the medical community. As we have seen these as especially important because, deeply imbedded tacit influences as a result of medical socialization, they potentially involve all clinical decisions, hence, like all tacit beliefs and comitments, are manifest largely without conscious thought. Science has also brought scepticism concerning the reliability of the patient's account of illness, to which clinicians have responded by a tending to favour the more 'objective' test findings over those of the clinical examination.

There is no doubt about the importance of psychological and social factors on doctors' decisions, although they have been little studied in clinical practice. It is a matter of common observation that some doctors are 'doers' while others, thought of as 'thinkers,' are more reflective about their actions. Some clinicians are aggressive, others more circumspect. Some are gullible in the face of new evidence particularly in the best journals; others maintain a more skeptical attitude. Other pervasive attitudes, easy to observe in practice but difficult to prove, are captured by the common aphorisms: 'better to be sure than sorry,' 'leave no stone unturned' and 'a stitch in time saves nine.' Such attitudes are reinforced by the inevitable regret or chagrin over an opportunity missed. Of the individual characteristics related to decision-making, among the more obvious are the clinician's speciality. Clinicians also have a personal practice style. Individual personality traits of the physician also affect patterns of utilization of resources and innovation (Eisenberg and Kleinman 1986). Thus some physicians pursue a suspected abnormality by follow-up and repeated investigations while others tend to shoulder the doubt in the interests of protecting the patient from anxiety.

There is some support for the widespread belief that physicians are more inclined towards medicine and surgeons towards surgery (Wennberg, 1982), a bias which is undoubtedly complex in origin but not too hard to understand - 'to the hammer, all things look like a nail.' Surgeons can also be identified by their routines of practice known as 'surgical signatures.' The specialist also depends for continuing referral of patients on the capacity to deliver specific services, surely a disincentive to a conservative attitude to intervention. Time since graduation, place of training and influence of the chief of service have also been found to correlate with the tendency to order more or less tests. An important and pervasive influence widely acknowledged but difficult to prove is cultural difference between countries. In general, British physicians are regarded as more cautious and pragmatic. U.S. clinicians, on the other hand, are regarded as more aggressive and more oriented towards both laboratory investigation and surgical intervention.

The Two Paradigms and the 'Thorough' Doctor

A prime example of the paradigmatic clash of art versus science is when a mistaken idea of 'thoroughness' leads to excessive hence inappropriate intervention. Thus doctors are seen by some as excessively concerned with the 'technological fix' as opposed to the social exploration of clinical problems, with the pursuit of diagnosis as an end in itself (the 'diagnostic imperative'), and with intervention rather than prudent observation (the 'therapeutic imperative'). It should be kept in mind that aggressive intervention was also an outstanding characteristic of medicine in the immediate premodern era before such technology had appeared. The view that intervention is preferred to prudent 'watchful expectancy' was nicely encapsulated in whimsical form by the clinician who confronted his residents with: 'Don't just do something, stand there!' (Jonsen 1987). A narrow view of 'scientific objectivity' can lead to downgrading of important 'soft data' from the clinical assessment and to neglect of the social transaction. Thus detailed and authentic information obtained by interview of doctors or patients may be dismissed as 'subjective.'

The rationale of favouring action over inaction is, of course, easier to explain to a concerned patient or family than is that of 'masterly inactivity' - especially in the event of failure - 'at least we tried'! In medicine, blame is more likely to attach to a sin of omission, a problem of neglect, than it is to positive action which goes awry when there is always the rationalisation of bad luck or refractory case, unfortunate side-effect or accident. In cases of doubt, confronted by a patient with equivocal or obscure symptoms, the therapeutic imperative may be bolstered by pressure from patient, family and referring doctor. This is particularly so if an investigation has demonstrated pathology even though the pathology may not be the cause of the symptoms. Thus there might be pressure sooner or later to remove or dissolve the gallstones found incidentally by an ultrasound test, even when the abdominal discomfort is much more likely the product of anxiety responsible for the 'irritable bowel syndrome.'

The best known demonstration of the therapeutic imperative in clinical medicine was a study of New York schoolchildren (Glover 1934). Following 3 successive clinical opinions following which those rejected for operation were re-presented to another doctor, tonsillectomy was recommended for all but 65 of the total of 1000 unselected children! This bias towards action is not confined to surgery or high technology. The tendency to favour 'the technological fix' can be linked to the excessive prescription of drugs, the focus of many primary care consultations. It applies too to the excessive ordering of diagnostic tests – 'the currency of the out-patients department' (Jennet 1982), and to the vogue for intervention in the asymptomatic in the form of screening and routine 'health checks' following the 2nd World War. This reflected the simple appeal of 'a stitch in time saves nine' logic, perhaps encouraged by the inappropriate mechanical model of the body projected by biomedical science and the superficial analogy with regular servicing of one's car.

The 'technological imperative' has often been related to the death-defying use of intensive care in the terminally ill elderly patient when ensuring the patient's comfort and relief from pain should be the prime consideration - so-called 'futile' intervention. Specialists in internal medicine may deviate from Hippocrates' dictum 'primum non nocere' when they imprudently use powerful diuretics to clear fluid accumulation in a patient's lungs following a heart attack, when a period of bed rest would achieve the same result physiologically, gently and more safety. Similarly, wisdom does not always prevail when excessive use is made of a tube in the heart (Swan Ganz flow guided catheter) to monitor progress in terms of pressures and blood flow in the seriously ill. Close clinical observation with a watch on the charts for trends in blood pressure, pulse rate, respiratory rate, venous pressure and urine flow may often be a safe and more satisfactory alternative to the passage of a monitoring catheter into the heart. In a hospital setting, in particular, it takes more self-confidence and some effort of will to withhold intensive treatment in the face of pressure and threat of criticism, than it does to intervene. A physician is much more likely to be criticised or sued for not ordering a test should something be missed. Accolades for prudent parsimony are rare. Small wonder then that doctors tend to err on the safe side. Unfortunately there is a vicious circle involved. Doctors who constantly rely on tests may suffer atrophy of clinical skills and erosion of their confidence, so that they become even less willing to back their clinical judgement.

An unwarranted stress on diagnosis, the 'diagnostic imperative' is an important example of a paradigmatic influence on clinical judgement. Given that diagnosis was all the physician had to offer until the advent of effective treatment in this century, it is perhaps not surprising that specialists in internal medicine place undue stress on diagnosis. Traditional medicine before the impact of science placed much stress on diagnosis as a guide to prognosis. The reduction of uncertainty by clarification of prognosis and failure to confirm malignancy, tuberculosis or syphilis in the past was undoubtedly reassuring. Moreover techniques of clinical examination designed to detect external evidence of disease, and diagnostic tests to probe the interior became available in the 19th century well before there was much in way of effective treatment, enhancing this fascination with diagnosis. There are still vestiges of this attitude in the sense that doctors tend to have a cavalier attitude to ordering diagnostic tests. This must have contributed to the tendency to view diagnosis as an end in itself rather than as 'a staging post on the way to treatment.' In fact, clinicians sometimes even fail to take note the results of tests which they had previously ordered. Another piece of evidence for this is that diagnostic tests have almost never been evaluated beyond measuring their accuracy. Few studies have even analysed the impact of a test result on patient management, especially an impact on patient anxiety even when this is the primary reason for ordering the test! No studies have been made of the impact of a doubtful or false positive result.

Is This Test Appropriate? – Well Sort of!

Most tests ordered in practice are generally related to the clinical problem at hand, and, in this sense, broadly appropriate. Thus an electrocardiogram is linked almost reflexly to the general objective of diagnosing a heart problem; the much more specific question as to whether clinical care would be enhanced and whether this patient would benefit or even be harmed by this electrocardiogam now is rarely asked. This loose connection between clinical problem and use of tests effectively conceals the problem of comprehensive overuse - the use of the test does not seem to be unreasonable but could have been avoided with a little critical thought. A study of the use of echocardiography, (ultrasonic imaging of the heart) concluded that two-thirds of the tests ordered could have been avoided in this way (McDonald et al. 1986). This is not to play down the clinical value of the test in selected patients. However, the fact is that medical teaching has not in the past insisted that students make the crucial link between the anticipated result of a test and the plan of clinical management.

Thus, while few tests ordered in clinical care can be branded as totally unnecessary, it is likely that only a fraction of the tests ordered in practice are actually necessary for patient care in the sense that we could possibly conceive that failure to perform them would have been likely to have had an adverse effect on treatment and on patient health. The science is inimical to the art when psychological harm and adverse social consequences follow a false positive, false negative or doubtful test result. A mistaken diagnosis of disease, even a doubtful test result can play havoc with peace of mind, creating anxiety and related iatrogenic illness, putting employment at risk, jeopardising insurance coverage. And this can be a life sentence.

Personal and Social Influences

Also important is the influence of peers and the opinions of colleagues who refer patients, and a test is performed in the interests of maintaining the referral network. A specialist is concerned to follow reasonable wishes for investigation or intervention, explicitly expressed or thought to be implicit - the 'your wish is my command' reaction. Similarly, in a competitive atmosphere, a specialist may use investigations as part of an aura of having ready access to the accoutrements of sophisticated diagnosis. It is common knowledge that an important contributor to excessive use of investigations in the teaching hospital setting is the 'hail to the chief' phenomenon - investigations are ordered by the resident doctor in case the senior clinician should ask for their results during a ward round.

There is overwhelming evidence that clinicians are responsive to financial incentives, as most of us are. There is evidence that physicians seek to reach a target income (Eisenberg and Kleinman 1986). Evidence supporting the influence of remuneration on practice pattern has also been obtained in situations when physicians' fees have been reduced when there have been what appear to be an increase in the volume of services provided or in the way these services are labelled or delivered (Eisenberg and Kleinman 1986). Evidence of response to financial incentives in no way implies that doctors are acting dishonestly. Most would accept that few doctors would order tests much less operate on a patient purely for personal gain.

Nevertheless, the influence can be much more subtle than this, operating when the likelihood of clinical benefit is marginal and when management is largely at the doctor's discretion. This is also when the risk is lowest. It is under these circumstances that subliminal incentives may become manifest as a form of bias. A special case of vested interest is the fear of being sued. Fear of litigation is therefore an understandable motivation for ordering additional investigations, and may influence the decision whether or not to operate. Although it is generally agreed that the spectre of litigation has promoted defensive medicine in the United States, the- extent of this phenomenon is not known. A well documented early observation was the difficulty in reducing the number of skull X-rays in the case of head injury even after a search had clearly shown this to be unjustified as a routine.

Patient characteristics including social class, age, sex, income, physical appearance and ethnic background have also been related to physician behaviour and decision-making (Eisenberg 1986). Social class may influence not only care but also diagnosis. Thus patients from lower social classes are more likely to be treated for organic disease than to receive psychotherapy when the problem is psychological. It has been suggested that women's complaints are more likely to be labelled as psychogenic, and the problem of gender bias in intervention is under scrutiny at the present. A patient's general appearance can influence management and doctors may make value judgements concerning societal worth (Schwartz and Griffin 1986). Differences have also been observed in the treatment of 'problem' and 'good' patients. Doctors also tend to be judgemental about noncompliant patients without exploring contextual factors which are important in determining adherence to treatment or advice (Schwartz and Griffin 1986). Controversy erupted in Britain with regard to a doctor's right to exercise a value judgment by refusing coronary surgery to a heavy smoker who subsequently died.

There are also professional pressures to which doctors respond. Professional leadership is certainly important in establishing patterns of drug prescription, setting patterns of surgery, use of diagnostic tests and particularly acceptance of innovation and new technology (Eisenberg 1986). In fact, attempts to change practice behaviour by introducing clinical guidelines will fail if they do not understand the importance of the clinical context and role of local opinion leaders.

Having explored the potentially large number of sources of error which can contribute to faulty clinical decisions, we now seek more direct evidence of their major effects. What other evidence is there which suggests that clinical practice is currently inefficient? We next consider direct evidence of inefficient practice, unexplained variations in practice and adverse events documented in hospital practice.

Direct Evidence of Inefficient Practice

Given the social sensitivity of the clinical consultation, the reluctance we all have to being graded, the opposition of doctors to external scrutiny, and the limited access accorded to health services researchers in the clinical field, it is hardly surprising that comprehensive studies of the quality of clinical practice in a real world setting have been thin on the ground. Surveys of practitioners conducted in ambulant care practice and the use of simulated case histories (Williamson 1965) have revealed inadequate collection of data, inadequate physical examinations, missing important problems, excessive prescription of drugs, neglect of preventive counselling and discussion of screening, failure to monitor abnormality (e.g., raised blood sugar) or progress of drug treatment (heart failure), failure to order tests and to note abnormal results among those ordered, and less than optimal treatment.

Direct studies have been few. What has been done is not at all reassuring. A pioneering study in the 1950s studied the quality of care in a university hospital outpatient department, employing surveys to monitor the recording of data and performance of health screening (Huntley et al. 1961). Many deficiencies were exposed. This was, at the time, a controversial step. Today it would be accepted as scientific clinical audit, now accepted as part of quality assurance activities. We now focus on less direct evidence of clinical inefficiency. This includes evidence of inappropriate use of specific technologies, unexplained variations in clinical practice to which inappropriate care is suspected to contribute, and documentation of adverse events in hospital practice.

Inappropriate Use

An intervention was appropriate for a given indication 'when the expected health benefit (i.e., increased life expectancy, relief of pain, reduction in anxiety, increased functional capacity - not necessarily in order of importance) exceeded the expected negative consequences (i.e., mortality, morbidity, anxiety of anticipating the procedure, time lost from work) by a sufficiently wide margin that the procedure was worth doing.' (Brook et al. 1987). An inappropriate intervention is the result of a treatment choice based on a faulty clinical judgement. Because inappropriate use of technologies is rarely obvious, and because such data is not collected routinely, elaborate methods were developed by the RAND Corporation to get this information from retrospective review of patient records. A formal method of expert professional consensus employing powerful statistics was used to generate a comprehensive list of 'legitimate' or 'approved' clinical indications. Trained non-medical reviewers then categorised the appropriateness of use of the intervention from the medical records of individual patients. A high proportion of cases were classified as 'uncertain.' Similar results were obtained for important procedures including coronary angiography, coronary artery bypass grafting, pacemaker insertions, carotid artery bypass surgery and upper gastrointestinal endoscopy.

Inappropriate use of a technology may stem from inability to critically evaluate the medical literature. Alternatively the ignorance often means lack of information concerning the pros and cons of a particular technology which reflects a lack of adequate evaluation or of dissemination of results. An inappropriate decision to intervene may be a marker for the operation of perverse incentives for use, errors of interpretation of patient values, lack of appreciation of relevant social context commonly coupled with failure to elicit the preferences of a reasonably informed patient, or the operation of undesirable social motivations such as self-referral or defensive medicine.

Mistakes in patient selection are inevitable if the extremely common distinction between organic disease and functional symptoms is not performed well. For example, if a patient with chest pain in association with anxiety over unemployment believes the pain to be angina, if the doctor's interview is superficial and misses atypical features, and if fee-for-service rewards intervention, then coronary angiography is likely to be undertaken. A lesion of doubtful significance, in turn, may then lead to inappropriate angioplasty. It is important for researchers to note that if the clinician describes the patient's pain as 'angina,' a subsequent review of the hospital chart will not usually lead to the slightest suspicion that an error with serious consequences has occurred.

Unfortunately, retrospective chart review and application of consensus criteria is a very blunt instrument. Despite the enormous effort and great expense involved it is, to say the least, highly questionable that information obtained from the medical record is sufficiently valid or detailed for the purpose of analysing appropriateness of clinical decisions. To get at the truth both patient and physician would need to be interviewed to allow such a complex judgement to be unpacked. This is probably why this method did not demonstrate that inappropriate use of technology correlated with excessive utilisation, an otherwise surprising finding. This negative finding is more likely to reflect the insensitivity of the method rather than the reality. Moreover, there are also sources of bias which can systematically distort the information in the records. Recording of reasons for decisions is scanty, patient and family perspectives are rarely documented, the determinants of the doctor's decision inevitably lack detail such as description of the nature of critically important symptoms such as chest pain. Hence the accuracy of the diagnosis itself cannot be checked. For all of these reasons, one would be entitled to be skeptical about the accuracy of retrospective survey of clinical indications which is not based on either discussion with the clinicians involved and interview of the patients.

Practice Variations

Practice variation is not a new topic. Witness the ten-fold difference quoted in the rate of tonsillectomy demonstrated between school districts in Britain in 1938 (Glover 1938). However its importance has been magnified by our current obsession with cost-containment. Interest in practice variations quickened during the 1960s and 1970s in keeping with the critical re-evaluation of health care and the rise of health services research, aided by modern information storage and retrieval. Marked variation in procedures and practice habits, health services, facilities and costs between have been documented between countries, geographical regions, institutions and doctors, Especially provocative were the 'small area' variations demonstrated by analysis of data bases serving specific regions of a health service (Wennberg 1982).

At all levels from small area to international, large variations have been found for procedures without any necessary relation to corresponding variations in health. Included are induction of labour, common operations such as prostatectomy, appendicectomy, hysterectomy, caesarean section and coronary artery grafting, non-surgical interventions such as cardiac pacing and lithotripsy, and unexplained variations in the use of diagnostic tests such as CT scans, magnetic resonance imaging and foetal monitoring. Thus the proportion of pacemaker insertions accepted as appropriate varied from 10% to 30% in hospitals in one city in the United States. In the case of coronary angioplasty what was disconcerting was that the indication was regarded as 'uncertain' in 38% of patients. On the other hand, differences between individual doctors and groups of doctors tend to cancel out in regions and nations. Hence these are more likely to reflect the nature of the health system and cultural attitudes to intervention. A large international difference was the almost forty-fold difference in the rate of renal dialysis in the elderly between the United States and Britain, and large differences in rates of coronary artery surgery between these nations.

Variation has been linked to excessive utilization and inappropriate use of technology. Availability of facilities can certainly explain regional differences such as the tendency for open surgery for kidney stones in areas far from the major centres which had a lithotripsy facility. Facilities are deliberately limited in the presence of a national health service. Lower surgical rates pertain generally in Britain and Scandinavia in comparison with those in the United States where there is fee for service reimbursement, and a more generally aggressive attitude to intervention and ample facilities for the insured. Marked variations involving potent technologies such as coronary surgery or renal dialysis, however, are more likely to represent excessive and inappropriate use of the technology or undesirable restriction in its availability.

Does variation necessarily mean clinical inefficiency? After all, clinicians rightly observe that each patient is different, and certainly each doctor and clinical context is different too. Given the complexity of modern treatment options and the extent of variation in the needs and wishes of patients, we should surely expect much variation in clinical judgements. Variation between regions could represent different local disease prevalence in the case of kidney stones or goitre, or patient characteristics in the case of differences in coronary interventions between countries with high and low rates of disease. It is equally obvious that there must be underutilisation related to lack of facilities in third world countries. So why the fuss? The fact is that inappropriate operation of the psychosocial influences involving habit or vested interest, and the fact that different practitioners are prone to different kinds of uncertainty and errors must surely account for some of the variation between doctors.

Unexplained regional variations without health implications are nevertheless suggestive of inefficiency, or at least should be explored. As one researcher put it 'if everyone is doing things differently, can everyone be doing them right?.' When there is uniform practice this is most often in a clinical situation in which there is little doubt about the most effective treatment and it certainly represents a consensus. For example, appendicectomy is universally regarded as the appropriate treatment of acute appendicitis. Conversely, practice variations imply lack of scientific consensus. Wennberg, a pioneer in the study of small area variations, has stressed the importance of an inevitable 'professional uncertainty.' Certainly there is a serious lack of information for the guidance of medical treatment because of lack of adequate research and evaluation of medical technologies, a problem first highlighted by Cochrane in the 1960s (Cochrane 1971). This must open up a larger zone of discretional use, hence a wider range of options in the individual case. At worst, variations mean ignorance on the part of individual doctors or the subtle intrusion of inappropriate attitudinal and social motivations into clinical decisions through the hiatus of uncertainty.

On the other hand, the absence of variation cannot be seen as evidence of uniformly good clinical practice. We have seen that many of the most pervasive problems are related to attitudes influencing most doctors as part of a shared medical culture based on a combination of the ancient Hippocratic and the new scientific clinical medicine. A more extreme example of conformity which is far from reassuring is the existence of fashion in diagnosis and treatment, a form of misguided consensus. This led to the acceptance of treatments such as radical mastectomy as the definitive treatment of cancer of the breast and gastric freezing as treatment of peptic ulcer. A false consensus of experts about the echocardiographic motion of the mitral valve lead to an epidemic involving the misdiagnosis of 'mitral valve prolapse,' when the real problem was failure to properly establish the range of normal of valve leaflet excursion on closure.

Adverse Events

An adverse event is defined as 'an unintended injury or complication which results in disability, death or prolongation of hospital stay, and is caused by health care management rather than the patient's disease.' (Wilson et al. 1995). Adverse events, inappropriate interventions, and appropriate interventions performed badly are all examples of clinical inefficiency as we have defined it. Adverse events might be thought of as manifestations of clinical inefficiency in a complex and hazardous hospital environment. An adverse event can be the result of appropriate and good quality care, inappropriate intervention or poor quality care, even negligence. All outcomes of an inappropriate intervention are adverse events. Even 'successful' unnecessary surgery is just a cluster of major adverse events.

The modern hospital is the womb of scientific medicine, and hospitals have made a major contribution to lowering mortality and reducing disability in this century. Once seen as dangerous places where people went to die, they became symbols of faith in scientific medicine. Recently, the pendulum has swung back somewhat. Hospitals are dangerous places. Their inhabitants are predominantly the sick and the old, often with multiple diseases, who have limited tolerance to high tech interventions and poor tolerance for the consequences of medical error. Given the frailty of human systems, the sheer complexity of treatment and of the organisation of its delivery is a powerful predisposition to medical error, and even more so as cost constraint chips away at the system's reserve capacity. 70 years ago, Barr wrote of 'the hazards of modern diagnosis and treatment' (Barr 1955). In 1964, Schimmel, a resident doctor at Yale wrote of 'the hazards of hospitalisation.' An important stimulus for the study of adverse events has been the increasing incidence of litigation in the U.S.A.

Adverse events are common and costly. The occurrence and impact of adverse events have been studied mainly in hospital practice. The issue is nevertheless important because hospitals are such an important community resource. We discuss the special problems of ambulant primary and hospital outpatient practice in the next chapter. A U.S. study found approximately 4% of adverse events as defined above, one-quarter of which qualified as negligence (Brennan et al. 1991). An Australian study which applied essentially the same methods and definitions reported a rate of 13% (Wilson et al. 1995). A high proportion of adverse events followed surgery (about one half). The other important categories were diagnostic error (wrong or delayed diagnosis), treatment error (wrong or delayed), drug-related, invasive medical investigations (angiography, endoscopy), anaesthetic complications, falls, obstetric and neonatal complications.

When a similar overall mortality is associated with a threefold difference in adverse events, undoubtedly a difference in the definition of an adverse event diagnostic event, involving a difference in measurement threshold for an event, must surely be the likely explanation. An adverse event may be classified as 'preventable' if it resulted from 'an error in management due to failure to follow accepted practice at an individual or system level.' (Wilson et al. 1995). Preventable does not therefore necessarily or usually imply individual fault. Most adverse events in medicine, like most accidents in aviation and industry, are located in system or organisational breakdown. Negligence is rare. It is 'care that fell below the standard expected of physicians in their community' (Brennan et al. 1991). Most adverse events in medicine, like most accidents in aviation and industry, are located in system or organisational breakdown.

The Measurement of Adverse Events

Even if we accept that adverse events are common and a serious repercussion of clinical inefficiency, we would be entitled to question the way they have been measured. Survey of medical records is useful but suffers from serious disadvantages. One is the need to apply criteria when information is often scanty. As we noted, the three-fold difference between adverse events recorded in major studies in the U.S. and Australia strongly suggests that an important difference in threshold for recording an event as adverse. This is supported by the finding that mortality was correspondingly higher in the U.S. study suggesting that the adverse events recorded were the more serious ones carrying a higher rate of adverse events. What is really in question here is whether it is possible to reconstruct clinical judgement and events accurately by retrospective survey of records. At the very least, such methods need to be compared to a gold standard comprising an on-line prospective study which includes interview of those involved. This might well result in a higher estimate of prevalence of adverse events! Such is the complexity of many clinical judgements.

Research into all of these areas of clinical inefficiency has been hampered by the use of surveys which, however elaborate, are not equal to the task if used alone. What are lacking are detailed prospective studies of clinical judgement based upon observation and interview of patients and clinical staff in the setting of day-to-day patient care. Only by talking to the actors can we access the meaning of the intervention and what influences were operative. Such an approach is difficult, the interpretive methods which are needed must include qualitative data analysis are not well accepted in health services research, and studies are intrusive, labour intensive and expensive. Yet, all of the problems notwithstanding, such studies are essential if we are to understand variation and draw conclusions about appropriateness of medical interventions. Even when we have convincingly demonstrated the extent of inappropriate intervention, of illegitimate practice variations and of adverse events, we cannot respond adequately to these manifestations of clinical inefficiency unless we understand the way in which the many potential influences interact in generating the flawed clinical judgements behind them.

Conclusion

In this chapter, we have explored the effects of error and inappropriate motivations as they impinge on the clinical process of diagnosis and management. We have documented the extent of this clinical inefficiency manifest as errors documented in clinical practice, unexplained variations in clinical judgements and inappropriate intervention, and adverse events. The methods used to document important aspects of clinical inefficiency, to whit inappropriate clinical intervention and adverse events, have been retrospective studies of patient records. There is an urgent need for prospective studies in clinical practice with emphasis on interview of players with analysis by qualitative data analysis. In each case multiple influences on clinical judgement are responsible.

We have emphasised the paradigmatic factors. Thus the nature of the art of medicine, remnant of the old classical medical paradigm, is important in perpetuating some old traditions, such as sole reliance on personal experience to the exclusion of scientific evidence - which is inefficient practice in the scientific era. The science of medicine has interfered with the prudent aspects of the ancient art when patients are subjected to excessive technological intervention, and when clinical judgement is seen as an entirely rational process rather than subject also to numerous psychosocial even emotional influences which are generally ignored. In the next chapter, we explore the complementary concept of consultation failure, the problems related to faulty communication and supportive care.

References

American Child Health Association., The pathway to correction. In Physical Defects. American Child Health Association. New York, 1934, pp. 90-96.
Armstrong D., Political anatomy of the Body. Cambridge University Press, Cambridge, 1983.

Barr D. P., Hazards of modern diagnosis and therapy - the price we pay. *JAMA* 159:1452-1456;1955.

Brennan T. A., Leape L. L., Laird N. M., Herbert L., Localio A, Lawthers A. G., Newhouse J. P., Weiler P. C., Hiatt H. H., Incidence of adverse effects and negligence in the hospitalized patients: results of the Harvard Medical Practice. I. *New Eng J Med* 324: 370-376; 1991.

Brook R. H., Chassin R., Fink A., Solomon H., Kosecoff J., Park R. E., A method for the detailed assessment of the appropriateness of medical technologies. *Internat J Technol Assessment* 1987;1:53-63.

Cochrane A. L., Effectiveness and Efficiency: Random reflections on health services. The Nuffield Hospitals Trust, London, 1971.

Eisenberg J. M., Doctors' Decisions and the Cost of Medical Care. Health Administration Press perspectives, *Ann Arbor*, 1986, p. 38.

Eisenberg J. M., Doctors' Decisions and the Cost of Medical Care. Health Administration Press perspectives, *Ann Arbor,* 1986, p. 30.

Eisenberg J. M., Doctors' Decisions and the Cost of Medical Care. Health Administration Press perspectives, *Ann Arbor,* 1986, p. 31.

Eisenberg J. M., Doctors' Decisions and the Cost of Medical Care. Health Administration Press perspectives, *Ann Arbor*, 1986, p. 48.

Evans R. G., Stoddart G. L., Producing health, consuming health care. *Soc Sci Med* 31:1347-63;1990.

Foucault M., Power/Knowledge: Selected interviews and other writings 1972-1977. Gordon, ed. The Harvester Press, Sussex, 1980.

Fuchs V., Who Shall Live? Health, Economics, and Social Choice. *Basic Books,* New York, 1974, p. 144.

Fuchs V., Who Shall Live? Health, Economics, and Social Choice. *Basic Books*, New York, 1974.

Fuchs. V., Who Shall Live? Health, Economics, and Social Choice. *Basic Books,* New York, 1974, p. 149.

Glover J. A., The incidence of tonsillectomy in school children. *Proc R Soc Med* 1219-36: 31;1938.

Habermas J., Legitimation Crisis. *Polity press,* Cambridge, 1976.

Huntley R. R., Steinhauser R,. White K. L., Williams T. F., Martin D. A., Pasternack D. S., The quality of medical care: techniques and investigation in the outpatient clinic. *J Chron Dis* 14:630-42; 1961.

Jennet B., High Technology Medicine; benefits and burdens. The Nuffield Provincial Hospitals Trust, London, 1982.

Jewson N., The disappearance of the sick man from medical cosmology, 1770-1870. *Sociology* 10:225-44; 1976.

Jonsen A. R., Teaching the ethics/technology interface. *Internat J of Tech Assess of Health Care* 3: 61-66; 1987.

Kahneman D., Slovic P., Tversky A., Judgment Under uncertainty: heuristics and biases. Cambridge University Press, Cambridge, 1982.

Koran L. M., The reliability of clinical methods, data and judgments. *N Eng J Med*:293:642-646, 695-700;1975.

Last J., 'Completing the clinical picture' in general practice. *Lancet* II:28-31;1963.

McDonald I. G., Guyatt G. H., Gutman J. M., Jelinek V. M., Fox P., Daly J., The contribution of a non-invasive test to clinical care The impact of echocardiography on diagnosis, management and patient anxiety. *J Clin Epidemiol* 41:151-161;1988.

Schimmel E. M., The hazards of hospitalization. *Annals Intern Med* 600:110; 1964.

Schwartz S., Griffin T., Medical Thinking: the psychology of medical judgment and decision making. *Springer Verlag,* New York, 1986.

Wennberg J. E., Professional uncertainty and the problem of supplier-induced demand. *Soc Sci Med* 16:811-24;1982.

Williamson J. W., Assessing clinical judgment. *J Med Educ* 40:180-6; 1965.

Wilson R. McL, Runciman W. B., Gibberd R. W., Harrison B. T., Newby L., Hamilton J. D., The Quality in Australian Health Care Study. *Med J Aust* 163: 458-471; 1995.

Chapter 10

Consultation Failure - Its Genesis

The art of medicine is the matrix of the consultation process. It comprises, on the one hand, the art of diagnosis which includes, on the one hand, the skillful interview, physical examination, the global clinical judgement, and categorization of illness in the individual patient. On the other hand, there is the capacity for doctor-patient communication, and empathic and sympathetic supportive care based upon understanding of patient and context. In this chapter, we discuss the problems which afflict this latter part of the clinical encounter. Failure of the communicative aspects of the clinical consultation, 'consultation failure,' can be a disaster since it often results in a dissatisfied patient, impairment or loss of the direct therapeutic effects on the consultation – the placebo effect – sometimes litigation, noncompliance with treatment recommendations, failure to accept appropriate reassurance, or defection to alternative medicine. The evidence for this failure of the consultation to achieve its communicative and supportive objectives, we discuss in the remainder of this chapter. The adverse consequences for patients and their care we deal with in the next.

An important consequence of the rapid shift of the foundations of medicine from the classical clinical tradition and humanities to technology and science has been dissonance between medical and lay paradigms of health care, decried as a loss of 'humanism.' Deleterious comments heard socially, obtained in opinion polls, elicited in academic studies, reflect concern about communication difficulties and a lack of personal support, professional self-interest, high cost of care and problems of access. What patients want most of all is an explanation of illness that they can understand, a feeling of being in control, reassurance which they can accept, and relief from disability. And often they are not successful. Doctors, on the other hand often focus on disease and its mechanism in biomedical terms. To restore the lost balance between the art of medicine and relatively new science is what is required and must be the primary objective of health care reform in the postmodern context.

The family's interpretation of illness is naturally based upon their own experience, on lay beliefs, family wisdom and advice from friends. The lay interpretation of the nature of illness and its appropriate treatment often diverges from the medical, and patients want these differences to be respected. All too often, the patient perspective is overlooked or dismissed. This clash of paradigms, this mismatch of expectations, often leads to a conflict of interests and to consultation failure as we have defined it.

Communication and the Doctor-Patient Relationship

It is ironic that just when medicine developed a new and potent scientific dimension to its effectiveness with a greatly enhanced ability to provide a valid explanation for illness and to deliver specific treatment, the doctor's ability to support them in their distress was blunted. This was no fluke, as it coincided with friction between art and science. This is important because many more patients nowadays present with symptoms related to psychological distress and problems of living than from the effects of organic disease. In such patients, communication, reassurance, support and the placebo effect are of overriding importance. Technological diagnostic interventions play an important supportive role by excluding disease and allowing reassurance. Thus the modern doctor has, by dint of professional training and socialization, has to a considerable extent lost the commonsense approach to 'dis-ease,' as human suffering and uncertainty, and as a result become less able to understand and relate to the patient's experience.

The modern obsession with disease diagnosis and technology has, we argue, distracted doctors from the crucial importance of the personal and social intercourse with the patient. We see consultation failure due to failure of the social transaction as dwarfing technical iatrogenesis in overall importance to the community. Given the regularity with which people visit their doctors and the dependency of the elderly on the profession, the risk of this variety of consultation failure is cumulative. It is therefore a pressing problem for public health as well as for clinical practice. This crucial connection will not be adequately addressed by health services research focused on clinical care, preoccupied by quantitative measurement of health outcome and patient satisfaction. At risk is respect for clinical judgement itself, the only conceivable way of handling the psychological and social effects of illness and treatment.

Newton showed, in mechanics, 'to every action, there is an equal and opposite reaction.' It is tempting to interpret the 'patient advocacy' movement as the social equivalent of this second law of mechanics! Health care retirees, doctors, nurses and lawyers have been recruited to accompany patients at medical consultations, to assist them in framing questions, to watch out for medical errors, to obtain second opinions, to handle financial issues and paperwork, to resolve misunderstandings, to anticipate misunderstandings and more. This response is scarcely apparent in Australia but is a game played for high stakes in the U.S., arranged privately, or through companies or managed care, and has emerged in Britain.

Tension between Medical and Lay Paradigms

At root, this breakdown of communication is a product of tension between lay and medical paradigms with the doctor invoking science, the patient preoccupied with meaning and wanting explanation in their own terms. As a result, the doctor tends to view patient decisions such as noncompliance, delay in seeking help and unwillingness to accept reassurance or seeking alternative medicine as irrational responses. In fact, they can be seen as rational when viewed in the richer context of the patient's life. If the doctor fails to understand precisely why the patient has presented for treatment now, and is unaware of psychological context or an important aspect of social context, then the patient and doctor pass like ships in the night, and the consultation will fail. Small wonder that there is dissatisfaction all round. Moreover, appreciating the patient's point of view is an ethical requirement, as well as resulting in better health outcomes.

In order to expose the problems of the social transaction in clinical care, we consider the problems in more detail. We do this by drawing upon the insights of several writers. One is a philosopher who suffers from multiple sclerosis. An account follows from three enlightened doctors, one providing an honest appraisal from the medical perspective, one stressing the paradigmatic conflict, although not using this term, and sketching the outline of a solution which is postmodern in essence although not proposed in these terms. We then summarise the academic models of sociology which provide in-depth theoretical understanding of the doctor–patient relationship.

Biological Explanation or Lived Experience?

A first hand account of the communication gulf which separates doctor and patient has been provided by Toombs (1992). A philosopher suffering from disseminated sclerosis. This account, based on phenomenology, clearly illustrates the 'incommensurability' of the patient's lived experience and the physician's understanding so strongly coloured by biomedical explanation. This is at the heart of the clash between lay and medical discourse, so often putting patient and doctor at cross purposes. This is the indigestion that medicine has suffered by swallowing 'science's fillet steak' whole! So difficult is it now to construct a shared world view of meaning between them. In fact, they cannot be said to share the same world view. Physicians interpret illness through scientific data analysed objectively. The problem is then to make a diagnosis rather than to find out what is the matter. Patients, however, encounter illness more immediately as a disturbance of a lived body and the meaning of illness in terms of frustration and limitation of social goals rather than as biological dysfunction.

An Alien World

Of prime importance is the impact of illness on life, difficult to incorporate if it is unexpected or unexpectedly serious, a threat to integrity and control over one's affairs. Commonsense interpretation is based on a limited source of unique personal as well as a shared knowledge base of lay people the lay perspective built into their paradigm. In the case of serious chronic illness, the body may become the centre of attention, a negative awareness which can be profoundly alienating as a portent of inability to achieve goals, shrinking of possibilities fof action, a world which looks different, unfamiliar even frightening. The web of associations on which the sufferer's life has been based has been shattered, generating a fear which is difficult to communicate, and refractory to the doctor's well meaning attempt to reassure by asserting that there is no cause for concern.

The Devil Is in the Psychosocial Detail

Eminent British physician Fletcher wrote a landmark review (1979) in which he cites many reports of patient's dissatisfaction, and requests by the Patient's Association for greater participation as consumers. He found that clinical teachers do have inappropriate confidence in their own skills, and do not see the need for specific training of students in this area. One study in general practice found that the most common complaint was that more than three-quartes were doctor-centred rather than patient-centred with a tendency to overlook psychological and social problems. The importance of counselling as therapy was stressed in light of the high proportion of patients presenting with psychological problems. The difficulties identified were identified as the dominance of doctors attributed to insecurity, a need to maintain a distance from the patient, difficulty dealing with emotional matters, and even a tendency to see their patients as deranged biological machines.

Even more of a difficulty was the 'exposition' interview when the diagnosis of disease or normality was explained to the patient together with the implications and need for treatment or otherwise. Fletcher documented evidence in the literature that patients complained of difficulty in getting information about illness, and related this to treatment noncompliance. Conventional medical training he saw as blocking improvement. Fletcher also considered doctors' attitudes as measures to reduce anxiety. He also considered problems of patient attitudes, those who do not wish to know, the role of anxiety and also medical use of jargon, brevity of interview, mismatch of lay and medical beliefs, and conflicting information. Fletcher was critical of the attitude that patients' failure to understand is 'sad but inevitable.' He particularly lamented the lack of teaching in this area: he might also have expressed the absence of clinical research into bedside teaching! Finally, he did discuss a range of more modern teaching aids, including the use of videotaped interviews.

Honest Negotiation between Equals

Brody (1992) emphasizes the interpretive or hermeneutic character of the clinical interview which he conceptualizes as a conversation. The consultation should be patient-centred, that is the doctor's management of the patient's problem should be grounded in the way that the patient defines, that is in accordance with their basic health beliefs and values. Part of the process of honest negotiation of a mutual understanding involves determining the extent to which the patient wants to be so informed, and wishes to participate in their own management. A postmodern perspective is that, according to Foucault, it is not possible to separate the sharing of knowledge and the exhibition of power (chapter 4). An ethical relationship which most benefits patients is one in which power is balanced, appropriately shared between the two parties. This allows for legitimate persuasion by the doctor but acknowledges the gap in knowledge and often social status between the two parties and the special vulnerability of the sick person. This approach has been presented as the physician's 'narrative competence' which requires empathy (Charon 2001). In the last chapter, we discuss the importance of the physician's capacity for what Schon called 'reflection-in-action,' involving accruing and access tacit learning, and 'reflection-on-action, the act of ruminating on and extracting lessons from daily clinical experience.

Illness and Loss of Control

An important part of a physician's role is to dismantle barriers to patient autonomy, enhancing the patient's ability to gain some control over the illness. The physician should be expected to manifest certain virtues such as those proposed by the American Board of Internal Medicine – integrity, respect and compassion. This justifies the trust which is so important to the success of the consultation. The key to good communication is honesty and openness to further patient questioning. Physicians 'empower patients by creating an atmosphere that encourages participation and dialogue; by following carefully the cues provided by the patient, and placing the new information in the context of the patient's life experience in the most meaningful, encouraging and health-promoting way'(Brody 1992). The legal requirements of informed consent have promoted an adversarial atmosphere, and a lip-service defensive response by doctors, and can also encourage disclosure of more than the patient desires. The second distraction has been a narrowly construed and potentially harmful idea of increased patient autonomy.

Provision of Information

Katz (1984), a legally trained academic considers that quality of information is crucial to the success of the clinical consultation, to medical ethics and to the public image of the profession. He too is critical of the concept of informed consent but shows how it has probed to the heart of the doctor-patient relationship, exposing powerful historical forces. These extend back as far as Hippocrates who advised that treatment should be carried out while 'concealing most things from the patient while you are attending him.' Katz's thesis has been that doctors have been socialized by their training to oppose free exchange with their patients. This ideology he attributes to the conviction that trust in the doctor, essential to the art of medicine, is central to the healing process. Thus, to some extent that non-disclosure in part reflects caring for the patient's confidence and well being. The legal has therefore collided with deeply rooted tacit assumptions of clinical practice.

However, according to Katz, the reluctance of doctors to divulge information has been projected onto patients or obfuscated by such fatuous claims as prohibitive cost and lack of time. He argues that, in the modern era, trust requires full disclosure delivered with compassion and appropriate acknowledgement of uncertainty, and with recognition that patients make judgements that are subject to irrational forces which 'shape all thoughts and actions' (Katz 1984). In order to tackle this basic issue, it will not be enough to graft a broader education in the humanities onto the current overloaded medical curriculum. What is required is research into the intricacies of the clinical process itself such as is advocated in the last chapter. A genuine trusting relationship would mean that the doctor will not have to fall back upon traditional authority and orthodoxy. A critical patient agenda for finding the real problem will frequently be revealed to the patient, empathetic doctor.

Telling the story can frequently act as a cathartic, which catalyses disclosure of much needed social or contextual information, central to understanding the real problem but previously withheld because of human respect. Patients value information but few, including most doctors wish to participate in decisions related to their own case. In the transitional early life of a new postmodern paradigm, there has been an increase in consumerist attitudes which include sensitivity to cost, seeking health information and exerting independent judgements but more in theory than in the deed! Communication breakdowns are a major factor in litigation, as one might expect.

Patient Stereotype

Rota and Hall (1987) found that doctors who reacted differently to patients because of legitimate social and cultural differences, may fail to notice such differences or may respond inappropriately to stereotypes as all of us are wont to do. Evidence has been obtained documenting an influence of age, gender, social class and other personal characteristics, including the 'difficult' even hateful patient and a tendency to prefer the well to the sick patient. Gender and race bias in selection of medical students has changed dramatically of recent years but representation of the lower class remains small. Differences have been found in relation to doctor gender, social class, political ideology and personality characteristics. Medical education is characterized by students who have made an early career choice and often by aggressive competitiveness needed to reach medical school and to succeed there.

Domination of the curriculum, first by the sciences then by scientific medicine in the hospital setting severely distorts the student's notion of the relationship between the symptoms of illness and those of organic disease, creating a serious problem for the management of the ambulant patient. They would never guess that that functional illness is, by far, the commonest cause of all important symptoms and many doctors never seem to reflect and to learn this crucial lesson from their own experience.

Education and the Product

Mizrahi describes how the medical course militates against humanistic medicine. The doctor dominates the interview, interrupting early and doing the bulk of the talking (Misrahi 1986), using closed-ended questions and controlling the agenda. The doctor's agenda seems to be variable but inflexible, that is, not modulated according to differences between patients. Patients were more satisfied by a patient-centred consultation, and doctor satisfaction seems to mirror patient satisfaction. There is a 'communication conspiracy' whereby doctors behave as if they understand, and patients as if they do. Sociological explanations are paternalism, and need to maintain status and control. Doctors underestimate patient information needs, withholding information ostensibly in the patient's interest. Patients are reluctant to question, and not all wish to ask questions. A prescription can be used in lieu of examination or information exchange, and patients know it.

The View from the Patient's Perspective

Doctors rarely elicit the patient's explanatory illness framework, so that there are two parallel monologues. Concordance is low between what doctor and patient think that the problem is. Satisfaction is enhanced by a partnership style with provision of information, good nonverbal communication, patient-centred interviewing with attention to pschosocial concerns, when doctors like the patient, and also technical competence. Communication skills are related to quality of care and accurate diagnosis, both technical and psychosocial, to patient satisfaction and cooperation, as well as to treatment compliance. The patient resumes control at the door of the doctors' surgery.

Meetings between Experts

Tuckett et al. (1986) undertook a monumental field study of general practice in Britain by tape-recording counsultations. They describe these graphically as 'meetings between experts.' Patient satisfaction was related to evidence that the patient was liked, allowed to tell their story, and given information they could use. Doctors gave information but often did not elicit what the patient felt, exchange ideas, attempt to persuade or to attempt to tailor treatment in such a way as to locate and resolve doubt and illuminate areas of misunderstanding. Even in the case of providing information, factors such as time constraints, social class or gender, good or bad news loomed larger than the need for clear patient comprehension. Moreover many patients were passive, inhibited in light of past experience, had difficulty their thoughts in light of conflict between their understanding and medical explanations. They were afraid of antagonizing their doctor. Questions or issues tended to be raised in a covert manner. The G.P.s tended to be unaware of the extent of their patients' rumination about their illness.

The Lay Interpretation of Illness

Patients understood their illness mainly on the basis of the agreement or otherwise with their own initial ideas, hence the importance of lay models of illness. Problems of communication were commoner for the one-third to one-quarter of illnesses in whom there was no physical abnormality found - those with functional illness. When interviewed, some doctors argued that exploring patient beliefs was impractical with some doubting the wisdom of doing so. There appeared to be two unstated assumptions – that the doctor's priorities were to make a diagnosis and to be in control. The reasons for doctors' failure to communicate were identified as the problems of medical education, their methods of dealing with their own insecurities and the counterproductive way in which patients often responded. It is important that the doctor appreciate the patient's view of illness. This is why it is important to know what underlies the patient's attribution, so that lay and medical may be compared (Stoeckle and Barski 1981). Cultural beliefs and folk wisdom may determine the response to illness and perception of benefits, and there may be discordance with the medical paradigm of which the doctor should be aware (Fitzpatrick in Scrambler 1984).

Cultural Understanding and the Interpretive Model of Illness

Conflicting beliefs may result in patient noncompliance or reluctance to accept reassurance. Hence the correction of misattribution or removal of inappropriate labelling may be important for a successful consultation. Meaning of an illness in a culture can be punishment for sin, a sign of weakness, relief from social burdens, part of a coping strategy, an opportunity to earn divine grace or as a feeling of loss (Pfifferling 1981). Barriers to successful communication lie at different levels involving meaning of words, emotive connotations or implications of cause. Not good enough is a reductionist approach, attempting to graft a modern biomedical interpretation onto a decoding of psychosocial and cultural interpretation (Good and Good 1981). The genuine hermeneutic or interpretive model needed for the full understanding of illness demands the seamless incorporation of the scientific explanation into the broader context of the illness.

'The Sick Role' – The Sociological Perspective

Attempts to address paradigmatic and cultural differences between doctor and patient, and to address the thorny problems of the doctor-patient relationship can be planned and prioritized best if we have a sound theoretical grasp of their basis. There has now been more than half a century of study which we can draw upon. But medicine and sociology remain far apart. The infant sociology in the 19th century was preoccupied with 'macro' issues related to the emerging state and social stratification, linked to industrialization and urbanization. Not until the fourth decade of the 20th century was attention turned to the doctor-patient relationship. Indeed, as we have seen, there was no such thing as an ongoing relationship until medicine rose to a dominant position in personal health care in the second half of the 20th century.

The Systems Model – Henderson and Parsons

During the early days of sociology, biology and physiology had presented the organism as a powerful model for the complexities of human interaction. This metaphor of what was later referred to as the 'complex dynamic system' was exploited by Pareto, a political economist. The capacity of an organism to maintain equilibrium of body chemistry was an interest of L.J. Henderson, Professor of Biological Chemistry at Harvard University. In an interesting twist back in the direction of Hippocratic medicine, he supported the idea that illness as a disturbance of social equilibrium: 'a physician and a patient taken together represent a social system. In any social system the interaction of the sentiments is likely to be as important as anything else' (Henderson 1935). He was also obviously aware of the importance of a medical interest in the human side.

Talcott Parsons, a junior colleague of Henderson, took up this idea. He brought together the systems model, the related the related notion of structural fuctionalism in anthropology, and Freudian psychoanalysis to forge a model of the doctor-patient relationship which dominated thinking for decades (Parsons 1951). His scheme viewed illness as a breach of social as well as bodily equilibrium. Hence the role of the patient was socially constructed, and that the doctor was 'homeostatic' - equilibrium restoring - in both a personal and a social sense. This opened the way for a long and productive debate about the nature of the relationship between doctor and patient, and between and the state. The essence of the model was that because patients were functionally disabled by illness, they were not blameworthy provided that they sought appropriate medical assistance, and made every effort to get well. Implicit was that illness could be used to evade social responsibility as a form of 'deviance.'

Parson's sick role model was broadened in other ways. There will also be variation over time as context and circumstances change. Thus a patient may be passive in the early stages of recovery from an acute illness, cooperative and accepting guidance during early recovery and more interested in participation during convalescence (Szasz and Hollender 1956). In addition, patients go on modelling, particularly if illness persists, so that the patient's understanding is not static but evolves over time. That if significant events occur, they may change their attitudes, their perspective on the illness and their trust in and their opinion of the doctor. Illness experience is then best conceptualized as an illness career in the course of which a patient often makes a series of judgements and decisions. Patients with chronic illness often become very knowledgeable about their condition, and often harder to satisfy as they struggle to maintain control of their lives in the face of adversity.

Illness Behaviour

Mechanic (1972) shifted this model in the direction of social psychology by studying what influences underpin 'normal illness behaviour' when they are troubled by symptoms. Patients go through a process of attribution of symptoms, following which they decide either to dismiss them as trivial or to act on them. The decision will also depend on the resources available at the time. Noting that three out of four people have symptoms about which they take action in any given month, he raised the question whether that action will be to seek medical assistance. Thus he stresses the importance of psychological, social and cultural influences of which patients are unaware or which they may deny. These influences included neurotic beliefs, family history and advice, occupation (especially that of medical student), recent medical experience, chance events and media publicity.

What symptoms cause most concern is part historical, part fortuitous and part learned behavior. What many clinicians learn from experience has also been confirmed – that patients present with symptoms or dissatisfaction with treatment when their real concern is a problem of living or a manifestation of a psychiatric disorder. It is also clear that the personal or social context are crucially important in determining action or lack of it, even in life threatening circumstances. Even in the case of a heart attack, some patients take a surprising length of time to consider diagnostic possibilities and the threat posed by the illness, aided by personal and lay theories, to put their affairs in order, to maintain appearances, to avoid loss of face, to adhere to social norms, as well as exhibiting a variety of mechanisms to create the appearance of normality (Dracup et al. 1997). Family members are often important in the decision to seek help.

Doctor-Patient Communication – A Synthesis

If we put all of this together, we can paint a fairly coherent picture. At the core is a sick role model which postulates that illness interferes with our functional status and personal activities but also curtails or prevents our customary social role. Those who take up the sick role by seeking medical help are those who are disabled or concerned to a critical extent - the great majority; and those who do so primarily as an expression of social pressure (somatization) or in association with a pathological fear of disease (hypochondriasis) – an important minority. The influences which interact to determine whether or when an individual will seek medical help, to decide what constitutes unacceptable disability or justifies release from social obligations, are intensely personal. They are a unique tapestry into which are woven together personality, life experience, family wisdom and myths, lay beliefs, cultural norms, attitudes to and ideas about illness, advice and reactions of friends, chance happenings, unsettling publicity – and more.

Trust is an unfashionable word these days vis a vis the doctor-patient relationship. It was part of Parson's model but has been extensively criticized. Has the bay been thrown out with the bath water? Thus Galen observed: 'He cures the greatest number in whom most men have most faith' (1984). Trust was central to the Hippocratic ethic. It remains central to the modern clinician. Trust is held to be important if the patient is to validate the doctor's interpretation of the illness, plan of treatment and its execution. Trust is also important to the direct healing effect of the physician, the placebo effect and of the clinical context. Erosion of trust in the doctor by the rise of consumerism and of managed care could therefore be damaging to the healing process.

Meetings between Experts

The postmodern consultation will reflect a balance between medical and lay paradigms, Tuckett's 'meeting between experts.' It will be a dialogue, a conversation in which the patient sets the agenda, and the nature and extent of their involvement. The objective is a fusion of their horizons, a negotiated mutually shared interpretation of the illness seen in its personal and social context, as well as in biomedical terms. In this iterative hermeneutic exercise, the doctor's role is to interrogate sensitively and supportively, to listen, inform, persuade and interact. The major obstacles are paradigmatic dissonance impacting on the the art within medicine subtly affecting the clinical interaction, and potentially creating a clash of perpectives between doctor and patient. No sharp distinction can be drawn between diagnosis and treatment because of the operation of the direct healing effects of the 'placebo' and 'Hawthorne' effects, discussed in detail later. The interpretation of patient symptoms ultimately reveals that most are 'functional,' that is, not explained by organic disease. In fact, only a miniscule faction (0.1 %) of these patients will be referred to that bastion of biomedical science, the university teaching hospital.

Functional Illness

Early in the 19th century, following the French Revolution, the shift of medical paradigm precipitated by the dramatic discovery that was the result of organ damage lead to a new disease taxonomy. An achievement of the correlation between the manifestations of illness in the sick and findings at post-mortem, it quickly became apparent that some conditions, for example some mental illness and fevers, were not necessarily so linked. The term 'functional illness,' that is 'not organic on post-mortem examination' was first used for these cases. With the advent of comprehensive modern diagnostic testing, the meaning of the term 'functional illness' shifted to meaning 'not due to organic disease,' meaning that clinical examination and investigations had not discovered an organic problem to account for the clinical illness. The modern name is somatization or 'somatoform disorder' as defined by the American Psychiatric Society (1985). The definition is thus: 'Disorders having the presence of symptoms that suggest the presence of a physical condition bur are not fully explained by a general medical condition, by the effects of a substance, or by another mental disorder. The symptoms must cause significant physical distress or impairment in social or other areas of functioning.'

Functional symptoms can suggest involvement of the body as a whole or of any organ system. For example, common symptoms are tiredness, breathlessness, insomnia, chest pain, palpitations, aches and pains, sore tongue, lump in the throat, abdominal pain, bowel disturbance, headache, dizziness and many more. Patients may present with single symptoms or multiple symptoms. Since individual symptoms and their combinations are so common, it is not at all surprising that they can mimic serious organic disease for which no specific treatment might be available. The mechanisms of such symptoms are poorly understood. At root is psychic or social distress related to loss, strife, interpersonal conflict, work stress, marital disharmony, difficulties with children, maladjustment, failure and isolation. In other cases there is a cultural basis to expression or when left inframammary chest pain is a harbinger of cardiac neurosis. Alternatively it may be 'atypical' – an unusual pattern, or 'bizarre' – not fitting any disease or pathophysiological category. In the case of 'atypical chest pain' in being felt on the let side of the near the palpable thrust of the apex of the heart, and is usually aching often sharp and stabbing, sometimes both. Pain arising from the heart or lung (pleura) is quite different. In some cases, physiological abdominal rumblings or palpitations may trigger alarm bells for the patient. In other cases, a minor abnormality often discovered in a screening test, an 'incidentaloma' may get the blame.

The following mechanisms probably account for most symptoms. In some cases, it may be a symbolic expression of concern, as when chest pain is accompanied by fear of heart attack in somebody who has had their heart queried, lost a loved one this way or who is being rehabilitated following such an attack. In other cases there is a cultural predisposition. It is important to accept that a patient with associated organic symptoms may present with a functional syndrome; organic disease is frequently associated with related or unrelated functional symptoms. Females are more prone to functional symptoms and somatoform disorders. There is sometimes a family history, and the diagnosis is commoner in those with lower socioeconomic status.

In all of these circumstances, there tend to be vicious circles operating, whereby the symptoms provoke anxiety and anxiety the symptoms; heightened concern and specific attributions increase sensitivity to particular symptoms. Symptoms may sometimes be exacerbated by attention from others and by the prospect of gain. An important and common aggravant is referral for a test which appears to give confirmation to the patient's fears. Worse is a doubtful test result, and worse still a false positive finding causing doubt which is usually very difficult to assuage. In addition, the low prevalence of organic disease statistically favours doubtful and false positive results, especially in the context of screening tests. The message is to keep testing to a reasonable minimum, recognising the possible difficulty of legitimate reassurance. The degree to which a patient adverts to a symptom, misattribute it, and the likelihood that they will seek medical clarification depends on many variables, personal, social, contextual as well as chance events.

Fortunately, the shrewd clinician can perceive with considerable accuracy, patterns of events and symptoms suggestive of functional illness, atypical descriptions, personal history and mien, and social and cultural context. This is a positive approach to diagnosis, although it is accepted that an appropriate approach to investigation will be taken to exclude organic disease. Unfortunately, doctors trained in the modern era tend to be focused on organic disease. Hence they have difficulty recognizing functional symptoms and neuroses and, especially in the specialty of internal medicine, a tendency to relentlessly pursue the organic disease diagnosis. The lack of reasonable emphasis in medical textbooks does not help. Nor does lack of patient satisfaction and the possibility of litigation in the event of 'missing something.'

Prevalence of Functional Illness

Many studies have shown that patients presenting with functional symptoms, especially in general practice, also in internal medicine, even in specialty practice, are common, a trap for the unwary, their medical records growing thick with the impact of 'false alarms.' A study in Britain found that two-thirds did not have serious organic disease (Kellner 1987). In a clinic offering primary care in the U.S., common symptoms were joint and back pain, headache, fatigue, chest and abdominal pain and dizziness. Less than 16% of patients with new symptoms had an organic cause, in 10% they were considered 'psychologic,' and in the remaining three-quarters they remained unexplained. The response of unexplained and psychological symptoms to treatment was poor (Kroenke and Mangelsdorff 1989). Tumulty (1960), writing about patients selected for referral to an internal medicine clinic, estimated that one-quarter had presented with functional symptoms, and that in 80% there were both functional and organic complaints.

Reid et al. (2001) found that a high proportion of frequent attenders had medically unexplained symptoms, and this included most specialities. Even in specialist medical practice, patients presenting with functional symptoms are very common; thus 'irritable bowel syndrome' was the diagnosis in 20 – 40% of patients seen by gastroenterologists (Walker et al. 1992). Even in a specialty cardiology clinic, patients with chest pain and palpitations received an organic diagnosis in only 50% of cases. In about one-third of patients seeking heart disease as the cause of chest pain were negative, that is, they showed no evidence of coronary artery disease at coronary angiography as the cause. There is a high incidence of panic attacks in such patients and pain often persists despite treatment.

That surgical treatment is not immune from such exigencies is suggested by terms such as 'post-cholecystectomy syndrome' describing relapse of symptoms following surgery to remove the gall bladder. In some cases, symptoms might have been functional, and since gallstones are often an incidental finding, the symptoms were probably functional and the remission of pain due to the placebo effect. The following figure gives some idea of just how common functional illness is attested to by the high cost. Patients with 'multiple unexplained symptoms' had multiple procedures and hospitalisations, adding up to $4700 annually, nine times the amount for other patients (Smith et al. 1986).

'Biomedicalisation of Illness'

Such is the domination of medical discourse by the biomedical paradigm of illness that there is a deep reluctance to accept the reality and legitimacy of functional symptoms. This narrow view of illness creates difficulties by impairing the mainstays of supportive care, disowning the contextual impact of caring, the positive impact of the healer, and often ignoring the personal and social milieu of illness. Especially striking is the 'biomedicalisation' of illness. This is a confusing tendency to classify and label symptom complexes according to a biomedical mechanism when it seems a priori unlikely that there was an organic disease at play causing the symptoms. Thus we have repetitive strain injury, chronic fatigue syndrome – also known as 'myalgic encephalitis' which bears a close resemblance to the 'neurasthenia' of the last century. Then there is 'irritable bowel syndrome,' temporomandibular joint syndrome, syndrome X - standing for chest pain with normal coronary arteries, mitral valve prolapse syndrome, fibromyalgia and multiple allergy syndrome. These modern diseases are only one step removed from the floating kidney, gastroptosis, acidosis, retroverted uterus, colonic toxaemia and chlorosis - denizens of the last century. Patients severely incommoded by symptoms often prefer to have their illness validated by the dominant paradigm since it is more socially acceptable, more likely to be handled with sympathy and understanding, more justification for adoption of the sick role. As American baseball umpire Yogi Berra once said: 'They ain't nuttin' till I calls 'em.' This seems to to be the attitude of the biomedical part of the modern paradigm!

Also revealing of the strong influence of the scientific biomedical discourse is the awkward way in which functional illness is handled by doctors. It is rarely discussed, seldom taught and almost synonymous with neurosis. Clinicians frequently appear embarrassed with the subject. A particularly unfortunate response, commoner among resident staff is to blame the victim, so that patients with functional symptoms are pilloried by such regrettable epithets as 'pills, crazies, nutters, gomers,' often with a wink and a nod. The use of abusive pejoratives is an aggressive defensive response to those whose illnesses have bemused them and resisted their therapeutic offerings, a response by a frustrated doctor ill equipped to deal with such problems. Meanwhile, the journals refer to 'symptoms not due to structural disease,' to 'patients with multiple symptoms,' or with negative investigations' or of 'non-specific symptoms,' or of 'undifferentiated illness.' Medical textbooks also betray the priorities of the medical paradigm. Standard disease classifications relate to hospital disease not ambulant care. The symptoms of functional illness are not covered by the sparse detail provided, especially unfortunate given their capacity for mimicry of organic disease.

The Two Zones of Clinical Practice

Over the last century, the focus of health care has shifted from self help and family assistance to the medical consultation (Shorter 1991). People used take time off work or sought help only for alarming symptoms or major disability, that is, the entry threshold for the sick role was much higher. They either treated themselves or consulted a healer. The doctor simply could not be afforded by most. Younger people and young people in particular children rarely received medical attention. When the threshold for seeking medical treatment declined, the result was an avalanche of symptoms. A useful concept for analyzing the impact of this burgeoning of medical practice is to consider medical practice as comprised of a 'Central Zone' where organic disease predominates and a 'Peripheral Zone' where most symptoms are classified as functional after organic disease has been ruled out.

The Central Zone of Care

The Central zone of medical care is essentially where the primary aim of treatment is to apply the 'new' scientific medicine in the form of technological intervention. Here the doctor as medical feels most at home. Here we think of biomedicine, of acute illness, of hospital care, of cure, and of medical specialties. Thus medical technology based upon and guided by biological models is applied to the management of trauma, to replace heart valves or hips, to treat infection or prevent by vaccination, to the correction of hormonal or vitamin deficiency, to the drug treatment of peptic ulcer, of asthma, of schizophrenia, to organ transplantation, treatment of leukaemia, the technical aspects of safe childbirth, and the safe use of agents such as antibiotics and antihypertensive drugs in ambulant patients. It must also include diagnostic tests without which surgery would be out of the question. Thus removal of the gallbladder would not be feasible without visualisation of the gallstones by diagnostic ultrasound. Selection of patients for coronary angioplasty would not be possible without prior detailed imaging of the coronary anatomy and pathology by angiography.

This is the high ground of medical practice where the problems are well structured and the variables relatively few. The application of science and managerial efficiency is relatively straightforward. The disease or problem to be treated is clear cut. Here Weber's 'instrumental rationality' holds sway as the relationships are essentially causal. In such cases there is no mystery as to why the patient sought help. About the desirability of intervening, the impact is generally obvious to all, clear cut and easily identified, and can even be predicted at least in statistical terms. The treatment is often a 'technological fix'the value of which is either obvious or well established. The determinants of the doctor's decisions are basically technical with a minimum of psychosocial input, and the patients respond in a predictable fashion, are generally satisfied, and their cooperation can generally be taken for granted. During this period, the supportive attention of the contextual doctor may be beneficial but is generally subsidiary to the benefits of the intervention, and the contribution of supportive care is less. Technical interventions reflect a technological rationale which can be subject to peer review.

This Central Zone is our contract for a safer birth, our hedge against premature death or disablement, protection against unwarranted fear of disease. Death can at least be made more comfortable. In the modern state, we insist on the availability of this 'insurance policy' as a basic right. We are born only once and die only once and serious illness is uncommon in between. Hence we call upon scientific medicine as 'catastrophe insurance,' and only infrequently when we are young. The Central Zone for all that it offers us is small. Just how small was shown by White et al. (1967). Of 1000 people in the general population over one month, 75% reported ill health or injury about which they took some action. 25% attended a doctor, 9% were referred to another doctor, only a tiny minority (0.1%) were sent to a university medical centre. A study of middle class American males 20 to 45 years over 20 years disclosed an average of one life-threatening illness, 20 causing disability, 200 which did not cause disability, 200 which did not disable and 1000 asymptomatic episodes (Hinkle 1960). Thus for all its importance to the individual and interest to the medical scientist, the fact is that serious organic disease is uncommon in early and middle life, in contrast to the plethora of functional symptoms.

The Peripheral Zone of Care

The Peripheral zone, fraught with uncertainty and human problems, surrounds the Central Zone like a vast penumbra. It is the medicine practised in general practices and in the hospital outpatients departments. Moreover, seriously ill patients whose treatment has been successful still suffer serious problems of social disengagement and frustration of goals. Hence the Peripheral Zone aso includes the convalescence and rehabilitation after serious illness. It is in this zone, comprising the bulk of medical practice that we see the most serious consequences of the clash between the art and science of medicine, and between the perspectives of lay people and scientific medicine. Thus polls and surveys indicate that the proportion of Americans satisfied with their health declining but the number reporting ill-health has more than doubled and to number of days restricted or confined to bed has increased since the 1950s. Barsky attributes this finding to reduced tolerance for symptoms, greater willingness to accept the sick role and to seek medical help for symptoms.

Pursuing a 'healthy lifestyle' encourages a growing fascination with diet, nutrition and weight loss' and is exposed to a growing 'physical physical fitness boom,' an increased body awareness and a tendency to amplify and react to symptoms. This is enhanced by commercialization and the media stressing the dangers of living. Between the 1930s and 1980s, the average rate of medical consultations has doubled in the U.S. and 30 to 60% of consultations reveal no serious medical diagnosis to explain symptoms. On top of all of this are unrealistic expectations. Such has been the success of medicine that the public believes that more of their ill-health is curable, and the effects of aging preventable.

The Classification of Illness

Almost unnoticed has been that little attention has been to the problems of decisions in ambulant practice where the classification of illness on the basis of organic disease is unsatisfactory. Apart from early McMaster initiatives, the setting of general practice or the hospital outpatients, the problems of the ambulant population have been comprehensively neglected. This has been in keeping with the longstanding anomaly that almost all scientific medicine is still practiced, students educated and research conducted in the rarified atmosphere of the university teaching hospital. This delivers a misleading message that the clientele and problems of ambulant care were similar which they clearly are not. This 'high ground' delivers the technologies upon which the community relies for greater longevity and freedom serious illness or incapacity and it is here that almost all clinical epidemiology is taught and practiced. However, as Kerr White has so cogently argued, it is nevertheless not where most illness is treated and most symptoms managed! Nor is it where most certainty resides, most variation in care and most error occurs. The end result is roughly tantamount to learning to fly in a flight simulator.

Like it or not, the low ground of primary care is where most medicine is practiced and where the problems of iatrogenesis and inadequacies of supportive care are greatest and most costs are incurred, especially the indirect ones stemming from misdiagnosis, inappropriate intervention and the consequences of overlooking the roots of problems in problems of living. Ironically, it is where most medicine is practiced that the quantitative methods of heath research are seriously limited in their capacity to probe the meaning of the symptoms linked to functional symptoms, and help patients to cope with their need to understand their experience. We shall return to this theme because it has been a more onerous task for dence-based medicine which has been attempting to sell its approach in general practice. We believe that there will be a need for a much closer liaison in this venture into 'tiger country,' recruiting the social sciences as guides.

A Perverse Effect on Medical Practice

How did this predominance of functional illness in the Peripheral Zone come about? Medicine, by its links to science and by its manifest success has prevailed in competition with other healers, and has attracted patients like moths to a light, convincing government and claimed a patient's democratic right to its ministrations. A large proportion of patients attracted were and still are in the Peripheral Zone, comprising largely those with anxiety and problems of living. It is ironic that the seeds of trouble were sown by the very success of scientific medicine. Throughout history, the elite or their slaves have been be attended by a practitioner of physic which therefore has been a badge of social success.

Virtually all of medicine was supportive or palliative care until the second half of the 19th century, so that treatment consisted of invoking the placebo effect and taking credit for the healing powers of nature. The American and French Revolutions provided the models of the democratic state, established just before the shift from the classical to modern paradigms of medicine. As we have already suggested, one of the myths of the time that scientific clinical medicine and public health would return society to its pristine state of good health by abolishing disease. Moreover, events in medicine and public health and improved living conditions did deliver a marked improvement in life expectancy and quality of life.

However, as Dubos (1960) pointed out, the ambition to conquer disease foundered upon the failure to have the same impact on chronic disease as was achieved for acute infection. Indeed in part some of the early gains are proving illusory with the emergence of bacterial resistance and with viruses proving refractory. In addition, the functional symptoms related to stress and problems of living and mental disorder have increasingly being taken to the doctor for diagnosis and treatment. An important factor lowering the threshold for seeking medical help has been that the welfare state has developed a national health scheme or health insurance which would allow easy access to medical care. Thus medical care became an integral part of the social wage, the safety net essential for the legitimacy of the modern welfare state and considered necessary for social harmony. Thus encouraged by easy access and culturally conditioned – 'if the pain persists see your doctor'- and egged on by breakthroughs, not surprisingly, patients visited doctors with increasing frequency. However of the patients directed towards the doctor, most are those stand to gain least from scientific medicine and who are most prone to iatrogenic harm and dissatisfaction. The innovation which spawned scientific medicine was the teaching hospital. What followed was a mechanical model which could be fixed by a specific technological intervention. The paradox here is that this kind of disease is relatively uncommon as a cause of symptoms but a potent threat to peace of mind.

Reefs in a Sea of Symptoms

The Peripheral Zone of medical care is therefore enormous, a sea of symptoms most of which are functional. The organic diseases are relatively uncommon, lurking below the surface like reefs to trap the unwary practitioner. Yet the ideology of modern medicine has managed to conceal the obvious, arranging funding, research and funding to be concentrated in the teaching hospital. This is an example of the ideological force of a dominant scientific paradigm, operating in large measure at least in an unconscious manner. The process was so obvious that we did not notice during the period of 'hegemonic stability' towards the end of the modern era. The great majority of those who present in the Peripheral Zone have no serious disease but fear that they have, or are troubled by symptoms. They look to the physician to call upon diagnostic technologies to confirm or to deny their fears, and seek reassurance and allay anxiety. Those with incurable chronic disease or handicap often complicated by old age, social disadvantage, poverty gender or ethnicity will often need prolonged support in order to have their symptoms alleviated, and to live in a state of constant adjustment to their limitations and fears.

Here it is absolutely essential that the illness be understood, as far as is possible in all of its complexity, including its meaning for the patient. We all have obscure symptoms from time to time for which we consult a doctor to exclude serious disease. This is the case only rarely so that reassurance and symptomatic treatment is on offer. This is when the art of medicine, especially clinical judgement is at a premium especially for those with problems of living and marital discord, sometimes drug addiction or alcoholism, or psychiatric illness or neuroses manifest as anxiety, hypochondriasis or depression. All of us have symptoms some of the time, the transients of the worried well, some have symptoms most even all of the time. These are the somatisers who express their stresses in the language of symptoms. These permanent residents of the Peripheral Zone present again and again with the same or different symptoms. A small minority cannot be convinced of the absence of disease. In the aged, functional symptoms can be hard to distinguish from organic disease or the impact of aging.

Many doctors regard functional symptoms which dominate the Peripheral Zone as trivial by virtue of their training in a teaching hospital serving predominantly the Central Zone of care. A skewed medical education and socialization has also blunted the doctor's ability to deploy the art of medicine and the direct contextual effect of healing, thereby robbing care of important contributors. The outcome is clinical inefficiency and consultation failure with patient dissatisfaction and diagnostic error with unnecessary costs, consultation failure, breakdown of the doctor-patient relationship and a poor health outcome.

Paradigms in Tension

Medicine and the patterns of illness in the Peripheral Zone of care have been moving in opposite directions. By the end of WW II the university teaching hospitals had become bastions of medical science. They continue to function as though the cure of organic disease, important as it is for us all, is the only or major problem confronting doctors – it is not and never was. By the 1950s medicine had become thoroughly obsessed with organic disease. Most primary medical care in the U.S. was delivered by specialists in internal medicine. They were not lacking in humanity but many were obsessed by the technicalities and bad at detecting and handling emotional distress. To doctors trained in the rarified atmosphere of a university hospital, a university, the 'worried well' and the symptomatic without organic disease are often seen as presenting with trivial complaints.

The same science which had delivered so much to some was often inappropriate when dealing with the many. This generated the self-image of a scientist. In the modern era, medical training was exclusively in the 'basic' sciences. The second half of the curriculum, in a university teaching hospital, powerfully reinforced that image and inculcated a mixed message. Exposure to scientific medicine certainly reinforced the ethos of science, and was separated by a chasm from the initial years. However in those hospital years, indoctrination of the student tapped into a marvelously rich clinical tradition, as a brotherhood, dating back to Pythagoras. Thus Flexner's medical curriculum developed in the U.S. and spread worldwide had the unexpected side-effect of guaranteeing that the clinician product would be 'schizophrenic' in the lay or popular sense of the word!

So the paradigm was in conflict with the unresolved competition between science and art, and this, in turn was manifest as tension between medical and lay perspectives. Patients sensed this from their own experience and were becoming alienated from doctors and mistrustful of medicine. Illness became synonymous with disease, diagnosis was decontextualized objectified, and in extreme cases was promoted as a mathematical algorithm. The clinical examination, interviewing and observing, was denigrated in favour of more 'objective' diagnostic tests and the preferred treatments became technological interventions. Medical research was biomedical research even in a clinical setting, a situation perpetuated by the granting bodies.

Uncertainty and Error in the Peripheral Zone

Uncertainty is rife in the Peripheral Zone. With biomedical science came potent specific treatment options for the patient, provided that the diagnosis was accurate. The problem was that intervention was useful only if the doctor had framed the question correctly in the first place, especially with regard to whether the illness was functional or organic disease. As it has turned out, most of those with symptoms might have been treated at home with less risk of adverse effects and inappropriate intervention. The doctor now runs the risk of being seen as just another technocrat. There are some doctors who would prefer it that way – free to treat 'real diseases' and not get lost in the swamp. But then who would decide what was 'real' or not, that most difficult of clinical judgements?

The community and public health have a problem in the cumulative effects of unwise interventions and their sequelae. These indirect costs arise from clinical error. Such 'diagnostic toxicity' can result in unwarranted disease labelling or in appropriate disease labelling. Evidence that this is so comes from our friends most of whom can recount a war story or two related to an incidental finding found on a routine examination or arising from a false positive mammogram or elevated blood cholesterol. Diagnosis can be even more difficult in patients who already have serious disease and who become depressed and anxious resulting in a subtle mix of functional and organic symptoms. Alternatively, a patient worried about heart or lung disease may complain about 'breathlessness' which on close interrogation turns out to be 'inability to get a deep enough breath,' or 'the breath stops there' (gesturing towards the mid-chest) or is 'not satisfying' – often illustrated with a sigh. This description provided with an absolute minimum of direct questioning, is virtually diagnostic of psychogenic breathlessness. These things are given a minimum of coverage in medical textbooks, and even less in the medical literature. The alert meticulous clinician can nevertheless usually dissect the functional from the organic symptom.

Then there is the psychosocial problem whereby an unrelenting search for organic disease leads the physician astray. Lack of awareness or misinterpretation of personal motivations and pressures can lead to misattribution of functional symptoms hence failure to spot the role of problems of living, anxiety and depression. Both can lead to ill-advised interventions and to missing the real problem. More subtle is failure to adequately reassure patients with unequivocally normal test results because of factors unknown to the doctor such as heath beliefs, past experience, family influence, media coverage and a host of other 'wildcard' influences (McDonald et al. 1993). Lack of communicative skill and deficiencies of supportive care can also be blamed for impairment of the placebo effect, patient dissatisfaction, lack of treatment compliance, doctor-shopping and the growing popularity of alternative medicine.

The Peripheral Zone is a swamp of uncertainty where there is a substantial element of discretion in the decisions of both doctor and patient hence much space for the intrusion of personal and social issues which may dominate their motivations. The severity of symptoms may not be compelling for the patient, either to seek medical help or to fully cooperate with treatment. That is to say that there is often a large discretional space in both cases. Here the doctor's decisions may be made under the influence of a wide variety of interacting variables, some of a non-technical kind such as the technological and diagnostic imperatives, single-minded pursuit of organic disease, seeking certainty beyond any patient benefit, bostering of confidence, fear of litigation, subtle influence of remuneration or fear of inhibiting referrals. Such influences as these can have the net effect of encouraging unnecessary intervention in a class of patients who are already vulnerable. It is also possible that misattribution of symptoms will result in a perfectly reasonable indication for intervention by a procedure of established effectiveness, but - for the wrong reason.

The diagnostic imperative may lead to overinvestigation by the 'thorough doctor' – the very thing that exposes the patient to the risk of iatrogenic illness resulting from a false positive or doubtful result from an unnecessary test, incorrect attribution of symptoms, loss of insurability or employment. Thus a doubt expressed about a heart valve after hearing a murmur in a patient who has been having panic attacks with chest pains, palpitations and breathlessness can lead to a disastrous exacerbation of anxiety. The finding of a harmless arachnoid cyst in a patient who had an unnecessary C.T. scan for headaches may lead to mounting pressure for its removal in the face of persistent headaches. On the other hand who ever heaped praise on a doctor for 100 consecutive tests appropriately not ordered, or for the judicious avoidance of an unnecessary investigation? But a single missed organic disease diagnosis can bring approbrium, and failure to act can look like negligence, especially if the means of intervention were to hand. In the case of chronic disease, the major clinical objective is its cure or palliation. Simply providing a diagnosis such as 'high blood pressure This has been called the 'labelling effect' by Haynes et al. (1978). This this study found a morbidity following the event. If there is onset or aggravation of illness as a result of a screening test seeking disease with no effective treatment, this is particularly regrettable.

Since people consult their doctor five or six times per year, there is a cumulative risk of iatrogenesis, posing a serious public health problem. The therapeutic imperative also operates. It probably accounts for some of the regional variations observed for hysterectomy. Persistent symptoms can also lead to major intervention. This is most likely when there is a non-invasive alternative to surgery such as lithotripsy (ultrasonic dissolution of galltones or kidney stones), or balloon dilatation of a coronary artery for angina. Not surprisingly, there is a tendency to try these less traumatic procedures when a patient has long suffered abdominal or chest pain, especially when an anxious family 'turns up the heat' for 'something to be done.' If the operation is unnecessary, it is an additional burden which the patient could have well done without. Costs attributable to clinical inefficiency and consultation failure contribute the lion's share of the blow-out in health services expenditure. The problems of high technology, abuse of 'big ticket items'such as computerized tomography, positron tomography and magnetic resonance imaging counterintuitively are not the main culprits of escalating costs, rather it is the cumulative cost of a multitude of flawed day to day decisions, the 'little ticket items,' and decline in the art of medicine causing consultation failure which has never been factored into economic evaluations.

These problems of the Peripheral Zone can traced to clashes of paradigm. There is tension between art and science, epidemiology and the social sciences, a wide rift between evidence-based medicine and many clinicians within the paradigm of medicine – too much biomedical science, not enough social or statistical science, the divorce of the social sciences and humanities are all evidence of a splintered paradigm. What modern medicine has to offer in the Peripheral Zone of care has led to widespread dissatisfaction, and tarnished the public image of the profession. A gap has opened up between lay expectations and the realities of what is on offer in the Peripheral Zone has led to dissatisfaction even recrimination. If they can regain the necessary balance between scientific intervention and the characteristic support of the traditional art, they too will regain some satisfaction in their practice, reduce current alienation with frustrated patients and often a feeling of being misunderstood so that a more rewarding atmosphere of practice could be restored.

Navigating the Swamp

Rather than blame the vulnerability of a sick population, the sheer complexity of the hospital environment or the hazards of the Peripheral Zone, we would do well to acknowledge all of these problems and aspire to gradual but progressive improvement in the quality of the health system. Continuous quality improvement would be the answer to some concerns. Damage to the art of medicine is a much more pervasive scourge. The only answer here is a root and branch reform of research and education to generate a new more balanced postmodern medical paradigm. Of course, not a few feathers would be ruffled and some could be edged to the limits of their tolerance but the future otherwise is too bleak to contemplate.

A New Postmodern Paradigm

These problems cannot even be researched under the old paradigm so that we need radical change, a new paradigm that we have been calling 'postmodern' which will overcome the obstacles and usher in a new era. The contribution of epidemiology and all of the arms of health services research will be involved but the methods cannot be just quantitative and scientifically controlled. We argue that the social sciences and humanities with qualitative interpretive 'hermeneutic' interpretation must be integral. In chapter 16, we describe a structure in which a unit will unite clinical research on the art of medicine aiming at multidisciplinary 'continuous clinical practice research' the humanities and social sciences to intellectually refine the art of medicine, conventional scientific methods, evaluation research, also supporting a repository of research methods for research and education for hospital and university departments interested in participating (chapter 16).

The objective of current epidemiological health services is to bring more science in to drain the swamp. A more credible alternative would be to learn to navigate it using a compass provided by both epidemiology and the social sciences. The swamp can be more easily negotiated with difficulty using the barge and pole of the interpretive paradigm when the power boat of the analytical paradigm of science is liable to break down. The treatment of psychiatric illness, common in the community and a potent cause of symptoms in the Peripheral Zone occupies an awkward middle position. It has been caught between the paradigms. Determined efforts have to explain mental illness in terms of biomedical tradition and analytical tradition as a Central Zone problem. But these have failed. In the cases of depression, schizophrenia and anxiety, this approach has enjoyed a good deal of success. The alternative is to view the eyes of the alternative hermeneutic interpretive tradition as related to psychiatric disturbance interacting with social influences; accepting this, it should marshal personal forces and cognitive recognition is the key to management. It would seem obvious that both approaches should be used.

Medicine as a Social Science

Louis in Paris in the early 1830s showed the way. He studied the effectiveness of bloodletting, de rigeur at the time, using a controlled experiment but his message was not heeded. More recently epidemiology has made its debut as 'clinical epidemiology' acting as a resource of scientific application of quantitative research methods to the evaluation the health system. More recently, this discipline has narrowed its focus to transmogrify into 'evidence-based medicine' which we deal with later in more detail since it has become increasingly at odds and controversial. However, Rudolph Virchow, pioneer of public health as well as scientific cellular medicine was right when he digressed to argue with passion that medicine is 'above all a social science' in its relationship with the community. This is true since most disease out there is functional not organic, and always will be so.

Some of the greatest early 19th century physicians, Osler, Peabody and Cabot, bemoaned their perception that, educated to follow the scientific way, were losing the ability to relate to their patients. But the liaison with science and robust clinical traditions has meant that so far clinical medicine has remained aloof from the highly relevant scholarship of the social sciences and the humanities. It is of interest to governments that the main drivers of rising costs of medical care is the result of what some might call a 'pie in the sky,' involving all aspects of medicine – clinical practice, education and research. Hence the answer to the central problems of health care means high quality medical judgements, satisfied patients especially in the Peripheral Zone of care and the revolution described involving the entire process of care. There is no alternative. Then let the dance begin.

Conclusion

The success of a medical encounter implies clinical efficiency and a successful consultation. This in turn means implies an accurate biomedical and psychosocial evaluation as the basis for treatment, patient understanding and recall, reassurance and counselling, increased patient control and satisfaction, optimal technical health outcomes and maximization of the placebo effect. Persisting tensions within the paradigm of medicine between the art and the science, and dissonance between lay and medical perspectives of illness are potent contributors to both clinical inefficiency and consultation failure. Thus the paradigm of medicine must be balanced for good clinical judgement, and lay and medical paradigms likewise for a successful consultation. Lack of clear understanding contributes to the frustration of doctors, cumulative damage to the image of medicine and unnecessary cost of care. The problems afflicting the clinical consultation between the art and science, and dissonance between art and science are potent contributors to clinical inefficiency and to consultation failure.

The problems with the doctor-patient relationship and information blockade are ultimately traceable to unresolved tensions between the art represented by the residual Hippocratic paradigm and the new biomedical science. The current training of students under the biomedical model emphasizing the scientific understanding and technical intervention has deskilled the profession with regard to the ability to offer the human understanding, social support and contextual care which so often elicits the placebo and Hawthorne effects. Externally, there is a cultural shift stressing individual autonomy. It is this hidden paradigmatic conflict which has soured the clinical and personal relationship between the modern doctor and patient, and tarnished the image of the profession. The problem has clearly been aggravated by the expansion of the Peripheral Zone of clinical care, comprising the ambulant patients with chronic disease and the worried well. The modern physician is obviously not equipped to provide a diagnosis and to provide the necessary supportive care. The problem is the schism is now between the patient's pressing needs and the lack of support.

The New Public Health Movement (Martin et al. 1989) represents a substantial response to criticism despite the fact that the discipline is directly in the firing line because their discipline tends to probe the political context of ill-health. We could speak of a 'new clinical medicine' to include a raft of band-aid solutions to the deeper wounds concerning patient dissatisfaction and declining public image, and government impatience. At least these concerns are out in the open. Since the Second World War medicine has responded to criticism but in a defensive, ad hoc and fragmented manner. Clinical epidemiology has made inroads with a few clinicians involved in trials, and evidence-based medicine has stressed scientific appraisal of the empirical research literature but is increasingly bogged down in controversy.

Lip service has been paid to Engel's 'biopsychosocial' model (Engel 1977) but more significantly, movements such as 'patient centred care' (Levenstein 1986) have appeared in response to public disquiet and to some extent as a reaction against the narrow base of evidence-based medicine (Chapter 14). These movements have proliferated like rabbits and are a potent testimony to medicine's Peripheral Zone blues. However, in general only in psychiatry and general practice have warnings been heeded the about poor communication with some action on the complaints. This is no coincidence since these are the very specialities which rely on the art of medicine and the healing power of the consultation. Ad hoc changes have been made to the medical curriculum and in some schools more extensive changes involving teaching methods and student selection. However the Mills of God grid slowly but they grind exceeding fine. Sacrosanct have been biomedical research and applied biology. Most doctors practice as they have been taught and observed in hospital practice. There has been much talk of change with no coherent direction or guiding philosophy. We continue to flounder between the well established modern and the emerging postmodern paradigms.

This problem of lack of understanding of the patient's perspective is a fundamental factor in patient dissatisfaction and an important contributor to diagnostic and therapeutic error hence to clinical inefficiency. We can only begin to build bridges if we clearly understand this. Even worse, subjective experience, the stuff of life, is often denigrated as 'soft data' (Reiser 1978). In order to understand this mismatch of expectations, we need to talk to patients, to analyse relevant texts, even consult accounts of death in the literature of the humanities to plumb meaning,. To access meaning means gaining access to qualitative data analysis to interpret narrative accounts of illness. This will require better integration of the dominant analytical and subjugated interpretive paradigms of research and appropriate modifications to medical education. This, in turn will allow students to tap into their own experience in order to cultivate empathy, and to respect and to accept stories of illness suffered by their patients.

References

American Psychiatric Society on Nomenclature and Statistics Diagnostic Manual of Mental Disorders, ed 4. Washington DC, American Psychiatric Association, 1985.

Barsky A. J., The Paradox of Health. *New Engl J Med* 318 414-8; 1988.

Bass C., Chest pain and breathlessness: relationship to psychiatric illness. *Amer J Med* (suppl 1A;92; 12S- 17S. 1992.

Brody H., The healer's power. Yale University Press, New Haven, 1992.

Ibidem., p 136.

Charon R., A model for empathy, reflection, profession, and trust. *JAMA* 286: 1897-1902, 2001.

Conrad L. I., Neve M., Nutton V., Porter R., Wear Eds., The Western Medical Tradition. 800 BC – 1800 AD. Cambridge University Press, Cambridge, 1995.

Dracup K., McKinley S. M., and Moser D. K., Australian patients' delay in response to heart attack symptoms *Med J Aust;* 166 (5): 233, 1997.

Engel G. L., The need for a new medical model. A challenge for biomedicine. *Science* 1977; 129-296.

Fitzpatrick R., Lay concepts of illness. In: Fitzpatrick R., Hinton J., Newman S., Scrambler G., Thompson J., The experience of illness. Tavistock, London, 1984. p. 27.

Fletcher C., Towards a Better Practice and Teaching of Communication Between Doctors and patients. Introduction in 'Mixed Communications,' Nuffield Provincial Hospitals Trust, Oxford University Press, Oxford, 1979.

Ibid., p. 23.

Foucault M., The Birth of the Clinic. An archaeology of medical perception. Tavistock, London, 1976.

Good B. J., Good M. J., The meaning of symptoms: a cultural hermeneutic model for clinical practice. In: The Relevance of Social Science for Medicine Eds Eisenberg L., Kleinman A. D. Reidel, Dordrecht, Holland 1981.

Guba E. G., Lincoln Y. S., Fourth generation Evaluation. Newberry Park Sage, 1989, p. 35.

Gutting G., Michel Foucault's Archaeology of Scientific Reason. Cambridge University Press, Cambridge, 1989.

Haynes B., Can it work ? Does it work? Is It worth it? The testing of health care interventions is evolving. *BMJ* 319 652-3; 1999.

Haynes R. B., Sackett D. L., Taylor D. W. et al. Increased absenteeism from work after detection and labelling of hypertensive patients. *New Engl J Med* 299: 741-41; 978.

Henderson L. J., 1935. Quoted in In: The Relevance of Social Science for Medicine Eds Eisenberg L, Kleinman A. D Reidel, Dordrecht, Holland 1981. p. 7.

Hinkle J. B., 1960 Quoted Ibidem. p. 84.

Katz J., The Silent World of Doctors and Patients. Free Press, New York, 1984.

Ibidem., p. 4.

Ibidem., p. 24.

Ibidem., p. 122.

Ibidem., p. 200.

Kellner R., Hypochondriasis and Somatization. *JAMA* 258: 2718-22, 1987

Kroenke K., Mangelsdorf A. D., Common symptoms in ambulatory care: incidence, evaluation, therapy and outcome.

Kuhn T., The Structure Of Scientic Revolutions. University of Chicago Press, Chicago, 1970.

Levenstein J. H,, McCracken E. C., McWhinney I. R., Stewart M. A., Brown J. B., The patent-centred clinical method 1. Family Practice. A model for doctor-patient interaction in family practice. *Family Practice* 3:24-30; 1986.

Lindblom C. E., The science of muddling through. Public Administration Review; 1979-89 1968.

Martin C. J., McMcQueen., Readings for Public Health. Readings for Public Health. Edinburgh University Press, Edinburgh, 1989.

McDonald I. G., Daly J., Jelinek V. M., Panetta F., Gutman J., Opening Pandora's Box: the unpredictability of reassurance by a normal test result. *BMJ;* 313: 929-32.

McDonald I. G., Information technology as a challenge to evaluation: a blessing in disguise? *Telehealth International;* 1: 21-2, 2000.

Mechanic D., Social psychologic factors affecting presentation of bodily complaints. *New Engl J Med* 286:1132-9;1972

Mizrahi T., Getting rid of patients: contradictions in the socialization of physicians. Rutgers University Press, New Brunswick N.J., 1986, p. 72.

Ibidem., p. 86.

Parsons T., The Social System. Routledge and Keegan Paul, London, 1951.

Pfifferling J. H., A cultural prescription for medicocentrism. In: The Relevance of Social Science for Medicine Eds Eisenberg L, Kleinman A. D Reidel, Dordrecht, Holland, 1981.

Reid S., Wesserly S., Crayford T., Hotopf M., Medically unexplained symptoms in frequent attenders in Secondary health care: retrospective cohort study. *BMJ* 322:767; 2001.

Reiser S. J., Medicine and the Reign of Technology. Cambridge University Press, New York, 1978.

Rittel H., Systems analysis of the 'first and second generations.' In Laconte P, Gibson J, Rapaport A eds. Human Energy Factors in Urban Planning. NATO Advanced Study Institutes Series D. Behavioural and Social Sciences No. 12. Martinez Nitjhoff The Hague, 1982, 35-63.

Rota D. L., Hall J. A., Physicians interviewing style and information obtained from patients. *J Gen Intern Med* 2:325-9; 1987.

The Royal Australian College of General Practitioners., Integrative medicine. Curriculum for Australian General Practice 2011 Integrative medicine.

Shorter E., Doctors and their Patients: a social history. Simon and Schuster, New Jersey, 1991.

Smith G. R., Jr, Monson R. A., Patients with medically unexplained symptoms. Their characteristics, functional health and heath care utilization. *Arch Intern Med* 146:669-77;1986.

Stoekle J. D., Barsky A. J., Attributions: uses of social science knowledge in the 'doctoring' of primary care. In: The Relevance of Social Science for Medicine Eds Eisenberg L, Kleinman A. D Reidel, Dordrecht, Holland, 1981.

Szasz T. S., Hollender M. H., A contribution to the philosophy of medicine: the basic models of the doctor-patient relationship. *Arch Int Med* 97: 585-92; 1956.

Toombs S. K., TheMeaningof Illness: a phonological account of the different perspectives of physician and patient. Kluwer, Dordrecht, 1992.

Tuckett D., Boulton M., Olssen C., Williams A., Meetings Between Experts: an approach to sharing ideas in medical consultations. Tavistock, London, 1985.

Tumulty P. A., The approach to patients with functional disorders. *New Engl J Med* 263:123-8: 1961.

Walker E. R., Katon W. J., Jemelka R. P., Roye-Byrne P. P., Comorbidity of gastrointestinal complaints, depression, and anxietyin the Epidemiological Catchment (ECA) Study. *Amer J Med* (suppl 1a) 92: 26S- 34S; 1992.

White K. L., Williams T. F., Greenberg B.G., The ecology of clinical care. *New Engl J Med* 265:885-97; 1961.

Chapter 11

Consultation Failure - The 'Symptoms'

In the preceding chapter we discussed the causes of failure of the communication and supportive aspects of a clinical consultation. A successful consultation is one in which the patient's objectives have been met so that he or she is satisfied with both the process and the outcome of care. We must, however, add the rider that the patient's judgement should be based upon a reasonable understanding of the important events, and specifically that there is no adverse effect of which they are unaware. In this chapter, we discuss the consequences of consultation failure leading to patient dissatisfaction. Patient dissatisfaction, in turn, is likely to curtail or diminish the powerful direct healing effects of the context of medical care itself. This is a serious loss to the therapeutic process as we will see.

Expression of Patient Dissatisfaction

Patient dissatisfaction may also be acted out as noncompliance with treatment, by failure to accept reassurance, by failure to give up the sick role to return to health and to a productive social role, sometimes despite extensive attempts at rehabilitation, by premature termination of medical contact, by doctor shopping or by 'defection' to alternative medicine. Such behaviour puzzles health professionals since it often seems counterproductive, even self-destructive. What seems illogical to the doctor, however may make good sense to patients and their families. Behaviour which might seem irrational to the observer, may be deemed entirely appropriate with full knowledge of that person's objectives, knowledge, definitions, beliefs and values. In short, their actions may be reasonably explained if only we could know more about their commitments and values, and hence about the balance of decision vectors which contributed to their judgements.

We saw in the previous chapter that the problem of loss of good clinical communication skills and supportive care has been compounded by a major increase in ambulant patients who present to a doctor complaining of 'functional' symptoms. Such symptoms are unrelated to organic disease which the modern doctor has been trained in the hospital environment to detect and treat. In the management of such patients good communication and support are at a premium. In this setting, an important aspect of healing is the direct effect of doctor and the context of healing which often has positive therapeutic effect.

Patient satisfaction, predicated upon adequate information about the quality of intervention in relation to health outcome and on a satisfying consultation, is the desired primary outcome of clinical care. Political pressures driving measurement of patient satisfaction have included the consumer movement and health bureaucracies anxious to demonstrate maintenance of standards of care in the face of cost-containment. Measurement has also been necessary to link patient satisfaction with patient behaviour such as noncompliance. Much patient dissatisfaction can be traced to unsatisfactory practical arrangements such as waiting time and difficulty in obtaining after-hours care. However patient satisfaction really centres on the doctor-patient relationship.

Benefits from improved clinical communication include improved understanding and recall, greater patient satisfaction, increased compliance, reduction of anxiety, and quicker recovery in some settings (Ley 1988). Patient satisfaction is enhanced by doctor friendliness, understanding of patients' concerns, meeting their expectations, good communication skills and by the provision of information (Korsch et al. 1968). Patient satisfaction is also related to expectations of care, including perceptions of how long the doctor spent with them. Involving patients in management planning has also been linked to increased satisfaction, and to better health outcomes (Greenfield 1988). In any case it is an ethical imperative, and often a political imperative, as more patients express a wish to be well informed or involved in clinical decisions concerning their own health care. Patient satisfaction is therefore a central requirement for good health outcomes, and as a bonus, optimises the placebo effect.

Measurement of Patient Satisfaction

Measurement of patient satisfaction is not easy. Williams (1994) explores implicit assumptions and contests the idea that patients have a level of satisfaction waiting to be measured. He specifically disputes the assumptions that a simple connection can be made to patient expectancies and values, and that satisfaction necessarily implies that aspects of service have been explicitly approved by the patient. Many patients are reluctant to be critical, especially with respect to the technical sphere of medical care where most are not competent to judge the quality of the intervention. Carr-Hill (1992) argues that satisfaction is not a unitary concept, that it can be defined differently by the same person at different times.

In their study in a neurology clinic, Fitzpatrick and Hopkins (1983) found that patient goals were much influenced by expectations which 'were expressed tentatively and seemed often to emerge out of the interview itself and the experience of making sense of the clinic setting.' Expectations were 'fluid and emergent and revised in the light of past experience.' The emphasis in the consultation was on the patient's immediate concerns. Fitzpatrick and Hopkins (1983) argue that a questionnaire can trivialise responses. Hopkins argues elsewhere (Hopkins, 1990) that '(I)n general, the most convincing studies of satisfaction are those in which particular issues are explored in relation to a particular client group or service by tape-recorded in depth interviews. From such interviews can be generated ideas for exploration by less expensive interview techniques.' When qualitative methods are used, more dissatisfaction is found (Williams, 1994).

The Contextual Factor in Healing

Good communication not only favours patient trust, satisfaction, cooperation hence a good health outcome, it also often elicits the placebo effect, a healing response to the context of the consultation. According to Houston, '(t)he history of medicine is the history of the placebo effect.' The direct effect of the healer has been known from antiquity. Socrates was aware of the 'healing effect of fair words' (Katz 1984). In modern times it was linked to psychological mechanisms. The clinical consultation incorporated an element of psychotherapy. Thus psychological healing is common to the shaman, the complementary medicine practitioner, the doctor and the psychotherapist (Frank and Frank 1991). The effect was to lift morale, and to combat demoralising meanings attached to illness. Parsons too believed that '(i)t is highly probable that, whether the physician knows it or wishes it, he is always exerting a psychotherapeutic effect on his patients' (Parsons 1951), which was incorporated into the supportive part of the art of medicine 'just as one can use a language well without even knowing that it has a grammatical structure.'(Parsons 1951).

Shorter traced the history of relations between doctor and patient over the centuries. He pointed out that an ongoing relationship did not exist before the early 19th century (Shorter 1991). The healing power of the informal psychotherapeutic interview, in which patients could tell their story in an unhurried way and the doctor took an active interest, and on which clinical practice relied until well into the 19th century, is now being overlooked by doctors and patients no longer have the same trust. The modern patient became more tuned into the workings of the inner body, more sensitive to symptoms. They had more confidence in the doctor whose image as a gentleman was still being assiduously cultivated. The high proportion of emotional illnesses in practice was recognised, and the rich German tradition of 'psychosomatic medicine' was influential in the U.S. Persuasion was an important element in the popular 'moral therapy' which was simple psychotherapy, a talking cure with rest and dietary measures. Trust was invited and the success rate in the treatment of 'neurasthenia' was claimed to be good. Certainly the closely similar chronic fatigue syndrome does not yield well today to treatment! Currently, by contrast, Shorter sees patients as often alienated and mistrustful.

The Placebo Effect

The importance of the placebo effect is underscored by the fact that 30% to 60% of subjects, sometimes even more, have exhibited the effect with a variety of clinical and experimental interventions (Shapiro and Shapiro 1997). According to the modern paradigm, the phenomenon has also been narrowly construed as a nuisance factor which complicated the objective evaluation of the specific therapeutic efficacy of drugs, a factor to be cunningly eliminated by the technical advance represented by the double-blind clinical trial. What is now beginning to be appreciated is that this 'contextual care,' a function of the image and social skills of the clinician, of patient expectation and of the clinical setting itself is always at the core of successful medical treatment. To ignore it is to court patient dissatisfaction and to sacrifice a highly effective therapeutic instrument. This instrument is undoubtedly the most effective available to the clinician working in the Peripheral Zone of care wherein lies the great bulk of illness. Neglect of this contextual care by the modern clinician has been blamed for the poor image of the profession and for its failure to fully capitalize on its scientific success.

Here then was the key to the positive effect of the clinical consultation itself. Sympathetic understanding, empathic support, careful explanation of the nature of illness, promoting the patient's understanding of illness in his or her own terms, persuasion with regard to normality or need for treatment, assuaging of doubt and anxiety are all major factors in patient satisfaction. These effects, in turn, enhance treatment by promoting patient cooperation and contribute to patient well-being directly through the contextual factor. This contextual healing effect represents the impact of the art of medicine as it applies to treatment. The positive effect attributed to the giving of pill or potion regardless of any specific biological effect was the intervention originally referred to as the 'placebo effect.'

The placebo effect appears to occur in the course of any clinical transaction as well as in many contrived laboratory situations. In fact the placebo effect can involve a therapeutic instrument (syringe), the healer (doctor, nurse or charismatic figure), a medical environment (dispensary or hospital, ward or laboratory), or clinical ritual (protocol of administration, physical examination). Hence it is clear that the effective agent is not really the inert pill or similar intervention, rather the active agent should now be seen to be the interplay of numerous variables comprising the entire context of the act of healing (Balint 1955). The intervention itself should be seen as simply providing a focal point. This point was emphasized by Balint who organized discussion groups in the context of general practice which focused on psychological aspects of illness, functional illness, so common in outpatient and general practice. These discussions had beneficial effects which included the patient's dealing with the doctor, and increased personal satisfaction for the doctor. This procedure was an important leap forward in the management of functional illness. The term 'Hawthorne Effect' has been applied to the positive therapeutic effect of simply showing evidence of caring for the patient (Spiro 1986). In order to avoid semantic quibbles, we lump these effects of the healing context and simply refer to the 'contextual factor.' The vexed question of the mechanism of the placebo effect is comprehensively covered by Bausell (2009).

Many of the studies of the placebo effect have involved the relief of pain, but improvement has been reported for a wide range of symptoms and conditions. However the evidence for placebo-induced improvement in organic disease, particularly cancer, is unconvincing (Spiro 1986). One of the most impressive results was the improvement of angina pectoris in all patients who had a 'sham' operation instead of a procedure (internal mammary artery ligation) mistakenly believed at the time to do so by increasing blood flow to the heart (Cobb 1959). Although practically any treatment can elicit the effect, its anticipated potency can have an effect; thus an injection may be more effective than a pill, and a painful injection more than a painless one. The effects of a placebo are generally transitory but may last for months.

Although the placebo effect is pervasive, its occurrence in a particular patient is largely unpredictable. The search for personality factors which were pursued assiduously in the earlier years of research in the area and for an archetypal 'placebo reactor' has been largely unsuccessful (Brody 1980). The reason for this is that the effect appears to be related to the interaction of a variety of factors related to patient expectation which are specific to their own medical and life experience. On the other hand a high component of anxiety, patient dependency associated with illness and higher suggestibility all favour its occurrence (Brody 1980).

Clearly the placebo has been integral to the art which has been exercised with success by doctors for many centuries and by other healers for aeons. Nevertheless, in general, an intervention can generally be used more effectively if we understand it better. After considering the many explanations posed for the placebo effect in the literature, ranging from the biological through to the cultural, one is left with the impression that to attempt a strictly mechanistic explanation has been futile. Thus it appears that the entire clinical context - physician, patient, instruments, ritual and setting can have a holistic effect on an individual patient's response to treatment, and that this operates in relation to that individual's personality, past medical history, social and cultural influences and beliefs.

Clearly this effect involves an extraordinarily complex hierarchical system. Some believe that the phenomenon is related to socio-cultural meaning hence difficult or impossible to explain under the modern scientific paradigm alone. This has important implications for research but does not necessarily mean that it is futile to seek lower order biological mechanisms for higher order effects. Some of its effect may be in the form of subconscious conditioning influences based on past experience with the medical system; in addition there is the effect of vicarious influences such as information obtained from other people and from the media. It is likely that there is a variety of positive feed-back loops involved as well. Among them might be increased confidence, decreased negative introspection, sensitized perceptions to beneficial effects, and selective positive interpretation of symptoms, allaying of fear, diminution of anxiety and the corresponding amelioration of symptoms attributable to mental stress.

Primacy should generally be accorded to the highest and most holistic level of understanding. In this case, there is ample evidence of a strong socio-cultural influence, of the power of symbolic effects related to the ethnomedical constructions of the society (Morris 1997). Society and culture mediate by providing appropriate roles to be played by the sick person and by the healer as well providing influences which will either produce illness or favour healing. The basic features of faith healing in primitive cultures were the provision of reassurance, suggestion that healing would occur, transference of responsibility to an authority figure, support of the social group as well as manipulation of cultural symbols often in a ritual setting. These apply no less in the placebo effect which may be considered to be a subset of faith healing.

An adverse effect of science on the paradigm of medicine is that this gift of healing has been received somewhat churlishly. Even in the time of Hippocrates, physicians had over-reacted to the magic of the cults and mistrusted the power of the word (Spiro 1986, p189). What the early Greek physicians gave up, it seems, was not just the incantations of the priests but also the positive effects of words of comfort. While the good clinician nowadays does have a deep tacit understanding of this manifestation of the art of medicine, conscious consideration or discussion of the phenomenon is likely to be a source of embarrassment. Its mysterious nature, the aura of the charlatan and the overtones of faith healing do not sit well with the conventional view of scientific medicine based on the natural and biological sciences. The explicit use of the placebo medicament also raises ethical problems. In addition, the effect can be threatening because physicians do not own the exclusive rights to this kind of treatment. The placebo effect is, in short, unpalatable in the modern paradigm of medicine. The fact is that to fail to take account of such an important factor in treatment because the phenomenon is somewhat arcane or because the mechanism is unclear, is, of itself, profoundly unscientific.

Treatment under the biomedical model has stressed technological intervention to the point of losing sight of the importance of the healing context. So much is this so that the tendency of scientific research methodologists to denigrate the placebo effect as a nuisance variable, a bias to be included among the important sources of experimental error, an effect modifier to be factored out of a randomised controlled trial. The objective is to determine the 'real' therapeutic effect of medication. To exclude it required the development of the modern double blind clinical trial. Such trials incorporate blinding of patients and doctors in an attempt to get rid of any placebo effects. A placebo effect may also occur in patients in both control and treatment arms of the study. Moreover blinding is not always feasible or successful. To separate a specific effect and a placebo response in a clinical trial is therefore more difficult than it at first seemed.

A good consultation with skillful and caring exposition of illness according to the patient's own personal and cultural models of illness promotes better understanding in the patient by resolving doubt, by clarifying specific misunderstandings, by persuasion and by assistance with the interpretation of illness manifestations. Thus the good clinical consultation can be indirectly therapeutic by ensuring good information related to medical diagnosis and psychosocial influences, by promoting patient satisfaction and engendering cooperation. A trusting therapeutic relationship also maximises the placebo effect which has a direct effect. Since these direct and indirect effects are interactive and multiplicative, the quality of the clinical consultation emerges as the key to good medicine especially in ambulant care where most care takes place, where practice is most difficult, where symptoms are not usually due to organic disease, where scientific medicine is most limited and where the placebo effect is most important. The public knows this and are hostile towards medicine's neglect in this area.

Noncompliance

The astounding fact is that, in a community with such respect for scientific medicine, roughly one in two of patients who seek counsel on the care of a medical illness do not implement that advice by taking medication as recommended (Sackett and Snow 1979). The rate of noncompliance can be influenced by the method of measurement. However, across a wide range of clinical contexts and in many countries, there is a surprising degree of consensus on an average figure of 50% for chronic illness in adults and in children. This is surely one of the most important but least discussed conundrums in health, rarely alluded to by doctors or taught to students yet among the most researched of all clinical topics. There are cogent reasons why we cannot ignore noncompliance. It is a mortal enemy of effective clinical intervention. Obviously medication which is not taken cannot work. Why would patients stop treatment, 'self-regulate,' take 'drug holidays,' or 'top up' before their next appointment, especially when the penalty could be hospitalisation, blindness, rejection of a kidney transplant, recurrence of asthma, epileptic fits or relapse of a psychiatric illness! In addition, if the doctor should react to apparent patient non-responsiveness to treatment by increasing the dose, toxicity can result.

Noncompliance not only substantially reduces the overall effectiveness of clinical care, it also places an additional burden on health facilities, and wastes vast sums of money at a time when health costs are such a major issue. One estimate reported $100 billion annually in the U.S. - approximately 10% of the total health budget (Berg et al. 1993). Moreover, noncompliance can invalidate the results of clinical trials upon which the very evidence of evidence-based clinical treatment policies ultimately depend. There are public health ramifications too. Irregular therapy can lead to microbial drug resistance, a serious problem in the treatment of tuberculosis currently re-emerging as a threat. Even more serious than these immediate considerations, noncompliance is a breach of trust, damaging to the doctor-patient relationship and sending a powerful message that we do not understand such basic aspects of medical care.

There are obvious, mundane explanations for failure to take medication as ordered. For example, the elderly in particular, may forget, become confused, misunderstand, be unable to read the label or open the bottle. But noncompliance usually runs much deeper than that. The Federal Government in Australia is planning to pay pharmacists to undertake a 'medication check' which is likely to be yet another superficial response which is unlikely to be the answer to noncompliance. What is not widely accepted in medical circles is that much evidence locates the roots of noncompliance in the problems of the doctor-patient relationship in the clinical consultation. It is often a symptom of consultation failure, a bellwether of difficulties in doctor-patient communication, and linked to low levels of patient satisfaction (Ley 1988).

There is evidence that the patient responds to many influences of which health professionals would rarely be aware. Many patient characteristics, nature of the illness and aspects of the patient interview have been related to noncompliance. Clearly, however, There is much evidence that noncompliance is often intentional behaviour. To the extent that it is, whether or not to take treatment as advised or not is, at some level, the result of a patient judgement. Their judgement on treatment recommendations can clearly be influenced by personal traits, beliefs and attitudes based on life experience and past medical encounters, specific attitudes to drug-taking and to doctors, and their own interpretation of illness events, influenced in turn by advice given by respected others, family or friends (Tuckett et al. 1985). There may be, for example a clash between the medical interpretation of illness and rationale of treatment and that of a lay model of illness or a specific family myth, so that following consultation with their lay network they may reject the doctor's interpretation of the illness or choice of treatment.

Important relationships have been demonstrated between patient noncompliance and poor quality of doctor-patient communication (Blackwell, 1979), patient dissatisfaction, and lack of patient understanding and of recall of the clinical consultation (Ley 1988). Patients may be alienated when the doctor who is dominant maintains the focus on the manifestations of disease and its mechanism, while the patient's priorities are related more to understanding of the illness in the context of social predicaments and of problems of living. Almost all research has adopted the perspective of the health profession, of 'the system' as it were. Hence noncompliant patients in the hospital setting who have simply resisted accepting a totally passive role can end up with the label of 'problem patients' (Wright and Morgan 1990).

Further evidence of the clash between lay perspective and medical paradigm is the word 'noncompliance' which itself has come to be imbued with a pejorative meaning. The implication of the word is that the patient is a passive agent who is expected to follow without question medical advice handed down by a paternalistic doctor – 'he who must be obeyed.' Parson's sick role implied that legitimacy in the sick role depended upon following medical advice. Not to do so was therefore construed as deviant behaviour. The argument of the consumer movement is that it should ultimately be up to patients to make their own decisions without the imputation of disobedience if they do not follow medical counsel to the letter. More politically correct terms proposed include 'lack of adherence' and 'self-regulation' which acknowledge these demands for recognition of greater patient autonomy. However no such alternative has gained widespread acceptance, and changing the word does not alter the flawed conceptual assumptions on which the term currently rests.

The reason that there have been so few studies of noncompliance which have used interview to obtain the views of the clinical players is that the research agenda reflects the effects of Snow's Two Cultures (Snow 1964). In Chapter 4 we pointed to the unfortunate schism between those disciplines committed to quantitative methods, survey or trial using statistical analysis and those committed to interpretive methods, interview and observation using qualitative analysis. In the case of noncompliance, a clash between the analytical scientific paradigm and the interpretive humanistic paradigm has created an unbalanced research agenda which has failed so far to engage with the meaning patients attach to noncompliance. As Haynes (1987) has put it: '(u)nfortunately the wind seems to have gone out the sails of the compliance research enterprize.' The likely reason is clear enough. The extensive literature on noncompliance has so far exhibited a strong proclivity for analytical quantitative methods - surveys, randomised trials, and psychological modelling. An important result has been is a lack of clear understanding of the patient perspective, or rather the wide range of such perspectives. Interviews are an indispensable method for exploring the meaning of noncompliance for patients, and to explain their behaviour. Such understanding is also necessary for designing trials of interventions. Nevertheless only a handful of empirical studies of involving observation and interview in the clinical environment are to be found in the literature.

When seeking solutions, the tendency has been to blame patients (the victims) for their forgetfulness or perversity, to look to the packaging of medication and other external factors which might act as impediments to regular taking of drugs, or to attempt to modify patient behaviour according to the dictates of a variety of cognitive models. All have their place but none has proved to be a panacea. This should not come as a complete surprise, given most noncompliance is intentional behaviour, often reflecting unrecognized problems in the doctor-patient relationship or patients' own views or wish to experiment according to their own ideas. The upshot is that much noncompliance is a symptom of serious paradigmatic tension, and the cure will be a new postmodern medical paradigm which is closer to equilibrium with the lay culture. This, we believe, is true. However, perfection is the enemy of the good, and something has to be done now, in this awkward period of transition.

A Place for the Nurse Practitioner

It is commonsense nevertheless that every attempt should be made to understand the patient's ideas about illness and their social background, to clear the deck of doubts and misunderstandings, to inquire sympathetically about problems of compliance, to identify specific obstacles as they arise. This can be done without a paradigm shift. Nevertheless, for those with special problems, including the aged and the chronically ill, and those in whom life-style changes are important, a more intensive strategy may be required. Thus there have been moves towards having a doctor and nurse working in collaboration in primary care or hospital ambulant care. Given the constraints on the doctor's time and the biomedical focus of medical training, this makes sense, and has been shown to be one of the most effective methods of identifying and tackling the problems underlying noncompliance. Thus, in the case of chronic illness, a doctor sympathetic to the idea of the interactive and supportive consultation style can work in tandem with a nurse who is able to visit and or follow-up by telephone, who has established rapport and trust and is in contact with family.

A nurse can supply ongoing support, and is directly aware of the patient's social context, hence in a good position to detect, suspect, confirm, address and prevent noncompliance in ways tailored to the patient's specific needs. The patient can be referred back to the doctor for periodic review when there is lack of progress, new problems arise or complications arise. This is an especially attractive option in general practice in light of the importance of anxiety, age and chronic illness, of problems of living and social predicament in the genesis of symptoms. A patient advocate could subserve a similar function. It is here in the Peripheral Zone of care that a patient-centred, in-depth interactive and supportive style of relationship is of manifest importance. However organised, a therapeutic alliance which encourages frank discussion and cards on the table would allow barriers to compliance of the willing patient should be identified and cooperatively dismantled. Covert noncompliance should not then be necessary as a means of expressing dissatisfaction or disagreement, frustration or anger. Should patients wish to modify or discontinue medication, discussion of this as an option should be discussed, with continued support a possibility, and the door left ajar should they change their mind.

Failure of Reassurance and Functional Illness

We noted earlier that the bulk of patients who seek medical help have health problems for which an organic cause cannot be diagnosed. Such patients with functional symptoms are the majority of patients in the Peripheral Zone of clinical practice. Their symptoms, we recall, may be symbolic in response to stress, minor disorders amplified by anxiety of body phenomena misinterpreted as possibly a serious manifestation of disease, a tendency to express feelings via symptoms or an unshakable conviction of serious illness. Anxiety is often caused by a medical query such as a heart murmur or the identity of a breast lump, raised in the course of a result of a routine examination, or the finding in a routine electrocardiogram or X-ray which shows an equivocal appearance or suspected abnormality. How common this is can be deduced from the high proportion of medical consultations for symptoms for which no organic disease is found and from the prevalence of normal test results in laboratory files. Under these circumstances, it remains, of course, central to the task of medicine, and clearly expected by patients, that an appropriate effort will be made to find and to treat disease or to reasonably exclude its presence, allowing appropriate reassurance.

Surely patient reassurance must be the commonest of all medical transactions. A medical consultation will almost always result in one of two outcomes. When a patient goes to a doctor with symptoms, the key issue is what these mean. In a minority of cases, modern clinical diagnosis complemented by special tests will reveal organic disease which can be treated in some way. In the majority, symptoms are functional, manifestations of responses to stress and anxiety or attributable to some minor abnormality often amplified by specific concerns and fears. When a clinical examination or test raises a query about abnormality, most people have some anxiety. The usual outcome, however, is that testing reveals no serious disease. Hence the commonest of all clinical transactions is an attempt to explain and reassure (McDonald et al. 1993).

Playing for Big Stakes

Reassurance is therefore the primary need of the worried well, that majority of patients presenting with symptoms in whom organic disease has been excluded, as well as important in some patients with acute or chronic disease whose fears are worse than their condition. Reassurance often involves otherwise healthy people, so that the stakes are high. The penalty for failure can be the human suffering and cost associated with life-long anxiety. Given all of this, we would expect that the topic of reassurance, techniques for handling it and the pitfalls and results would be thoroughly covered in the medical textbooks, figure prominently in the medical literature and be extensively taught and demonstrated to medical students. So strong is the influence of the modern paradigm, however, that it is almost completely ignored in medical education! Students are more or less expected to pick it up by role modelling or to regard it as a matter of commonsense which does not require teaching. If they sought information of reassurance, they would be bound to be disappointed since it is not discussed to any extent in medical text books. Finally, if the text book wished to include it they would be frustrated by the extraordinary absence of information in the medical literature, or in the literature of any academic discipline for that matter.

The problem is that it seems to be the common assumption of doctors trained in the modern scientific paradigm that reassurance must follow careful disclosure of the fact that no disease was found, often with the offer of a plausible alternative. Unfortunately this quite logical assumption is often incorrect. In practice, reassurance is commonly either unsuccessful or only partially successful, leaving a legacy of doubt and residual anxiety. Even if reassurance is achieved at the time, increased vulnerability to anxiety may have been created in the event of a future query, say in the case of a heart murmur, or future disconcerting experiences such as the death of a friend or occurrence of new symptoms. This is particularly unfortunate if the anxiety was created in the first place by a query raised by a routine examination for an incidental complaint such as bronchitis or treatment for high blood pressure, or in the course of an insurance or employment health check, or as a result of a community screening for elevated cholesterol or breast cancer.

After a negative result from investigations, patients are particularly dependent on communication with their doctors to try to understand why they were queried in the first place. Under these circumstances patient-doctor communication is difficult especially if the doctor loses interest in the light of failure to find organic disease. We do not know what long term effect this has on the patients, or even to what extent it contributes to dissatisfaction with medical care. Once organic disease has been excluded, the illness is then traditionally placed in the category of functional illness with a strong emphasis on 'neurosis' as the likely 'cause.' Sometimes the patient is simply told that 'there is nothing wrong.' This is likely to be rejected outright by a patient with continuing symptoms or by the network of lay consultants drawn from family and intimate social circle.

On the other hand, few doctors are equipped with the knowledge or have the inclination to engage in the substantial dialogue often necessary to disclose, and hopefully to remove, the doubts and log jams of misunderstanding which prevent successful reassurance. This is especially so since patients may require much encouragement if they to disclose their crude lay models of illness to a highly trained health professional. The medical perception is that patients worried about underlying disease are reassured when they are clearly and unequivocally informed that they are well. In practice, we now know that reassurance often fails, although doctors are not often aware of this (McDonald et al. 1993). Even if the doctor offers some plausible explanation for symptoms and attempts to persuade the patient that all is in order, there may still be serious impediments to the acceptance of reassurance.

Wildcard Effects

According to the patient's understanding and model of the illness, however, the reassurance may simply have been unconvincing at the time or rendered so by subsequent events (McDonald et al. 1993). The patient with attacks of chest pain, palpitations, breathlessness, numbness, faintness even a sense of impending death - actually panic attacks as manifestations of severe anxiety - will be difficult to convince even with the help of a normal test. This is especially so if doctors have previously failed to spot this acute psychological response for what it is, and missed the underlying social predicament such as final examinations or inescapable marital discord. Similarly, the person with an 'innocent' heart murmur whose sibling died of unsuccessful surgery for congenital heart disease will require some persuasion of the innocent character of a murmur. The patient who is mistrustful of technology may not believe the X-ray or ultrasound machine's results.

Sometimes the impediments to reassurance are quite subtle, based on the totality of the patient's life history and medical experiences and on a rich tapestry of family, social and cultural influences. These interact such that the outcome of attempted reassurance often could not have been predicted prior to testing by doctor or by patient, hence we have named them 'wildcard' effects. In a minority of patients, there is resistance to reassurance related to symptoms which are expression of anxiety (somatisers), or to morbid fear of illness (hypochondriasis) when even good communication and patient support achieve only temporary reassurance or none at all. Nonetheless there is an especially heavy responsibility on the doctor to help to steer the patient through the episode which maximum understanding of what is going on, without the hazards of unnecessary testing, with adequate moral support with an explanation that can be understood so that there is no residual misunderstanding, doubt or residual anxiety.

Lacking feedback or misunderstanding the reasons for failure, there is no pressure to improve things. Yet all clinicians know that reassurance is not always successful although they are rarely conversant with the extent to which this is so. Confronted by the patient who is refractory to reassurance, clinicians are inclined to fall back on labelling the patient as neurotic or crazy rather than exploring the psychological or social background which makes it easier to understand if not explain. As with noncompliance, a trained nurse or patient advocate in frequent contact with patient and family may be an attractive option to reinforce the message of normality, and to achieve and maintain reassurance.

Conclusion

The current rate of patient dissatisfaction with medical care is an indictment of the modern medical paradigm. Its consequences are serious. It is an important contributor to some of clinical medicine's most intractable problems. Dissatisfaction impairs the contextual factor in healing, including the placebo effect, encourages noncompliance with treatment, failure of reassurance, and makes alternative medicine more attractive. Research as a basis for improving patient satisfaction, maximising the contextual factor, improving compliance or facilitating reassurance has not been very successful. Basic reasons for this have been a lack of interest from the health professionals, the difficulty sociology researchers have in obtaining access to the clinical environment, and paradigmatic prejudice of health services researchers in favour of quantitative epidemiological methods. Surveys yielding information about the average influence of a large number of individual variables do not do justice to the complex interaction of influences which can influence the judgements and responses of an individual person under particular social circumstances. A qualitative interpretive study was required (McDonald et al. 1996).

Humanistic care so-called is an issue important to patients, and an integral part of the healing process. Dismissively dubbed the art of medicine, it has nevertheless survived its bruising encounter with science. Their cooperation with potent modern treatment, hence its likely success, still depends on sensitive communication. Such skills, belonging to the art of medicine, were paramount in the traditional clinical paradigm up to the time of the impact of science (Jewson 1976). The wide spectrum of patient responses in these situations in relation to personality, life experience and social context cannot be studied without interpretive field studies which include interview of patients and probing of meaning by qualitative analysis. This hiatus in our knowledge of the patient perspective on the meaning of their actions is hampering the planning of interventions to improve supportive patient care. Hopefully, the introduction of multidisciplinary continuous clinical practice research will rise to this challenge (Chapter 16).

References

Balint M., The doctor, his patient, and the illness. *Lancet;* I: 683-688. 1955.

Bausell R. B., Snake oil science. The truth about complementary and alternative medicine. Amazon. 2009.

Berg J. S., Dischler J., Wagner D. J., Raia J. J., Palmer-Shevlin N., Medication compliance: a healthcare problem. *Annals of Pharmacotherapy* 1993; 27(9 Suppl):S1-24.

Blackwell B., The drug regimen and treatment compliance. In Haynes RB, Taylor DW, Sackett (Eds) Compliance in Health Care. Johns Hopkins University Press, 1979.

Brody H., Placebos and the Philosophy of Medicine. University of Chicago Press, Chicago, 1980.

Brody H., The Healer's Power. Yale University Press. *New Haven* 1992, p. 81.

Carr-Hill R. A., The measurement of patient satisfaction. *J Pub Hlth Med* 114: 236-49;1992.

Fitzpatrick R., Hopkins A., Problems in the conceptual framework of patient satisfaction research: an empirical exploration. *Sociol Hlth and Illness* 5: 297-311; 1983.

Frank J. D., Frank J. B., Persuasion and Healing: a comparative study of psychotherapy. The Johns Hopkins University Press, Baltimore, 3rd edition, 1991.

Greenfield S., Kaplan S. H., Ware J. E., Patients' participation in medical care: effects on blood sugar control and quality of life in diabetes. *J Gen Intern Med* 3: 448-57;1988.

Haynes R B., Wang E., Gomes M. D. M., A critical review of interventions to improve compliance with prescribed medications. *Patient education and counseling.* 10: 156-66. 1987.

Hopkins A., Measuring the quality of medical care. *R Coll Physic* London p. 55-60;1990.

Houston W. R., The doctor himself as a therapeutic agent. *Annals Int Med* 11:1416-25 1938.

Katz J., The Silent World of Doctors and Patients. *Free Press*, New York, 1984, p. 20.

Korsch B. M., Goxzzi E. K., Francis V., Gaps in doctor-patient communication. *Pediatrics* 42: 855-71; 1968.

Ley P., Communicating with patients: improving communication, satisfaction and compliance. *Croom Helm,* London, 1988.

McDonald I. G., Daly J., Jelinek V. M., Panetta F., Gutman J., Opening Pandora's box: the unpredictability of reassurance by a normal test result. *BMJ* 1996; 313: 329-32.

Morris D. B., Placebo, pain, and belief: a biocultural model. Harrington A, ed. Harvard University Press, Cambridge, 1997.

Parsons T., The Social System. Routledge and Keegan Paul, London, 1951, p. 54.

Parsons T., The Social System. Routledge and Keegan Paul, London, 1951, p. 55.

Sackett D. L., Snow J. C., The magnitude of compliance and noncompliance. In Haynes RB, Taylor DW, Sackett DL (Eds) Compliance in Health Care. Johns Hopkins University Press, 1979.

Shapiro A. K., Shapiro E., The Placebo: is it much ado about nothing? In: The Placebo Effect: An interdisciplinary exploration. Harrington A, ed. Harvard University Press, Cambridge, 1997.

Shorter E., Doctors and Their Patients: a social history. *Simon and Schuster,* New Jersey, 1991.

Snow C. P., The Two Cultures and a Second Look: an expanded version of The Two Cultures and the Scientific Revolution. Cambridge University Press, Cambridge, 1964.

Spiro H. M., Doctors, Patients, and Placebos. Yale University Press, *New haven,* 1986.

Spiro H. M., Doctors, Patients, and Placebos. Yale University Press, *New haven,* 1986, p. 189.

Tuckett D., Boulton M., Olssen C., Williams A., Meetings Between Experts: an approach to sharing ideas in medical consultations. Tavistock, London, 1985.

Williams B., Patient satisfaction: a valid concept ? *Soc Sci Med* 38: 509-16; 1994.

Wright A. W. L., Morgan W. J., On the creation of 'problem' patients. *Soc Sci Med* 30: 951-9; 2002.

Chapter 12

The Evaluation of Health Care

Thus far we have considered the impact of various perspectives or paradigms on clinical care. But the problems of paradigm do not end with those concerning the practice of clinical medicine. Equally important are the same issues capable of influencing its evaluation where similar paradigmatic road blocks threaten its effectiveness. Few would argue that there is no need for reform. But who or what is to guide that reform process? The concept which has evolved as one answer to that question is the concept of multidisciplinary top-down 'health services research' which we discuss in this chapter and bottom-up multidisciplinary 'continuous clinical practice research' discussed in Chapter 16. Intermingled with the powerful and potentially disruptive forces of paradigmatic diversity there are bound to be intrusions on vested interests, crimping of opportunity, encroachment on privileges and political pressures. There may be further conflict with patient advocates and conflict of professional and public interests. Equally important are those changes which involve clinical evaluation, medical education and research. But what form will it take and who is to undertake this extensive and delicate reform process diplomatically with minimum friction and heat?

Central to our argument has been the notion that clashes of paradigm have had a damaging effect on clinical care and diminished respect for the doctor in the community. However it is difficult to imagine issues more likely to encounter serious problems than the clashes of paradigm which must surely occur with evaluation of health care and in particular the processes of clinical decision making, the role of expert judgement and of expertise, and with the doctor-patient relationship perceived as under threat by the inroads of evidence-based medicine. Many clinicians point to the fact that evidence-based medicine has never been evaluated, and perhaps never will be, and that it distorts the realities of clinical management by its central naïve concept of 'evidence.' A more general objection is that evidence-based medicine reinforces the perception of a technocratic, disease-orientated, hospital-based health care system, distorted as a side-effect of the brilliant accomplishments of biomedical science, and currently under some pressure from evidence-based medicine.

Engaged under the umbrella of 'health services research' are a number of disciplines which have emerged separately but which are now tending slowly to coalesce. Hence we have the evaluand, clinical medicine, and the evaluators in the form of quality assurance, technology assessment, effectiveness and health outcomes research, clinical epidemiology, evidence-based medicine, public health, sociology and economics - each with its own distinctive paradigm contributing to its fundamental beliefs, skills and prejudices. Clashes of paradigm are therefore inevitable but their impact can at least be minimised if we understand them and are willing to engage in constructive dialogue. Unless such interdisciplinary tensions can be minimised there can be little hope for optimising the effectiveness of clinical interventions, for continuous improvement in the quality of care and containment of its cost.

There was no place for the notion of evaluating the effectiveness or cost of health care in the classical paradigm of medicine. Even after appropriate methods had been developed employing statistics early in 19th century France, and medicine was shifting to the new scientific paradigm, clinicians did not follow the lead offered by Louis, one of the pioneers of the new science (Chapter 6). The key role of context is evident from the broad similarity of circumstances surrounding the genesis of the abortive precursor of health care evaluation of in the first half of the 19th century - Louis' numerical method - and its revival in the second half of last century. Both its emergence and its re-emergence have occurred in times of instability when social and political change impinged on the delivery of health care as a key social institution. In each case, a contested space had developed at the intersection of clinical medicine, public health and government. Not to mention the eventual financial pressures on governments and their generally defensive response.

The first such contest was in France after the Revolution during the early growth of capitalism and emergence of a welfare state. The second was the early 1970s when capitalism was seen by reactionary forces to be threatened by the cost of the welfare state with medicine seen as one of the most profligate spenders. Medicine, fortified by links to science, was recruited by the post-Revolutionary government in France in a clash with the traditional Hippocratic medical perspective of the Societe de Medicin. The old order, elitist and wedded to the ancient model of disease was doomed. What saved the day for the medical profession was its new commitment to scientific medicine nurtured in the new teaching hospitals. Thus transmogrified by science, medicine swept to a dominant position in emerging health systems in the Western world, re-established its credentials with governments and spread its benefits to most citizens of the modern state. A similar drama is being played out today.

The main drivers of social, cultural and political change in the 19th century were easy to identify as Enlightenment thought with scientific rationality as a central thread, and the ideal of democracy linked to modern industrialism. Today the scene is not so clear cut. Since the 1950s at least, there has been intellectual ferment challenging the claims of science to objectivity, a renewed interest in language, discourse and social evolution, recognition of the complexity of systems in the natural and social worlds, increased scepticism and a challenge to authority of all kinds. This ill-defined phenomenon has been called 'postmodernism' (Best and Kellner 1997). One could argue that the coalescence of disciplines which has produced a challenge to conventional thinking about the mechanisms underlying the much maligned clinical judgement, and rejection of the role of emotions in decisions have the hallmarks of postmodern research attitudes.

A more visible influence has been the emergence of 'late capitalism' characterised by dry economics, economic rationalism, which has driven a reduction of welfare spending and privatisation, and integrative forces accelerated by information technology, part of so-called 'globalisation' (Castells 1996). A challenge to economic growth initiated by the oil crisis and recession of the 1970s set the stage for a call for greater accountability of social welfare services including the health services and medical practice.

The last development was the insight which led to 'clinical epidemiology.' Just as Morris and Cochrane in Britain the 1950s had seen that epidemiology provided the tools for the study of the delivery of health services, so Feinstein in the 1960s first spotted the lack of science in the methods of clinical examination of patients and diagnosis of disease (Feinstein 1967). He saw then that epidemiology also provided the empirical scientific methods required to connect the variety of specific patterns of illness which characterise a single disease in individual patients to prognosis and the choice of best treatment.

Closing the Circle

The field of evaluation of health care is a contest being played out right now between clinical medicine, clinical epidemiology and evidence-based medicine, and managerial authority in the form of government bureaucracy and managed care interests. Feminism, consumerism and environmentalism have also emerged as political players. Public health has once again been recruited, this time as managers of a changing health system, and as exponents of health services research. At the same time, clinical epidemiology and evidence-based medicine, representing the clinical adaptation of epidemiological methods, have become major contributors to health services research which is seen by some to have a coercive element aiming to rein in clinical autonomy, even to ration services by stealth by the enforcement of clinical guidelines.

Five main disciplines have emerged for the evaluation of health. The first was 'quality assurance' which began as a routine clinical activity under the aegis of doctors in the early part of the 20th century (Codman 1914). The second was the recognition by Morris (1957), in Britain, that epidemiological methods based upon empirical statistical science could be used not only to study diseases but also to study the methods of delivery of health care to the community. This was the birth of 'health services research' although he did not call it by that name. The name, much of the further development of the idea in the U.S., and certainly the realisation of the importance of the connection of health services research to clinical practice, we owe to Kerr White. Related is health outcomes research which utilizes indices of quality of life.

The third key development was the development of the research technology which has come to epitomise science in evaluation and health services research – the evolution of 'evidence based medicine' which has championed the cause of the randomised controlled trial. This discipline has evolved from a related progenitor - 'clinical epidemiology.' The application of the randomised controlled trial to the evaluation of drugs can be seen in retrospect as a response to specific events, in particular the sulphanilimide disaster of 1937. It can also be seen as societal and political resonance with concerns over the effectiveness of medical treatment and the issue of lack of medical accountability. In that sense it was a warning red flag shown to a profession previously accustomed to only in-house and less formal evaluation of its activities. It could even be seen as an early manifestation of the mood of economic rationalism and managerialism which had targeted health care.

The fifth development was the establishment of medical technology assessment which emerged in the U.S. during the 1970s as a systematic program of evaluation of new high cost technologies. It was a policy tool with an eye to containment of cost. Its base has been since broadened by the advent of 'effectiveness research' and related 'health outcomes research.' The historical evolution of each of these disciplines has forged a distinctive world view, specific assumptions, methods and research agendas, reacting to in quite different historical and political contexts. However they are now coming together under the umbrella of health services research, so that quality assurance or continuous quality improvement, and technology assessment currently share the burden of evaluating clinical services and interventions with major methodological input from clinical epidemiology and its progeny, 'evidence-based medicine.' These various disciplines which have evolved to study health care have distinctive historical roots, potentially conflicting commitments and different but complementary agendas.

Quality Assurance

The circle which eventually did link clinical medicine, public health and government in the evaluation of health care included quality assurance - an important discipline which began under medical aegis early in the century. It is now seen as one of the arms of health services research. As such it has forged strong links to clinical epidemiology. The idea of quality which began with the work of Codman, a surgeon and administrator in Boston in the early part of the 20th century (Codman 1914), focused on medical audit, extending later to self regulation activities such as accreditation. Over the years, medical audit became firmly entrenched in hospitals as, later spreading to encompass accreditation of hospitals. These activities made no claims to being scientific, were the exclusive province of doctors, part of the self regulation with which the profession is comfortable. Quality assurance activities are now undertaken by medical and non-medical experts, mainly in hospitals. Its perspective is primarily the standards of routine clinical care and its management, although information aggregated across institutions can be used to inform policy. Its aim is to monitor on-line the processes and outcomes of clinical care with the objective of detecting and correcting problems thereby achieving continuous improvement.

It is useful to see the process and general aims of our 'continuous clinical practice research' which we will describe in Chapter 17, as analogous to 'continuous quality improvement.' Both are continuous iterative dialectical processes, and they aim respectively for continuous improvement in the quality and safety of the clinical care environment and the quality of procedures of clinical care itself. In Europe, linkage of general practice, hospital and social services as a part of utilizing information technology to link these elements of the health system. Note that such networks are becoming common in European Union countries.

The basic philosophy of quality assurance has been influenced by 'systems thinking' (Donabedian 1966) which originated in sociology and in biology in the last century became widespread after the Second World War. The monitoring was done using methods and statistical techniques of industrial control based upon systems assumptions (Plsek 1990). Modern methods of corporate management, encapsulated in the concepts of continuous quality improvement and total quality management, were exported from U.S. to Japanese corporations, were then imported back into the health system (Blumenthal 1995). During the 1980s, the quality movement moved to centre stage, and developed a top-down perspective as the containment of care costs without the public perception of reduced quality became a basic objective of governments, health bureaucracies and of managed care (Health Care Quality Commission 1998).

The National Health Service in Britain's adoption of the principle of managed competition has driven a strong interest in quality of care, especially of clinical audit which involves management, nursing and allied health disciplines, and on the development and implementation of clinical guidelines. Later, following the demise of the conservative government and the accession to power of the Blair Labour government, the emphasis on competition switched to cooperation with the motif of 'clinical governance' which emphasises professional accountability (Quality Management Team, NHS Executive, Department of health 1999). Clinical epidemiology and evidence-based medicine (see below) have become key elements in the development of clinical indicators, monitoring of trends and planning and analysis of audit studies.

Quality assurance has traditionally been less concerned with evaluating specific technological interventions. Quality assurance is therefore a variety of 'formative' evaluation in that its primary aim is to incrementally improve the clinical system evaluated rather than to simply pass judgement upon it. Much of the data is qualitative. It is therefore liable, like other forms of qualitative research, to be denigrated. A variant, 'continuous quality improvement' has gained recognition. This variant tends to be more supportive and collaborative, and less adversarial. A variety of techniques for monitoring quality of care have evolved under the influence of industrial quality control and of scientific thinking in general. Most of these methods are relatively simple. They include methods for flagging potential problem areas (indicators), for tracking trends in statistics and indicators (graphs with confidence intervals), for locating difficulties (flow charts, Pareto diagrams, clinical indicators), for obtaining feedback on-line from participants (informal discussions, meetings, surveys, formal consensus methods), and for identifying specific problems as they arise and solving them by consensus (clinical audit studies), all supported by appropriate statistical analysis. These methods overlap with those of clinical epidemiology and epidemiological skills are increasingly being used to refine the methods of continuous quality improvement.

The paradigm of quality assurance has not clashed much with the clinical paradigm. The reason is that, until quite recently, its activities were practised by clinicians who conducted audits and developed the indicators which flagged adverse events. Since clinical epidemiology follows the methods of empirical statistical science, its major thrust differs from the paradigm of quality assurance which is strongly committed to the systems approach. The latter aim for continuous quality improvement which tends not to blame the individual for most error. Indeed a good case can be made in the future for quality assurance and centres for the study of clinical practice to be merged because their eclectic approach to research method is very similar, albeit that the former has its focus on continuous quality improvement in the standard of facilities and efficiency of procedures, while the latter has an analogous focus a is about research and evaluation involving continuous improvement in clinical diagnosis and management interventions.

In both cases, ongoing evaluation research predominantly utilizes formative methods with on-line feedback leading to prompt action (Scriven 1967). Summative evaluation methods are used much less, when trials and cost efficiency issues can capture this information from a stable and better understood pattern of utilization of an intervention. Having the imprimatur of approval of management and government, of course, quality assurance is already well established. At present, the widespread application of clinical practice research awaits the establishment of centres for the study of clinical practice, and availability of 'reflective' physicians as defined and discussed in Chapter 16.

Technology Assessment and Effectiveness Research

Health services research from the community perspective dates back to Morris' 'Uses of Epidemiology' (Morris 1947), but was named and driven as a movement by Kerr White in the United States. It subsequently developed in a fragmented manner mainly in response to specific problems. Medical technology assessment emerged first with its sights set on the financial threat posed by high cost medical technologies (Foote 1987). In the U.S. during the 1960s, a systematic program of evaluation of social institutions appeared which was called 'evaluation research' or 'program evaluation,' largely in response to increased welfare spending of Johnson's Great Society and the cost of the Vietnam War. The drive for cost containment was exacerbated by a subsequent oil crisis and economic recession in the early 1970s. Thus, against a general concern about the societal impact of new technologies, Congressional interest in technology assessment was stirred by cost developments in the Space Program. Subsequent interest in medical technology specifically began in the mid-1970s, stimulated by the cost of renal dialysis to the Medicare Program, the prospect of the artificial heart and the advent of CT scanning, the first of the high cost imaging technologies (Banta and Luce 1993).

Other countries followed the U.S. lead by establishing formal arrangements for the evaluation of health technologies (Banta and Luce 1993). In retrospect, these developments can be seen also as an early manifestation of dry economics and economic rationalism. The emphasis of medical technology assessment has been on synthesising information. Clinical epidemiology and health economics have provided information for estimations of cost and benefit, in particular the results of randomised trials, and construction of outcome measures including quality of life and patient satisfaction.

Medical technology assessment, primarily an instrument with the objective of providing objective evidence of the impact of new high cost technologies, has been supported by governments world-wide. Its chief orientation is therefore top-down, towards the policy perspective. Its main aim has been to synthesise information on specific medical technologies with an emphasis on the new and the expensive. The conduct of such studies is the mandate of health services researchers calling mainly upon the methodological skills of clinical epidemiology, evidence based medicine and health economics. Information used is mainly in the form of formal scientific studies of efficacy, trials of performance under ideal conditions of use, and studies of cost-effectiveness. Medical technology assessment is therefore a form of summative evaluation, an aid to the establishment of priorities in the allocation of scarce resources by informing political decisions. Missing we note is representation of those with most at stake - clinicians!

Costly Judgements, Costly Interventions

It was soon recognised during the 1980s that, even in hospital practice, high unit cost technologies such as CT scanning and renal dialysis were not the main problem in the escalating cost of medical care. The focus therefore shifted from the specific big ticket technologies to the effectiveness of day-to-day decision making and to the evaluation of the efficiency of clinical care itself. This undertaking should surely have been mainly the responsibility of clinicians. A shift of emphasis from specific technologies to problems more intimately associated with routine clinical care was heralded by Congressional support for a program of 'effectiveness research.' Its main foci of interest have been the appropriateness and effectiveness of medical interventions. These interests merged with a closely related activity which was focused on the measurement of health outcomes expressed in terms of functional status, quality of life and patient satisfaction.

These initiatives included attempts to measure quality of hospital care and of that delivered by individual medical practitioners. These activities have been focused on obtaining information from administrative and clinical data-bases. Again clinical epidemiology has played a key role in the construction of outcome measures, and in the methods of analysis of data-bases. All of these evaluation activities, linked together under the umbrella of health services research, have therefore called upon the skills of clinical epidemiology and, more recently, evidence-based medicine as part of their methodological tool box. They do not, however, enlist interpretive methods as well such as underpins our idea of clinical practice research nor do they examine the clinical tools of patient evaluation, history and physical examination.

Technology assessment has presented a low profile vis a vis clinical medicine. Few doctors are aware of its activities which are directed at government and health policy issues. Its publications are read by very few clinicians. Hence there was no paradigm clash with clinical medicine. Proponents of effectiveness research and health outcomes research were more critical of clinical medicine, especially in the context of variations in clinical judgement (Chapter 12). Nevertheless there has been little engagement between these paradigms and that of clinical medicine. There has been some controversy surrounding the validity quality of life measurement, particularly to the need to augment patient input (Gill and Feinstein 1994). The discipline which has clashed with clinical medicine has been a stripped down version of clinical epidemiology called 'evidence-based medicine' which has had a major impact on thinking in health care. Hence we will critique it in more detail later.

The first application of science to the evaluation of clinical care occurred in Paris early in the nineteenth century when C-P-A Louis conducted a scientifically controlled study of the popular therapy of bloodletting. It was shown to be ineffective. The basic idea of a scientific approach to evaluation of medical treatment subsequently lapsed for 150 years! I have already pointed to the application of science to clinical care in the form of epidemiological methods of research. Adroitly applying his training as a mathematician, Feinstein made two proposals. Feinstein first introduced the idea of dealing with the complex interaction of variables determining patient presenting signs and symptoms of illness, patient treatment preferences, prognosis, choice of treatment and recording of the response, and many more, as 'patterns' of such variables needed to scientifically summarise a patient's and the illness manifestations required a scientific classification based on taxonomy, analogous to the scientific classification of plants and other living things. Feinstein's aim was computer storage of these individual patients' patterns of illness as 'thumb-nail sketches' representing the complex interaction of many variables to produce the specific 'clinical picture.' To achieve this, he proposed the taxonomic approach to classification to be expressed in terms of Boolean logic, mathematically expressed as Venn diagrams. Perhaps not surprisingly, this important but admittedly rather unfamiliar even somewhat esoteric idea did not catch on with clinicians.

Around 1970, his other insight notion of using epidemiological methods for the evaluation of health care did finally emerge again, the second side of Feinstein's idea. This was in the form of a new evaluation discipline he called 'clinical epidemiology.' By this he meant the application of scientific methods based on epidemiology, the science of public health, to generate empirical statistical clinical medical research. (Feinstein 1985). In order to pre-empt possible confusion, we note in passing that the name had been used first quite differently by John Paul (1938) also from Yale, to describe the study of disease ecology in families and small communities, a part of what would today be called 'community medicine.'

Clinical Epidemiology and the 19th Century Shift of Paradigm

The development of clinical epidemiology has been described as a 'paradigm shift' (Feinstein 1983), but empirical statistical science did make its initial appearance in medicine through Louis in the early 1800s at the same time as did the new biomedical science (Chapter 6). Hence its second sortie into the inner citadel of clinical practice should be seen, not as another paradigm shift, but rather as a much delayed completion of the same shift which produced scientific medicine just 200 years ago. Feinstein was a clinician to his bootstraps so, not surprisingly, his original concept of 'clinical epidemiology' was entirely faithful to clinical traditions which focus on bedside medicine and on the individual patient. Clinicians think in terms of the patterns of evidence of individual cases of illness, and these clinical pictures are the vehicles of their communication with one another. Based on Feinstein's conception, when empirical statistical science emerged within medicine in the 1960s, the methods used were the empirical study designs and statistical methods used by epidemiology. This was well accepted by clinicians but has been an issue with evidence-based medicine as will be seen.

In his ground-breaking 'Clinical Judgment,' Feinstein (1967) also showed how scientific thinking could be applied to improve the clinical examination of patients, and developed a taxonomy of disease presentations. As a clinician, he called for a broad program of clinical epidemiology which applied a range of epidemiological methods to study the relationships of these clinical patterns of illness to treatment and patient outcome. The importance of clinical medicine's reliance on the experience of individual cases, given structure by a taxonomy of illness, is reasserting itself since information obtained under controlled conditions as in a clinical trial, yielding abstracted and averaged data, is oftentimes insufficient for the clinical practitioner who must deal with the illness of the individual patient in a specific context. Moreover, as we will suggest in the last chapter, advances in information technology will make it possible for the patterns of illness in individual cases to be stored not only in the memories of clinicians, in the literature and in textbooks but in data bases of patterns, taxonomic patterns including patient symptoms, signs and test results, illness details, estimates of prognosis, details of treatment and outcomes, a resource built up in the course of routine clinical care, but also accessible locally and worldwide as aids to diagnosis, prognosis and treatment response accessible to clinicians wherever they be.

Feinstein freely acknowledged that clinical pictures of illness based upon empirical observation had been used by earlier clinicians - by followers of Hippocrates in ancient Greece, and by Sydenham in 17th century England. We have noted also that attempts had been made by French clinicians who used combinatorial probability and the analogy with language and with chemical compounds, to develop a more scientific interpretation of these patterns just before the scientific revolution in medicine. Feinstein's claim was, nevertheless, that 'the therapeutic decisions of clinical judgment require valid evidence, logical analyses, and demonstrable proofs. Their scientific quality can be discerned, assessed, and improved by the same rational procedures used for any other act of experimental science' (Feinstein 1967).

In short, a taxonomy of illness pattern could be linked to outcomes using empirical scientific methods. At the same time his respect for the long evolved traditional procedures of clinical practice was manifest, and he freely acknowledged the limitations of science in the 'environmental' issues, that is the social context of the patient. Feinstein's brilliant insights thereby narrowly missed the opportunity to initiate our idea of multidisciplinary 'clinical practice research'!

Clinical epidemiology and biostatistics started out with a broad base and initially at the burgeoning department of Clinical Epidemiology and Biostatistics at McMaster University. This new department, the first of its kind in the world, set up with Dave Sackett as founding Chair with the assistance of John Evans, founding Vice-chancellor at McMaster and with the support of the influential Fraser Mustard. Sackett was inspired by Feinsein's pioneering work on the application of Boolean algebra to clinical diagnosis. Feinstein was appointed Foundation Director of the Robert Wood Johnson Foundation, and a Professor of Medicine and of Epidemiology at Yale. Feinstein took Sabbatical Leave at McMaster, and Sackett and he set up the innovative new department.

Clinical epidemiology was applied in the clinical context by other groups in the U.S. who emphasized its teaching potential, and its importance in the activities of a department of internal medicine. The movement spread worldwide. In this setting, it engaged with the need of general internal medicine to re-establish its identity in competition with the medical specialties which had strong roots in biomedical science. Clinical epidemiology also exploited a window of opportunity provided by managed care and related cost-containment measures. It was clinical epidemiology according to this broad formula which was spread around the world by the Rockefeller Foundation through the International Clinical Epidemiology Network supported by the Rockefeller Foundation (White 1991). Kerr White aimed to use clinical epidemiology as a kind of Trojan Horse to try to get clinicians to first take on board epidemiological methods, then to direct their attention outwards towards health services research and the study of disease from the population perspective. The hope was that this initiative would therefore build a bridge across the chasm between clinical medicine and public health. Thus far, as suggested previously, this has been a lost cause.

What we should note at this point is that the key requirement for connecting clinical illness to prognosis and treatment is a systematic taxonomy which covers, not only the different patterns of illness which are the manifestations of different diseases, but different patterns manifest by patients with the same disease. This is crucial because a different clinical presentation and clinical course of a disease frequently means a quite different prognosis and a different plan of treatment. Even the early development of clinical epidemiology had already left behind this crucial ingredient of Feinstein's initial agenda for introducing taxonomic science into the methods of clinical practice. We therefore need to keep this hiatus in mind when we summarise the evolution of clinical epidemiology up to the present time, and discuss the emergence of the variant known as evidence-based medicine.

We return to this important question of taxonomy when we consider the important issue of clinical data-bases and the current state of play in evidence-based medicine. We have proposed that in his judgement, Feinstein, trained initially as a mathematician, had invented clinical epidemiology, as well as what he called 'clinimetrics'; this was essentially a method of operationalizing or coding clinical evidence to allow creation of taxonomic patterns which can summmarise such data scientifically so as to allow its critical contribution to diagnosis alongside scientific evidence. Regrettably, clinimetrics did not take off, probably because few clinicians or epidemiologists understood his argument which applied Boolean algebra (Venn diagrams) which many clinicians would find somewhat arcane for bedsise application.

Now clinimetrics could bridge a gap which has developed between evidence-based medicine and clinicians who object to the downgrading of clinical experience and expertise in 'league tables' of strength of diagnostic evidence. Essentially clinimetrics confers scientific validity upon clinical 'soft data,' hence the ability to manipulate it to potentially allow research data to be generalized to the management of individual patients in a doctor's medical practice. This was a return to the taxonomic botanical classification of the individuals' clinical manifestations of illness, a technique dating back at least to Linnaeus, perhaps even to Hippocrates! The world has now moved on. There has been a steady increase in combining quantitative data with qualitative, 'mixed methods research' giving access to both numbers and meaning extracted from a combined data-base.

A few clinical variables are obviously already expressed in quantitative form – to whit heart rate, blood pressure, respiratory rate, temperature, body weight, duration of illness. Nor have clinicians been entirely remiss with regard to developing the necessary definitions and ordinal grading scales comprising 'clinimetrics.' Severity of pain is usually quantified according to the common 'mild, moderate, severe' scale, as would be symptoms such as limitation by angina of effort and intermittent claudication. Nevertheless, the quality of such instruments should be evaluated using psychometric indices of reliability and validity, calling on experience in 'psychometrics.' Textbooks and research papers already contain many important definitions, classifications and grading scales. In 1939, Wagner and Keith produced a grading scale for severity of hypertensive retinopathy. Other well-known examples include the New York Heart Association grading scale for dyspnoea, the Apgar score for neonatal respiratory distress, grading of carcinoma (e.g., breast, colon) for prognosis and treatment, a classification of coronary events and the Glasgow Coma Scale widely used to express depth of unconsciousness and the Jones criteria for the diagnosis of rheumatic fever. No doubt many more clinimetrics could be developed for patient assessment. Quality assurance would also benefit from more precise data.

Clinical Epidemiology Gains a Foothold in the Clinical Scene

There was initially virtually no resistance to clinical epidemiology from within medicine, and certainly no political controversy. The name was becoming familiar to doctors. The discipline had worked its way into academic departments of general medicine, staked a claim at the edges of medical education, and was beginning to establish a modus vivendi with biomedical science by providing a useful window to skills in research method and biostatistics. Its existence was little known to those outside of health, to academics in other disciplines, or to consumers - nor had governments displayed much interest. Clinical epidemiology was therefore well on its way at last to successfully, unobtrusively breaching the ramparts of the traditional clinical paradigm by gradually introducing empirical science into clinical practice and research.

During the 1980s it could be said that clinical epidemiology was going about its business, spreading the word effectively with a low profile and without generating much controversy. Its agenda was not difficult to understand and certainly not easy to object to. Its scientific approach to clinical methods was clearly useful to clinicians who wished to practice more effectively, and useful to a profession which wished to improve its image while maintaining its commitment to science. A major critic was public health which saw it as a way of enhancing the power of clinical medicine under false pretenses by concentrating on clinical decision-making as a distraction from the central concern of that discipline - the delivery of health care and the welfare of the population at large. This was a clear paradigm clash between clinical medicine with its focus on the individual and public health which serves the community. Hence Last (1988) described the name of 'clinical epidemiology' as an 'oxymoron,' and the movement as 'a threat to health.' However this was never a dialogue which came to the notice of many clinicians.

From Clinical Epidemiology to Evidence-Based Medicine

Feinstein's original program of clinical scholarship with its emphasis on clinical patterns of illness was broad in that science was to be applied across the board to the refinement of clinical practice and research. This can be seen as the 'soft program' for the deployment of empirical science in clinical medicine. We should note that this is a form of clinical practice research - but differs in that Feinstein saw traditional clinical methods as informing the personal and social part of the consultation rather than an improved academic and practical understanding available from the social sciences and humanities. In this sense, his clinical research moves away from the biomedical to address the problems of 'clinical inefficiency' but not 'consultation failure' as we have defined it.

The McMaster department became the driving force for the further development and dissemination of clinical epidemiology with its emphasis on refinement of research method, strongly focussed on randomised controlled trials, economic analysis and quality of life measurement, and on developing an epidemiologically based critique of evidence in the medical literature. This became the 'hard program' in that it considerably narrowed its intellectual focus to the randomised trial as an experimental method for testing hypotheses, and to mathematical modelling as a direct aid to diagnosis. There was also a strong emphasis on the on-line evaluation of the quality of clinical evidence in the medical literature. It was at McMaster that the first move was made to connect the findings of clinical trials to health policy through links to health economics. It was this 'hard program' of clinical epidemiology which formed the core of evidence-based medicine, as first proposed and as it since developed.

Two primary forces have driven the evolution of evidence-based medicine - the idea of a critical approach to the evaluation of medical evidence –'clinical appraisal,' and the use of data-bases to collect the results of randomised controlled trials, pioneered by the Cochrane collaboration. The former,'critical appraisal,' emanated from McMaster University, the latter from Oxford University. Critical appraisal was defined as 'the application of certain rules of evidence to clinical symptoms and signs, paraclinical laboratory and other diagnostic tests, and published data (advocating specific treatment manoeuvres or purporting to establish the aetiology or prognosis of disease) in order to determine their validity (closeness to the truth) and applicability (usefulness in one's own clinical practice).'(Sackett et al. 1991). Guyatt had coined the term 'evidence based medicine' to describe clinical diagnosis which explicitly evaluates and incorporates such evidence from the medical literature. In the second edition of 'Clinical Epidemiology: a new science for clinical medicine,' Sackett et al. (1991) state that: 'Around our town, the incorporation of critical appraisal into clinical practice often is called "evidence-based medicine."'

The departure of evidence-based medicine from the original broader agenda of clinical epidemiology was explicitly acknowledged: 'Its shift in focus (from theory and explanation to tactics and clinical applications) provokes our growing ability to transform critical appraisals of evidence into direct clinical action.' (Sackett et al. 1997). Nevertheless the spotlight has shifted from Feinstein's central challenges for the 'clinical scholar' – to whit the development of a distinctive clinical taxonomy, vocabulary, definitions, and clinimetric tools, and a research program which would link clinical disease patterns and patient cooperation to treatment outcome. However, this broader agenda for clinical epidemiology has regrettably been a casualty of the strong current of evidence-based medicine. No one has so clearly articulated what is really at stake as Feinstein. While he acknowledged the importance of randomised trials which are at the heart of evidence-based medicine, he has expressed his concern about 'diversion of prime intellectual energy from the more basic scientific work that needs to be done..' Thus he complained that 'the meta-analysis of randomised trials concentrates on a part of the scientific domain which is already reasonably well lit, while ignoring the much larger domain that lies either in darkness or in deceptive glitters.' (Feinstein 1995). Evidence-based medicine soldiers on, albeit with some evolutionary modifications.

The Roots of Evidence-Based Medicine

When the importance of counting outcomes and statistical analysis surfaced again within health care during the 1950s, it was hardly surprising that these skills were imported from epidemiology, the basic science of public health, the sister discipline of medicine in the modern health system. Hence the interest in the evaluation of diagnostic tests such as the chest radiograph, in the randomised trial predominantly to test drugs and the blossoming of clinical epidemiology. The influence of science in our culture is still strong. The icon of science is the laboratory experiment. It is not surprising therefore that a form of clinical epidemiology has evolved - 'evidence-based medicine' - which focuses its attention on the randomised controlled trial and trial meta-analyses of treatment effects to the exclusion of the large number of variable influencing a clinical decision. The emphasis of evidence-based medicine is on collecting the results of trials, and using statistical meta-analyses and scientific reviews to synthesise them, then making this knowledge resource available to clinicians, patients and administrators as an aid to better decisions. This might not sound like a controversial activity but it has become so.

Clinical epidemiology had initially been a North American phenomenon, despite the beginnings of health care evaluation being credited to Britain. Evidence-based medicine then took off in Britain where public health has traditionally been much stronger. Thus 'evidence-based public health' had actually begun with Morris' 'Uses of Epidemiology' (Morris 1957). The time was ripe in that Archie Cochrane had already raised awareness with his widely publicised plea for the use of randomised trials to evaluate health interventions (Cochrane 1971). This was implemented as policy when the Peckham Inquiry placed increased emphasis on health services research, and supported the development of a new style of clinical epidemiology unit based on evidence-based medicine.

The Cochrane Centre

Also key was the existence of The National Perinatal Epidemiology Unit at Oxford, funded by the World Health Organisation and British Department of Health in 1978. Its founder, Iain Chalmers, an obstetrician at Oxford, had already appreciated the importance of making 'hard evidence' from randomised trials on the efficacy of interventions available to clinicians by gathering it into a computer data-base, the central task of the Cochrane Centre established by the NHS in 1992. Sackett moved from McMaster to take up a chair in the Research and Development Centre in Evidence-based Medicine, also at Oxford.

Other important ingredients in the evidence-based medicine stew was the concept of scientific synthesis, the generation of scientific reviews of the medical literature undertaken with statistical analysis, with special precautions to minimize bias and error, and developing interest in evidence-based clinical guidelines. The Cochrane Centre and this unit formed the nucleus of the Cochrane Collaboration, founded in 1993 when 77 people from 9 countries formed 'an international network of individuals committed to the preparation, maintenance, and dissemination of systematic reviews of research evidence about the effects of health care' (Chalmers et al. 1997). This initiative continues to develop as a collaborative effort to facilitate systematic reviews of RCTs across all major areas of health care.

The major contribution of evidence-based medicine has been its pioneering effort to make scientific evidence more readily available to clinicians, together with promoting critical appraisal of evidence. In medicine, synthesis of evidence has traditionally been informal in the form of personal experience, and collected in textbooks and as narrative reviews in the medical literature which were frequently biased due to the author's interests and affiliations. The main interface between the Cochrane Collaboration and those with a stake in the health system is through the Cochrane Library. Its core comprises The Cochrane Database of Systematic Reviews and The Cochrane Controlled Trials Register. The Cochrane Review Groups which generate and update these reviews concentrate their attention not only on diseases within medical specialties but also on the components of the health care system, that is the settings, providers, consumers, interventions and on the methods used in the empirical studies and process of synthesis. Other data-bases maintained include a Cochrane Review Methodology Database and The Database of Abstracts of Reviews of Effectiveness containing abstracts of reviews from a range of other sources. Input from consumers is actively sought - in line with Iain Chalmers' early commitment. Education and support are available from Cochrane Centres which have been established worldwide. Most support so far has come from governments and universities but more links to non-profit private agencies and support from industry are anticipated.

Narrowing the Focus of Clinical Epidemiology

Taking stock of these developments, we can now clearly see a spectrum of agendas for clinical epidemiology. (a) Kerr White's notion of more scientific clinical care linked to public health research in the community was the broadest of these. (b) Feinstein's program was a comprehensive injection of science into the techniques of diagnosis and treatment but he saw no sense in trying to recruit clinicians into the work of public health. (c) The McMaster program which evolved into evidence-based medicine drew the circle still more tightly still around the randomised trial and clinical appraisal. (d) Our objective is rather to broaden the concept into 'clinical practice research' which can address the problems of clinical inefficiency and consultation failure with the indispensable assistance of the social sciences and humanities.

It is difficult to imagine that anyone would argue against more intellectual rigour in clinical techniques or that better scientific evidence could per se be anything but a good thing. In any critique of this initiative, what must be at issue must surely be a question of balance of influences. The impact of biomedical science on the medical paradigm was obviously beneficial, providing insurance against early premature death or disablement, and protection against unnecessary suffering. However at the same time the biomedical disease model did tend to distort clinical care such that curative intervention was elevated over comforting support, and rational diagnosis of disease over understanding of illness in its social and cultural context. These have been unfortunate side-effects of the potent highly beneficial impact of the 'basic medical science.' So it is for clinical epidemiology and evidence-based medicine. Better decisions made on the basis of better evidence must be a good thing. But are there have been some side-effects.

What Is to Come?

It is much too early to study the history of evidence-based medicine. The discipline is still evolving. For example, it has softened its stance on the importance of patient values, the role of clinical expertise and biomedical evidence in response to criticism, and to some extent softened its stance on the primacy of randomised controlled trial evidence. In fact Charles' and coworkers' critique (2011) has analysed this as a series of 'versions.' They have drawn attention to a number of shortcomings in developing a model of how to implement an EBM practice. They point to a lack of scientific rigor in terms of failing to clearly define and operationalize each model variable, to justify the inclusion of each component, to showing how to how to weight and integrate each component of the model in order to apply evidence-based medicine in practice. Also, when the model is revised, the authors should justify the changes, explaining why certain components are added, deleted or modified, and most of all how the revised model is better than the previous versions. Charles et al. (2011) argue the fundamental requirement that evidence-based medicine must be empirically evaluated - the evidence-of-effectiveness challenge, an objection raised by others. How come that has this absolutely basic requirement has not been required until now? Then there is the authority challenge, essentially replacing the 'clinician authority' by that of evidence-based medicine gurus, the methodological problem of conflicting hierarchies, and the intolerably narrow definition-of-evidence controversy.

What has to be clearly spelt out is that clinical decision-making, like patient judgement, may require evidence for patient management which will then be applied with the guidance of a more comprehensive postmodern medical paradigm which encompasses some or all of the contributors to a clinical management decisions, to whit - the patient's social context, treatment environment, patient narrative, computer stored individual illness pattern, the clinician's experience, expert consultations, clinical appraisal of empirical evidence, basic biomedical science data, clinical epidemiology, clinical physiology, pathology and clinical biochemistry, as well as with currently neglected evidence from the social sciences and humanities. It must also be conceded that emotional forces must impact on both doctor and patient influencing their judgements, and the core skill of clinical judgement, a 'threatened species' needs a committed defence from its misguided detractors . If physicians do respond to the call for compromise, perhaps advocates of EBM would accept the central importance of clinical experience, and the 'soft' clinical data diligently made 'hard,' operationalized and contextualised by narrative.

There is not yet a vantage point from which to gain an overall perspective. We will, however, argue that to achieve balance between the many influences on clinical judgement and, to the program of clinical research, requires simply that clinical epidemiology and evidence-based medicine be incorporated with the social sciences and humanities into a broader framework of clinical practice research, the outlines of which we will sketch in the last chapter. These disciplines will also become part of the reflective physician's store of tacit knowledge, accrued unconsciously the hard way from clinical experience, and to be deployed and consciously in clinical decision-making and in clinical practice and research together with explicit knowledge garnered from books, the literature and from verbal presentations.

In order to discern the requirements for such a framework it is necessary to look carefully at the perceived shortcomings of clinical epidemiology and of evidence-based medicine.

These are more cogent in the case of evidence-based medicine because it has accentuated some of the problems by both narrowing its focus and by acquiring a much higher political profile. It is in this form that the paradigmatic clashes with clinical medicine have taken place. The emphasis on the scientific analysis of the technical outcomes of intervention has been sharpened, and the focus on hospital interventions increased by increased concern about the quality of evidence for scientific clinical intervention.

Evidence that the supportive role of clinical care and art of medicine has been a subjugated paradigm has been the tendency of clinical research to persistently ignore important questions related to patient and doctor behaviour, or to address them without recourse to appropriate interpretive qualitative methods. These are unfortunate side-effects of the more recent potent highly beneficial impact of a 'new science of clinical care,' one based upon empirical statistical science imported from epidemiology. The effect has been to hamstring a critical area of research, and to concentrate the research of clinical epidemiology and evidence-based medicine on the technological intervention in the hospital setting, the Central Zone of care, with a tendency to ignore the setting in which most clinical care actually takes place - in primary care practice in the Peripheral Zone of clinical care.

This is an unfortunate case of 'searching under the light.' The emphasis on probability-based quantitative data and clinical trials is also seen by some clinicians as denigrating the value of clinical experience, and its incorporation into guidelines raises the spectre of coercion of doctors to conform and of rationing based on data from trials. Thus evidence-based medicine is the pointy end of clinical epidemiology. In this form it has proved especially attractive to governments and to managed care which in itself sets off alarm bells in clinical circles.

The empirical statistical science which underpins both the original clinical epidemiology and the new evidence based medicine is quite compatible with the science of medicine but clashes with the art at some key points. A basic dissonance is that this new science presents results for groups of patients while the clinician must deal with individual patients, and this is the basic reason why the external validity of trial epidemiological is limited when applied to clinical problems. Another is that clinical diagnosis is a process of interpretation of the illness of a patient in social and cultural context. This complex system does not easily lend itself to splitting off the scientific and technological concerns which emerge in the clinical consultation from the problems and predicaments of the patient's life. Reliance on the methods of empirical science also means that the interpretive process of diagnosis is misunderstood, oversimplified models applied to it, important problems neglected if they do not yield to the quantitative scientific approach alone. Qualitative research is urgently needed as an integral part of our clinical practice research toolbox.

Conclusion

The health system has responded to pressures for integration. There has been a strong tendency towards the linking up of previously loosely articulating modules of health care delivery and related social services. A corresponding tendency for the various activities of health services research, which had developed in an ad hoc manner in response to specific problems, to converge into a more coherent activity. Of all these activities of health services research, there has been only one, evidence-based medicine which has had serious clashes with the clinical paradigm. These clashes are of the utmost importance to the success or failure of health services research at clinical level, to our 'clinical practice research,' as it were. We therefore devote the Chapter14 to examining the strong interaction of the paradigms of clinical medicine and of evidence-based medicine. The centre for the study of clinical practice reflects these same pressures, by playing a leading role in initiating and promoting clinical practice, and being involved in a full range of evaluation activities.

The development of the concept of an integrated and comprehensive program of clinical research should also contribute to the lowering of fences around individual subdisciplines of health services research - quality assurance, health technology assessment, effectiveness and health outcomes research, clinical epidemiology and evidence-based medicine. All of these need to work effectively – along with the social sciences! This underlines the importance of injecting the social sciences and humanities into the medical curriculum. This is turn would facilitate a more integrated approach to clinical research. This is not to be taken to mean that these activities can simply be merged. On the contrary, each has evolved to fill a particular niche. What is needed is to link them up, exploit their areas of overlap and, above avoid or at least paradigmatic conflict. Although postmodern thinking has brought with it some reaction against science, and more specifically a formidable challenge to an excessively positivist approach and to the reductionist methods of empirical statistical science, the influence of the physical and biological sciences has remained dominant in our culture welded as it is to the modern medical paradigm.

References

Chalmers I., Sackett D., Silagy C., The Cochrane Collaboration. In: Non-random reflections on health services research on the 25th anniversary of Archie Cochrane's Banta HD, Luce BR. Health care technology and its assessment: an international perspective. Oxford: Oxford University Press, 1993.

Best S., Kelner D., The Postmodern Turn. The Guilford Press, New York, 1997.

Blumenthal D., Applying industrial quality management science to physicians' decisions. In: Blumenthal D, Scheck AC eds. Improving Clinical Practice. Jossey-bass, San Francisco, 1995.

Castells M., The Information Age: Economy, Society and Culture. Volume 1: the rise of the network society effectiveness and efficiency. Maynard A, Chalmers I. Eds. London: BMJ Publishing Group, 1997.

Charles C., Gafni A., Freeman E., The evidence-based medicine model of clinical practice: scientific teaching or belief-based preaching? *J Eval Clin Pract.* 2011;17(4):597-605.

Cochrane A. L., Effectiveness and Efficiency: Random reflections on Health Services. The Nuffield Hospitals Trust, London, 1971.

Codman E. A., The product of the hospital. Surgery, Gynecology and Obstetrics 1914;18:491-6.

Donabedian A., Evaluating the quality of medical care. Milbank Memorial Quarterly 1966; 44:166-206.

Evidence-based medicine Working Group, Evidence-based medicine: a new approach to teaching the practice of medicine. *JAMA* 1991; 268: 2420-5.

Feinstein A. R., An additional basic science for clinical medicine: the constraining fundamental paradigms. *Ann Intern Med* 1983;99:393-7.

Feinstein A. R., Clinical Judgment. Kreiger, *Malabar,* 1967.

Feinstein A. R., Clinical Judgment. Kreiger, *Malabar,* 1967, p. 29.

Feinstein A. R., Meta-analysis: statistical alchemy for the 21st century. J Clin Epidemiol 1995;48:71-9.

Foote S. B., Assessing medical technology assessment; past, present and future. The Milbank Quarterly 1987; 65:59-80.

Health Care Quality Commission, Consumer Protection and Quality in the Health Care Industry. Quality first: better health care for all Americans. U.S. Department of Health and Human Services 1999.

Gill T. M[1.], Feinstein A. R., A critical appraisal of the quality of quality-of-life measurements. *JAMA*. 1994;272: 619-26.

Morris J., Uses of Epidemiology. Williams and Wilkins, Baltimore, 1957.

Plsek P. E., Resource B: A primer on quality improvement tools. In: Curing health care: new strategies for quality improvement. Berwick DM, Godfrey AB, Roessner J, eds. San Francisco: Jossey-Bass, 1990.

Quality Management Team, NHS Executive, Department of Health 1999.

Sackett, Haynes, Tugwell and Guyatt, Clinical Epidemiology: a new science for clinical medicine 2nd edition, 1991, p. 39.

Sackett D. L., Richardson W. S., Rosenberg W., Haynes R. B., Evidence-based Medicine: How to Practice and Teach EBM. Churchill Livingstone, New York, 1997, px.

White K. W., Healing the Schism: epidemiology, medicine, and the public's health. *Springer-Verlag,* New York, 1991.

Chapter 13

Tacit Knowledge, The Emotions and Their Role in Judgement

Evidence, Memory, Judgement, Decision and Emotion

The basics of good clinical and public heath decision making are valid evidence, understanding the strengths and quirks of the practitioners' memory for facts, sound judgement, and appropriate decision making. In this chapter, we discuss two topics which have long been anathema in medical academic circles. We focus on the issue of the respective roles of tacit or subconscious influences, then as a surprise packet – the emotions have emerged as important factors in decisions! Both have now proven to be crucial to clinical judgement and evaluation research so that we must strive to understand the underlying message. In fact the current evidence should prompt a radical comprehensive rethink of these determinants of a sound decision in clinical practice and for formulating public health policy, and for science generally! This is especially so as both influences have long been dirty words in this context.

Descartes' philosophy of 'mind-body dualism' has cast a long shadow since attitudes in our scientific practices have been in keeping with his argument that rational argumentation was its sine qua non . However two compelling trends in relevant research of recent years have turned earlier theories topsy turvy. Our remit therefore comprises an obligation that we examine the current evidence critically. It will become apparent the stakes are high for both clinical medicine and public health because of practical and financial implications. The foundations of important scientific intellectual commitments have shifted in a rather disconcerting manner so the issue has an important message for science in general as well. If rationality is not to be the basis of scientific hypothesizing, judgement and validity, then what is?

We will first address the broader issue of what constitutes valid evidence, the most basic of the requirements for a reliable decision. We will consider the respective roles of tacit knowledge and the emotions as important variables influencing judgement, the precursor of decision-making. We will pay particular attention the role of the emotions as contributors to judgement, sometimes its major determinant because they are a particular bete noir of the scientific community. First we must consider a basic consideration - what are the sciences impacting on medicine?

While it would obviously be the height of folly to deny the obvious overall benefits of science to mankind, to gain a balanced view of the impact of science on medicine we have to acknowledge two things. The first caveat is that 'science' is not a homogeneous entity. Such was the evolution of 'biomedical science,' the understanding of human biology in health and disease, that it has been an extremely valuable asset available to us all. There were, however other branches of scientific thought which had also put in an appearance. The science required for the evaluation of treatment, 'empirical statistical science' was also conceived by P-C-A Louis early in the early 19th century in Paris,' but was neither welcomed by the medical profession nor needed by government at that time. Fortunately the skills were preserved and developed by public health interests.

A branch of science vital to the clinician's accurate understanding of disease and its treatment is 'taxonomy,' a broad concept of scientific classification of living things by multiple attributes. Patterns are central to any kind of clinical practice and the idea was revived last century by Feinstein in the form of 'Boolean algebra' but it has barely rated a mention since. Hence over two centuries, medical 'science' has become differentiated into biomedical, empirical statistical and taxonomic varieties.

A New Concept of 'Evidence'

Another important development in science was that the conception of what constituted 'evidence' underwent a major shift. Earlier, it had meant that the information was 'concordant with beliefs of the ancients.' Later, it came to mean 'supported by empirical observation.' An important collateral development was the blossoming of statistics and analysis of empirical data, along with the beginnings of the discipline of public health epidemiology.

Many Influences on Every Clinical Decision

The number of influences – pieces of evidence which can make a contribution to any clinical judgement are surprisingly numerous, as all physicians must know at some level. Evidence-based medicine values empirical statistical data, the results of randomized trials. However the variables which influence a clinical decision could include some or all of:

- patient narrative account of illness
- treatment facilities available locally
- the patient's values and preferences
- the social context
- patients' and doctors' emotional reactions
- politics behind the distribution of facilities
- family advice
- computer storage of individual taxonomic illness patterns
- the doctor's own experience

- advice from expert consultations
- clinical epidemiology
- evidence-based empirical data from clinical trials
- contributions from clinical guidelines
- information from clinical science, physiology, pathology, biochemistry
- evidence relevant to the case from the social sciences and humanities

In a new postmodern paradigm of clinical practice, these kinds of evidence can all contribute empirical data to the management decisions, as appropriate for each individual patient. Hence aggregated information, stored in memory as interconnected items, used for a decision may be tacit, explicit or mixed with some aspects of selection and interpretation of information from these episodes being harder to explain than others, and the reasons given by physicians may even be partly influenced by post-hoc rationalisations. The picture becomes more obscure if we accept the dominance of the 'tacit' knowledge over the 'explicit' knowledge, and even if we accept the important input to judgements of the emotions which have for far too long been effectively sidelined.

Evidence-based medicine has concentrated on providing information which relates to the outcome of randomised trials of technical interventions, especially drugs, under highly controlled conditions of administration, usually in the hospital environment in the Central Zone of clinical care. A much wider range of evidence, as above is needed for doctors making clinical judgements, for patients making their decisions, for administrators and policy-makers making theirs. To privilege trial results in this way does seem rather futile. The relative importance of each of these will vary; those factors carrying most weight in the judgement will obviously depend on the specifics of the particular patient and details of each illness. The situation is like attempting to rate the usefulness of the tools in the shed – a hammer, a screwdriver, a saw, a chisel and an axe; this is a futile exercise because it is dependent on the task in hand! A plank cut with a saw is aesthetically and functionally better than one cut with an axe. However, the wood cut for kindling may be that cut with the axe! In addition, one should remember that these many clinical influences interact as part of a complex dynamic system, hence interact in countless unpredictable ways as the variables of a   complex dynamic system . Small wonder that clinical judgement is so demanding, a critical influence in decision making and that medical training takes so long!

The Power of Human Judgement

Not only does the current scientific medical culture underestimate the sheer number of decisional variables contributing to clinical decisions but, as it turns out, adds insult to injury by seriously underestimating the intricacy and computational diagnostic power of the expert clinical judgement itself. We must therefore review the theories which are relevant to the process of clinical judgement. It is of the greatest significance that there has been a quiet revolution in these ideas about the nature of clinical judgement and decision making over the past quarter century or more. Finally, we intend to consider the important role of the emotions in judgements. The scientific quality of evidence must be decided on well-established grounds but should be seen as just one important factor determining the magnitude of the clinical contribution. The value of a piece of clinical evidence must ultimately be judged by its specific contribution to patient management.

The Damage Inflicted By Science on the Art of Medicine

The damage inflicted on the art of medicine has been blamed on the 'science,' largely attributed firstly to the dominance of the biomedical model which reduced the centre of gravity of health care to a focus in the teaching hospital, equipped to handle organic disease, but a far cry from meeting the medical needs of most patients in the community. Indeed, the negative influence of the biological and natural sciences has been profound, and much to the detriment of the clinical role of the social sciences and humanities and in teaching in the curriculum. All too often the doctor is seen as a technocrat whose skills and interests are in scientifically based intervention, and often as lacking skills in supportive care and the art of medicine.

Knowledge, Judgement and Memory - Resurgence of the Tacit Dimension

Descartes' theory of a mind-body split had cast a powerful spell over philosophy. Only over the past two decades has its impact begun to clear. We turn therefore to a remarkable rather silent intellectual revolution which has occurred with regard to knowledge, judgement and memory over the past three or more decades. In particular, what had been overlooked or discounted was the rapidly emerging role in judgements and decisions of the comprehensively overlooked tacit dimension of clinical judgment. As a result of a remarkable intellectual revolution which has occurred with regard to knowledge, judgement and memory, the basic mechanisms responsible have been effectively transformed root and branch.

Tacit, implicit or gist unconscious knowledge is enjoying a strong resurgence in the debate over the determinants of decision-making, including those of patient management. The major insight has been a result of a somewhat belated better appreciation of the roles of 'tacit' unconscious versus conscious 'explicit' knowledge as propounded by Michael Polanyi (1967, 1969), polymath physician, scientist, philosopher and social scientist, of a similar distinction between unconscious 'reflection-in-action' and conscious 'reflection-on-action' by educationist Donald Schon (1988), a similar one between 'Personal Practical Knowledge' and 'routine knowledge' by John Dewey (1916), and of the 'fuzzy trace' theory of psychologists with its contrast between unconscious 'gist' knowledge and conscious 'verbatim' knowledge described by Brainerd and Reyna (1990). These developments are also consistent with Hammond's 'cognitive continuum' theory of judgement which has unconscious 'implicit' knowledge at one pole and conscious 'explicit' at the other (Hamm 1988). This interpretation has therefore enjoyed strong support, coming from four quite different sources and a wealth of empirical research.

The centre-piece of the modern scientific paradigm with its assumption of judgement is at odds with this evidence, simply holding that explicit reasoning refined by expert judgement must obviously be superior to intuitive or tacit judgement hence should be the basis of all sound reasoning. Little has been done to reconcile the variety of concepts which has emerged. A partial exception has been the idea of 'intuition' in clinical medicine and related research, especially in fuzzy trace theory. This crucial element of 'clinical judgement', a process viewed with suspicion and de-emphasised by evidence-based medicine, seen because of its apparent lack of an overt scientific basis, even seen as exhibiting a despised aura of the occult!

The reason for this transformation in thinking is that there has been a confluence of research in the related disciplines of neurophysiology and neuroanatomy, neurology, psychology, management science and computer science which have contributed invaluable supporting evidence on the mental mechanisms involved, and there is a contemporaneous intense interest in the role of the tacit knowledge and emotions in judgement (vide infra). When applied in an appropriate environment, simple decision heuristics can exceed the accuracy of more sophisticated, classification and prediction tools, including that of regression models or neural networks (Goldman 1990). Changing conceptions of diagnosis have evolved accompanying changes in culture. In premodern times, diagnosis was based upon simply an unselfconscious dialogue between doctor and patient which was not subjected to detailed analysis. In the modern era, the traditional clinical examination incorporated scientific models, and narrative accounts of illness earned respect (Greenhalgh 1999). Researchers outside of medicine also took an interest.

The result has been like the three blind men and the elephant. So in psychology, diagnosis was modelled as hypothetico-deductive reasoning, artificial intelligence emphasised the linear algorithm by analogy with the computer, while the neural network computer added the important idea of generating and recognising patterns. Economists supported the maximization of expected utility model, the ultimate in rationalist modelling. Psychologists developed the notion of 'dual pathway' models with unconscious and conscious elements operating in parallel.

The scientific view emphasised by Feinstein's clinical epidemiology is that diagnosis and treatment is about hypothesis testing and experimental intervention (Feinstein 1963) but clearly rapid unconscious pattern recognition is also central. While Feinstein's experimental model is partly true, it has recently been persuasively argued that such a process must be seen as a fundamentally interpretive process more appropriately residing with the humanities (Hunter 1991). Thinking along similar lines at an earlier time, master physician William Osler had already likened the patient to a text which is interpreted by the doctor (Hunter 1991). Indeed the clinical examination is inherently a hermeneutic activity, an iterative process of interpretation which always stays close to the context of the illness, the individual patient and the specific clinical context, and is presented as a narrative in history taking in the clinical notes and at meetings.

As we shall see, unencumbered by any consideration of tacit knowledge, formal decision models hold a special attraction for health care policy makers. Despite this mounting body of evidence, undoubtedly health policy makers will continue to rely upon computer-aided decision theory and cost-management systems when determining the conditions and efficacy of clinical practice. Protagonists of the old view could be said to perceive no difference in principle between the clinician's thought processes and those of a sophisticated computer software program (Goldman 1990). Fuzzy-trace theory encompasses memory, reasoning, judgment, and decision making. Reliance upon intuition increases with development from childhood to adulthood, along with experience in life, analogous to the development for adults from novice to expert in a domain of expertise (Reyna & Lloyd 2006). It has been shown that children reason rationally in the classic sense but that adults forego rational reasoning in favour of the representations, which support deployment of fuzzy tacit 'gist,' unconscious knowledge, and of superficial 'verbatim' representations of information, which support precise analysis. Hence, as development progresses, judgement and decision making become more streamlined and better integrated, rather than more detailed and elaborate (Reyna et al 2011). A partial exception has been the idea of 'intuition' in clinical medicine and related research. This crucial element of 'clinical judgement,' a process viewed with suspicion and de-emphasised by evidence-based medicine because of its somewhat mystical nature and lack of an overt scientific basis. This might be because we have all experienced it.

Knowledge, Judgement and Memory

Over the same period there has been a confluence of research in the related disciplines of neurophysiology and neuroanatomy, neurology, psychology and computer science which have contributed invaluable supporting evidence on the brain mechanisms involved, and there has been a contemporaneous intense interest in the role of the emotions in judgement (vide infra). Few attempts have been undertaken to reconcile the variety of concepts which has emerged.

Changing conceptions of diagnosis have evolved accompanying changes in culture. In premodern times, diagnosis was based upon simply an unselfconscious dialogue between doctor and patient which was not subjected to detailed analysis. In the modern era, the traditional clinical examination incorporated scientific models, and narrative accounts of illness earned respect (Greenhalgh 1999). Researchers outside of medicine also took an interest with a corresponding proliferation of models based on their professional preconceptions as stated above.

Clinical Care as an Experiment

The scientific view emphasised by Feinstein's clinical epidemiology is that diagnosis and treatment is about hypothesis testing and experimental intervention (Feinstein 1963) but clearly rapid unconscious pattern recognition is central as we shall see. Michael Polanyi's astute exposition of the relative contributions of 'tacit' subconscious and conscious 'explicit' knowledge does seem to be prevailing in the clinical judgement debate. Another potentially unifying concept is the model of dual processing whereby unconscious (tacit) and conscious (explicit) thinking, including intuitive knowledge, operate harmoniously together in judgements such as the clinical diagnosis, with the dominant one in the case of the expert being the unconscious one (Brainerd and Reyna 1990). When applied in an appropriate environment, simple decision heuristics can exceed the accuracy of more sophisticated, classification and prediction tools, including that of regression models or neural networks

(Goldman 1990). The cumulative results of their investigations threatens to invalidate the currently held rationalistic nature of judgement, including the currently endangered clinical species!

Can a Computer Do the Job or Are We Sending a Boy on a Man's Errand?

Clinical judgment refers to the totality of the mental processes involved in all stages at which the clinician collects and interprets data, formulates a problem statement, confirms and refutes diagnostic hypotheses; considers, plans, and implements possible diagnostic and therapeutic options, tests, and interventions; and evaluates likelihoods and outcomes (Goldman 1990). As much research has affirmed, the tacit component of this knowledge could never be reduced to even the most sophisticated software programs. Without question, however, the explicit theory is the most widely held view of the nature of professional judgment, especially clinical judgment. It may boil down to being another example of the 'rule of numbers', the prevailing quantitative scientistic thinking in health care.

Sustaining this seriously misguided view, the dominant view among physicians and educators, which is basically the only view acknowledged by professional policy makers and cost analysts, is one that characterizes clinical judgment as a fully explicit process, involving in all respects the conscious application of defined rules and explicit knowledge. It contrasts with the neglected alternative view that tacit, implicit unconscious knowledge does, in fact, play the dominant role in clinical judgement. This neglected view, while not formally acknowledged by many practising clinicians, nevertheless is likely to be partly the basis for their increasing unease with the current rejection of clinical judgement by evidence-based medicine. A formal system which can explicitly identify and quantify all relevant data, options, and outcomes is quite mistakenly believed to have a greater potential ability than intuition for dealing with the complexity and uncertainty which is inherently part of clinical practice.

The tacit dimension tends to be portrayed rather as a nebulous even ethereal concept, rather than an integral aspect of everyday human knowing and judgement, seemingly unusual only because of our modern focus on science and its apparent reliance upon explicit knowledge. This fact seems odd only because our society takes for granted that true, scientific knowledge must be wholly explicit - which it could never be. Medical knowledge can be classified as both scientific and practical - both types of knowledge which are similar in that they are explicitly known by the clinician. The scientifically proven portion comprises that medical knowledge which has been validated by scientific research. Practical knowledge - that is, knowledge which has been established by previous clinical experience (Goldman 1990) and empirically thought to be useful, but which has not yet been subjected to rigorous scientific analysis for confirmation or refutation.

The Algorithmic Approach

Explicit theory is a widely held view of the nature of professional judgment, especially in clinical judgment. Indeed the explicit theory provides much of the theoretical basis for the impressive edifice of decision analysis, artificial intelligence expert systems, and applications for clinical prediction rules, algorithms, and judgment theory. The dissenting opinion - the theories of tacit knowledge or of professional judgment as knowing-in-action (Polanyi 1969), 'gist' knowledge (Brainerd and Reyna 1990) and reflection-in-action - involve tacit knowledge which is out of conscious reach. On this second view, it is a gross error to expect or assist the clinician to make fully explicit and quantifiable the entire range of data and rules he uses in clinical judgment. Much of the knowledge that the clinician uses is not explicit, could not be made explicit, and does not need to be because it is deployed as tacit knowledge. Although we make many decisions at an explicit level, a wholly explicit system of knowledge is impossible. Tacit integrations of information underlie our conscious deliberations; indeed their speed and complexity permit our explicit operations to function. 'Verbatim' is memory for surface form, for example, memory representations of exact words, numbers and pictures.

Tacit Thinking Underlies the Most Advanced Thinking

According to this view, the knowledge employed in any skill, physical or mental, can be divided into two partnered components: explicit and tacit. The use of the explicit component of knowledge, the "knowing what," actually depends upon the underlying tacit component, the "knowing how." We have all experienced an intuitive insight allowing us to arrive at a conclusion in a flash. Packaging of an element of rhetoric in such a way as to encourage certain interpretations and to discourage others is common. People build a series of mental 'filters' through biological and cultural influences; they then use these 'frames' to make sense of the world. 'Gist memory' is memory for essential meaning, the substance of information irrespective of exact words, numbers, or pictures. 'Intuition', in this view, relies on the meaning-based gist representations. Advanced decision making relies mainly on gist-based intuition in law, medicine and public health. In fact, contrary to what most scientists believe, intuitive thinking underlies the most advanced of thinking processes. The current traditional modern scientific view of judgement strongly emphasizes an exclusive role for explicit knowledge in such enterprises, and relegates tacit unconscious knowledge to the realm of non-professional, irrational thought!

Two Partners Yoked Together for Judgement – Explicit and Tacit Knowledge

The knowledge required to interpret and decide the relevance of explicit conscious information, and used to recognize and apply the appropriate explicit rules to a given problem is therefore tacit knowledge. On the one hand, the teacher deliberately communicates explicit information to the student by instruction, which consists of conveying specific, impersonal, hard, isolated facts and rules. Tacit or implicit knowledge, by contrast, is imparted by example. This being so, in principle, no amount of scientific validation of practical clinical expertise, no degree of systematization of clinical rules into formal systems, no enhancement of our ability to achieve precise measurement and quantification of probabilities, however important all these achievements may be, can eliminate the permanent and important role of tacit knowledge in judgment, clinical or otherwise. This debate appears to be one more recycling of the age-old, recurring controversy over whether clinical practice is predominantly art or science. On the other hand, as discussed above, dissenters have raised concerns that the fundamental obstacle to the success of formal models may be the extent to which such thorough identification and processing of information is possible. Furthermore, it may be the decision theory, not the clinician is in error when discrepancies arise (Goldman 1990)! And so we turn our attention to the importance of the emotions in decision making.

Serendipity Supervenes -
The Sad Story of Phineas Gage

Time to act in an emergency has never been shorter than in this case. A major advance in thinking about the role of the emotions in judgements and decisions was the result of an accident in Cavendish, Nebraska, U.S.A. involving a railroad construction foreman. Phineas P. Gage, 25 years old, was 'setting a blast' at 4:30 p.m. on September 18 1848. He was clearing rock from a railroad in Vermont using a 'tamping iron'. 'This involved boring a hole deep into an outcropping of rock; adding *blasting powder*, a fuse and sand.' But his assistant did not insert the sand in time. Impacting this charge into the hole using the 'tamping iron' presumably generated a spark against the rock, possibly because the sand was omitted. When the powder exploded, the large iron rod, custom made for Gage, 1 m long and 3.2 cm in diameter, weighing 6.0 kg penetrated, through the left side of his face, under the zygomatic arch directly below his left eye passing out through the the top of his skull. The large missile destroyed much of the brain's left *frontal lobe* and destroyed the left optic nerve. The tamping iron, "smeared with blood and brain", landed some 25 m. away! Gage "was thrown onto his back by the explosion, made a few convulsive motions "then, remarkably, "spoke in a few minutes", then walked with little assistance. There was no paralysis or sensory deficits except for the loss of vision in his left eye, which was directly damaged by the rod. His manual dexterity was intact, and there was no noticeable difficulty in his speech, language, or capacity for rational thought.

What was impaired, however, was his personality. Specifically, Gage was no longer able to behave appropriately as a social being, and instead made choices that were consistently inappropriate or disadvantageous to him, so that that his friends and acquaintances said he was "no longer Gage". Nevertheless, he subsequently improved and did hold down a responsible job driving a team of six horses pulling a stage-coach for long distances in Chile - but was not offered his previous job! The case received a large amount of study and public attention, and initially much scepticism until its veracity was confirmed by Doctor Bigelow the vice-chancellor at Harvard University. A much delayed outcome over the past 25 years has been a great deal of research into localisation of specific functions in the brain. This has borne much fruit. One such recent investigation studied Gage's skull, and used radiographic and nuclear imaging to confirm the iron bar's trajectory so long ago [Damasio 1990]. These findings confirmed the initial diagnosis of gross damage to the orbito-frontal region which fits with his behavioural change. Thus has the role emotions in judgements been consolidated.

The Emotions as Central to Judgement

For many years, cognitive science took what could be seen as the commonsense view that rational decision makers would make normative objective decisions based on the time and information they had available. However, studies of judgement and decision making in 'naturalistic' models of human decision making have advanced greatly over the past few decades. In fact, deviations from this model were in the past called decision making biases. However, research conducted outside of the laboratory has discovered that for decision making in natural environments, research has shown that emotion and value-based judgments can change the way decisions are made in a fundamental way.

Sometimes when time is short, selecting a solution that is satisfactory but not optimal may be a better approach, a heuristic strategy called 'satisficing' by Herbert Simon. Thus experts may be more likely to employ an unconscious pattern matching process based upon availability, defined as having a large number of templates stored in memory to match problem and context, in order to make judgements that have yielded satisfactory results in similar contexts in the past. In ICU, a treatment protocol that worked successfully in the past is chosen and adapted and updated according to the patient's responses. What the rational cognitive completely overlooked was the powerful impact of emotion, often a determining element in judgement.

Emotion may be defined as a complex state of feeling that results in physical and psychological changes that influence thought and behavior. Some emotions emerge as personality traits which are durable tendencies, 'moods' operate medium term, 'sentiments' longer, and 'emotional bursts' are brief. All four have an impact on perception, attention, and decision making. Emotion is not a bias at all, rather a legitimate and important judgement vector, sometimes conscious but often not. In fact, the more complex a decision making context, the more useful emotion may be in complementing and even governing decision making and judgment. Emotional arousal can lead to the identification of new and better solutions because emotional intensity leads to rapid selection of intuitive responses. In general, emotional influences tend to increase creativity, flexibility and efficient decision making (Raddatz, Werth, and Tran, 2007). On the other hand they can increase optimism and decrease risk perception (Xie et al, 2011), which can lead to overestimation of positive outcomes and underestimation of negative outcomes (Hudlicka 2010); on the other hand negative emotions can lead to pessimistic predictions, and thus higher risk perception.

The Somatic Marker Hypothesis

Just one of the important questions which we must confront is - should the impact of emotions on decision-making be accepted as part of clinical 'evidence' or not? It is hard to make a case for ignoring such a compelling effect of affect in the light of recent debate in the relevant academic disciplines, as we shall see. The other area where science has been party to inadvertently misleading us has been in downplaying the role of the emotions in judgement. Emotions, as defined by Damasio (1994), are changes in both body and brain states in response to different stimuli. Physiological changes such as muscle tone, heart rate, respiratory rate, endocrine release, posture, facial expression, bowel motility, muscle tone and urinary continence occur in the body and are relayed to the brain where they are transformed into an emotion that delivers to the individual information about the stimulus that they have encountered.

Over time, emotions and their corresponding bodily changes become associated throughout life with particular situations and their past outcomes. When making decisions, these physiological signals, 'somatic markers' and their evoked emotion are consciously or unconsciously associated with their past outcomes and bias decision-making towards certain behaviours while avoiding others. The emotion may therefore act as an internal early alarm system warning the individual to avoid a hazardous situation or course of action or an alert to seize an unexpected opportunity. Such was apparently the case in the incident recounted by Greenhalgh et al. (2014), and which will resonate with all clinicians. A male patient who set alarm bells ringing during a home visit died soon afterwards.

These situation-specific somatic states, based on past and present experiences, help to guide behaviour in favour of more advantageous choices and therefore are adaptive in nature. Thus the brain stores scenarios of life events and their outcomes as 'images' in the ventromedial prefronatal cerebral cortex over an entire lifetime (Damasio 1994). These are generated and stored, and are activated together with the emotion when a matching pattern is encountered. This process begins at birth, such that storing of patterns continues through childhood and adulthood, and is responsive to the joys and sadnesses, the personal traumas and social exigencies, as well as to the judgements of clinical practice.

According to Damasio's 'somatic marker hypothesis,' two distinct pathways can activate such responses. Direct access to the storage system can elicit a 'gut feeling', that visceral response that provides the early warning of trouble brewing or the appearance of an opportunity. In this first pathway, the emotion can be evoked by the changes in the body that are projected to the brain—called the "body loop." In an alternative response, a second pathway, cognitive representations of the emotions can be activated in the brain without being directly elicited by a physiological response—called the "as-if body loop." In this way, over time, emotions and their corresponding bodily change(s) become associated with particular past situations and their outcomes. Thus one could explain the impact of intuitive stimuli as the basis for a patient's reactions; encountering a repulsive object like a large hairy spider is likely to cause fear, and may initiate the fight-or-flight response.

An Emotional Guardian Angel

Thus the somatic marker hypothesis proposes a mechanism by which *emotional* processes can guide *behaviour* continuously through their influence upon decision-making. Emotions, as defined by Damasio, are changes in both body and brain states in response to different stimuli. Physiological changes, as just described are relayed to the brain where they are transformed into an emotion that informs the individual about the stimulus encountered. When making decisions, these physiological signals and their evoked 'somatic markers' emotion are consciously or unconsciously associated with their past outcomes and bias decision-making towards certain behaviours while avoiding others. For instance, when a somatic marker associated with a positive outcome is perceived, the person may feel happy and motivated to pursue that behaviour. When a somatic marker associated with the negative outcome is perceived, the person may feel sad and the emotion may act as an internal alarm to warn the individual to avoid a course of action.

These situation-specific somatic states based upon and reinforced by past experiences help to guide behaviour in favour of more advantageous choices, hence the part played by emotion has survival value. Thus the influence of emotions on decision-making is a potentially strong, frequently determining contributor. Emotions during decision-making have been divided into two types: those anticipating future emotions and those immediately experienced while deliberating and deciding. Anticipated (or expected) emotions are not experienced directly, but are expectations of how the person will feel once gains or losses associated with that decision are experienced.

The influence of emotions frequently operates in a modulating role. The main emotions studied have been happiness, sadness, optimism, pessimism, fear and disgust. A large number of neurological structures have been implicated with progress accelerated by human studies applying PET and/or MRI scanning. Brain structures highlighted by imaging methods are located in the brain stem, hypothalamus, amygdala, cerebellum, basal ganglia and both of the cerebral hemispheres. Our daily choices and our life decisions, conscious or unconscious, are therefore made against a guiding repertoire of constantly updated stored resource of remembered patterns of previous life events.

The Intricacy and Unpredictability of Clinical Judgement

Unhappily, I have been able to locate only two papers analyzing in detail the clinical process of decision-making itself, both by Alvan Feinstein, published in the early 1970s (Feinstein 1973a, 1973b). This unique perspective covered essentially the clinician's reasoning processes and approach to diagnostic categorization. Not included in these papers were the clinical determinants of management decisions, a subject integral to the disagreement between evidence-based medicine and clinicians who, as Feinstein did, have a profound respect for 'clinical judgement.' As we have noted, this topic is often denigrated simply because most of the knowledge used is tacit, largely involving pattern recognition, employed subconsciously and therefore invisible - which effectively conceals the awesome intricacy of the intellectual processes involved.

This failure of past clinical research to even suspect this misunderstanding now poses all researchers with a serious problem requiring urgent resolution. The vectors which can make a contribution to any clinical judgement are numerous as shown above. The relative importance of each of these will vary; those factors carrying most weight in the judgement will obviously depend on the specifics of the particular patient and of the illness. The evidence needed for patient care should be applied to the clinical management decision with the guidance of a more comprehensive postmodern medical paradigm.

Inserting the Soft Clinical Data into the Pattern

Data from trials and tests is mostly considered 'hard.' A basic problem, however, is that patient presentations and health outcomes in 'real world' clinical populations are often much influenced by a large variety of uncontrolled, indeed generally uncontrollable 'soft' variables. Most important are the so-called 'psychosocial' variables with which patients often present, especially in general practice (Balint 1957). Such problems are generally related to the personal, family and social context, and are sometimes known to the managing physician - but often not. These include marriage disharmony, family disputes, employment problems, financial difficulty, examinations, fear of serious illness and many more. These 'problems of living' frequently cause symptoms which can closely mimic organic disease. To have clinically useful external validity, the patient's illness must therefore be fully specified as above by the taxonomic clinical pattern envisaged by Feinstein with its rather daunting array of component variables, and this must include the above 'soft data.'

The Impact of Emotions on Clinical Decisions – A Plea for Urgent Remedial Action

Changes in the direction of research in decision-making with some confluence of related disciplines, and the conspicuous absence of empirical 'bedside' studies has had the paradoxical effect of eventually emphasising the contribution of emotions to decisions. This is particularly so for clinical decisions which, by their very nature, are so often emotionally charged, often for patient, family and doctor.

Not only are the crucial emotions important for medicine's image community respect and continuing government support but they can readily related to the success or otherwise of each individual consultation! Doctors tend generally be unaware of possible emotional influences on clinical decisions. Moreover, their track record handling personal and social issues in patient consultations to date do not inspire much confidence for major improvement any time soon. But least doctors should know that such influences do impact on their decisions, and be sensitive to their existence, albeit as supposedly 'unscientific soft data', in their patients' narratives so that they can strive to address these to the patient's satisfaction. However these soft data influences are still more often than not overlooked or dismissed, leaving patients feeling that they have not been properly understood by their doctor. Sadly, the outcome is often 'consultation failure' (Chapter 11) resulting in a dissatisfied, oftentimes uncooperative patient and a physician who remains unaware or simply nonplussed by such subtle undercurrents.

Reactions to the Perceived Damage
to the Art of Medicine

To a limited extent, matters have come to head over the last two decades. The most constructive response to criticism has been the emergence of many 'social movements' representing patient interest groups, professional societies and governments, essentially based on George Engel's 'biopsychosocial model' of clinical care, an application of systems thinking pioneered by Ludwig van Bertalanffy. A prominent example of this genre is 'patient-centred care.' Their chief objectives revolve around initiating a revival of more supportive patient care, greater respect for patient rights and 'shared decision making' by doctor and patient insofar as this is the patient's wish. In addition, the clinical patient narrative also provides the only way to elicit the circumstances needed to interpret the illness in the patient's terms and the significance of particular symptoms. This is precisely the kind of information which could be recorded at the bedside by the physician with aid of a hand-held computer. Such patient-specific taxonomic patterns of illness manifestations and the clinical context, 'condensed' clinical experience as it were, could later be fed to a physician's personal data-base, and then into one programmed with local and even international experience.

Feinstein, as we have seen, proposed this notion of using the computer to store individual patient data as summary patterns of variables in order to overcome the external validity problem of the clinical trials. However, it is worth noting that a closely similar idea has recently been proposed whereby routine clinical data including illness outcome can be computerised and applied to inform local patient management. This can also be used to match the illness patterns of similar patients in the future. This procedure has been called 'evidence farming' (Hay et al. 2008).

The Spectrum of Evidence and the
Intellectual Paradigms

We observed in Chapter 4 that the 'Two Cultures problem' as a manifestation of the conflict between the analytical scientific and interpretive humanistic paradigms is alive and well in health research. We noted that the biomedical sciences, epidemiology, clinical epidemiology and evidence-based medicine, health economics and quantitative sociology have a strong commitment to science and quantitative analytical methods. Here the emphasis is on reduction of complexity by control of variables and by quantitation. Laboratory physics is the exemplar. Validity is defined chiefly in terms of internal validity, that is, demonstrable freedom of results from error, objectivity, statistical significance and freedom from value judgements. Other disciplines with a stake in the study of health care, such as qualitative sociology, clinical psychology and the humanities, are committed to interpretive methods based upon observation, interview and examination of records which requires qualitative data analysis of text or transcript. Validity for such qualitative data is defined in terms of careful collection of sound evidence, and on the rigor, coherence and credibility of an argument which draws appropriately upon theoretical principles. Currently, it remains one aspect of a 'subjugated paradigm' in clinical research. Technical and numerical information on the effectiveness and efficacy of technological interventions cannot alone provide all of the information needed for clinical judgements, patient decisions and administrative planning. Such decisions inevitably reflect personal attitudes, social, cultural and emotional influences.

We have observed that illness in the ambulant patient in the Peripheral Zone of care, in general practice and in the outpatient department - where most medicine is practised - frequently presents as ill-defined symptom complexes rather than as clear cut disease, and problems of living loom large. Technological interventions may have unpredictable effects on patient anxiety. Moreover, such is the uncertainty that treatment options are often multiple, supportive care is of prime importance and the patient's cooperation with treatment cannot be assumed. Thus patients often do not comply with treatment, delay seeking it, do not accept legitimate reassurance, or turn to complementary health care. Nor does the wide variation observed in doctors' practice habits seem to represent efficient practice. These are the realities which can nullify the potential of the beneficial effects of interventions demonstrated to be effective in randomised controlled trials.

Rational Decision-Making - Really?

'Homo economicus' is expected to follow the dictates of naked self interest as proposed by the rationalistic theory of 'maximisation of expected utility', the basis of the modelling of cost-utility analysis. This assumption, rarely questioned in the past, that only rational conscious considerations contribute to judgements, means that other influences such as tacit knowledge and emotions are seen as biases. This, according to much recent research, is quite seriously misguided. Decision-making in the real world is a great deal more complex and must recognise include the potentially powerful emotional and tacit influences. This applies to patients' decisions, and in the case of doctors is even relevant to limitations afflicting mathematical modelling of the process of diagnosis known as medical decision analysis. This model has never caught on as a practical diagnostic aid among clinicians. At societal level, according to Adam Smith, an 'invisible hand' regulates commerce by inexorably linking supply and demand. However decision-making in health matters frequently deviates from these prescriptive models. Even in simple situations in which personal preferences are elicited by survey, other social factors intrude.

Muddling Through

In management science, good judgement and experience have proved more important than quantitative modelling for the policy-level problems confronted by executives (Dreyfus and Dreyfus 1986). The same is true for in scientific research (Medawar 1984). Political decision-making has to be pragmatic and sensitive to social and cultural context. We have told of Lindblom's (1953) contention that administrators and policy analysts apply a process of iterative interpretation based on judgement and experience to problem solving, not the formal algorithmic approach taught at business school. Dubbed 'muddling through,' this pragmatic approach bears a close structural resemblance to medical diagnosis! Doctors would not take much convincing that a clinical evaluation is itself often a wicked problem, or that they were often muddling through! The upshot was first a move towards greater use of economic modelling, and more recently there has been a further push for evidence-based decision-making by health bureaucrats responsible for resource allocation (Gray 1997). They would be better served by studying the recent literature in the neurological and neurosciences arena, and taking note of the meteoric rise of evidence supporting a central role for the emotions in judgements.

How Do Doctors and Patients Make Decisions?

Even to consider corrective action for such problems, we must understand much better than we do how patients and doctors think in their clinical context. This requires a different kind of evidence - information derived by observing doctors and patients in the field, and interviewing them. Such interpretive studies applying qualitative data analysis are needed if we are to establish what is behind apparently perverse behaviour patients and doctors. So far such studies have been very few. The role of emotions relevant to clinical decisions of doctor, patient and family needs much more research. Evidence-based medicine, by placing emphasis upon explicit numerical evidence related to technical interventions, tends to discount the importance of these other kinds of contextual evidence which turn upon personal beliefs and preferences, emotional reactions, social attitudes and cultural values. Obviously, there is a need for more studies applying the humanistic interpretive research paradigm which produce evidence generated as argument in narrative form by qualitative data analysis.

A Critical Perspective on Approaches to Diagnosis

Studies with sociology and anthropology have been few until now because of the gulf which has separated these two basic analytical and interpretive intellectual paradigms. Only with their union will 'soft data' crucial to clinical management be to hand. Feinstein summed up what he saw as poorly directed clinical research thus: 'During the past 2 decades, these improvements have not occurred as extensively as expected because many investigators working in clinical forms of clinical research have not addressed these basic scientific challenges in data, taxonomy, and reasoning. Instead, the investigators have applied quantitative 'models,' derived from non-clinical domains, that focus on hard data, randomized trials, Bayes' theorem, quantitative decision analysis, and psychometric strategies for clinimetric measurement'(Feinstein 1994). Feinstein also wrote, tongue in cheek, of 'the ghost of Gauss, the haze of Bayes, the aerial palaces of medical decision analysis and the computerized Ouija board'!

Feinstein was essentially castigating clinicians for relying on such 'hand-outs' from other disciplines, especially when these do not fit well with the iterative interpretive or hermeneutic, way in which clinicians really work. Moreover, clinicians often juggle a number of such patterns simultaneously when considering differential diagnosis. Nor do the pieces of such a pattern of clinical variables convey independent information as the mathematical theory requires. Rather it is the interaction between the pieces of clinical information which make up the emerging clinical picture or pattern - as for a jigsaw puzzle, isolated pieces do not, initially at least, necessarily suggest the final picture. It is also believed to be the mechanism whereby the human brain has the ability to recognize, analyse and interpret clinical patterns of illness (scripts) in individual patients – the key word is pattern or picture, or perhaps often 'puzzle'!

How Other Professionals Think

Our argument about the excessively rationalistic conception of expert judgement in clinical medicine and the problems of mathematical formalisation under the analytical scientific paradigm is reinforced by a nagging feeling that we are re-inventing the wheel. Analogous confusion about the respective roles of expert interpretation and rational models has emerged in many fields. A prime example is the field of 'operations research' has proved useful in constrained, simplified contexts but unsuccessful in the more complex fields of the evaluation of social institutions, social planning and political decision-making. In social planning, the term 'wicked problem' was introduced for the poorly structured, context-dependent and socially contingent tasks posed by the evaluation of social institutions which was the rage in the U.S. in the 1960s and 1970s (Rittel 1978). In contrast were the 'tame problems' in the natural sciences where laboratory control of variables and mathematical modelling has been so successful. Wicked problems require for their solution an incremental iterative process of interpretation within a specific social and cultural context. As Schon (1988) put it, the operations research approach, which spawned a new breed of systems and policy analyst and management scientist and computerized formal models, has had a life of its own 'increasingly divergent from the real world problems of practice.'

Medical Education and the Refinement of Both Science and Art of Medicine

Diagnosis cannot be confined to the labelling of disease. It must take account of personal differences and of social context. The pioneers of clinical epidemiology did indeed take heed of these psychosocial aspects of illness. Feinstein suggested that knowledge of this kind is important in medical education: 'Instead of learning all of the details of cytology, microbiology, and biochemistry before starting clinical work, a medical student might just as profitably study anthropology, sociology, and symbolic logic as his pre-clinical subjects. The knowledge to be learnt in these subjects is often more basic and germane to the care of sick people than many of the clinically esoteric more irrelevant concepts of contemporary cytology, microbiology, and biochemistry.'(Feinstein, 1963). Similarly Sackett et al. (1991) stated: 'The clinician who takes pains to listen to the patient and to pay close attention to the physician-patient relationship is doing much more than practicing the art of medicine: the clinician is practicing good scientific medicine. An understanding of the impact of interpersonal and behavioural factors upon both diagnosis and management is central to the practice of scientific medicine.'

The view of these pioneers of clinical epidemiology has been that the science of medicine should be bolstered and the traditional art respected. Alas there has no provision for the scholarly refinement of the art to balance the contribution of science! This is in keeping with a tendency for researchers to work on the high ground of science and mathematics, while there was a need for many to work in the low ground, the swamp which is the messy reality. The art of medicine desperately needs an academic foundation and bolstering by the social sciences and humanities. It could be argued that we have to first learn to crawl before we can walk, that is to study clinical practice first in the easier hospital setting using simpler quantitative methods. However, the methods of evaluation applied there often encounter much more difficulty in the low ground of ambulant care. As we suggested earlier, health researchers must learn to navigate with barge and pole in the swamp rather than pretend they are on the open sea in a power boat!

Science and the Culture

Clashes of paradigms are inevitable since an old paradigm must eventually become incorporated so as to co-exist with the new, just as Newtonian physics has survived to be re-interpreted and nested within the new theory of relativity, remaining central to our practical understanding of the world. This is our common experience of cultural change. Whether we think of social attitudes, motor cars or of architecture, it is not difficult to identify elements of the premodern and modern worlds side by side with new and unfamiliar ones belonging to a new less familiar postmodern world. This co-existence of disciplines committed to different paradigms of thought must surely be true of the health system, which must reflect the culture of the current society in which it is imbedded and to which it is ultimately beholden.

In fact, there co-exist within clinical medicine the emerging postmodern clinical paradigm with its respect for experience, authority and clinical judgement, side by side and in tension still with the new postmodern scientific one which loudly proclaims the virtues of rationality and objectivity. It would be foolish to simply dismiss traditional clinical beliefs with such a long historical evolution as wrong-headed, obsolete or irrelevant. However it would be equally foolish to deny that some do need to be re-interpreted and re-aligned in response to new knowledge and social attitudes.

Indeed, as noted above the older holistic tenets and the link to the humanities are just now being revived as the humanistic movement within medicine. These include the original concept such as the basic 'biopsychosocial model' of George Engel and patient-centred care. Respect for authority based upon clinical experience is just as relevant today as it was in earlier days, provided that clinicians do not reject other valid sources of knowledge. Thus the clinician's attitude to what is acceptable knowledge for incorporation into clinical judgement needs to be extended and refined but not dominated by information from new sources – with contributions from academically appraised evidence in the medical literature, and with input from the burgeoning social, informational and neurosciences, with more weight now allocated to patient values, preferences and emotional states of all parties. Indeed we will argue that individual and collective clinical experience will return to centre stage in the future appraisal of clinical judgement.

The Art vs Science Debate Given New Light

Right at the core of the basic disagreement over the nature of clinical reasoning is the nature of the knowledge used. A valuable, well researched and balanced critical synthesis of the crucially important issues has been provided by Goldman (1990) which addresses major clinical and public health concerns and also addresses the basic issue of their theoretical basis. As we have observed, it has long been the view of the dominant paradigm in medicine that clinical judgment is a fully explicit process is compared to the relatively neglected view that tacit knowledge and emotion plays a substantial role in the clinician's mental operations. This older idea now flies in the face of a large body of research in many disciplines with a stake in clinical judgement as we have noted, notably in neurology, neurophysiology and anatomy, psychology and computer science. So much time, effort and money has been invested in decision analysis, expert systems, and computer-aided cost-benefit applications to medicine, despite the fact that there appear to be severe limits to the contribution of such applications to clinical and public health medicine (Goldman 1990) – not to mention possible patient public harm and opportunity cost. There is therefore a heavy price to be paid should this turn out to be so. The context of health care delivery is changing, and decision and cost-management theories are being increasingly applied to the administration and supervision of clinical practice.

Conclusion

The complexity of clinical judgement has been grossly underestimated. Specific components neglected have been tacit or intuitive judgement and the central role of emotions, either of which which can be determining variables in judgement. However, science and philosophy, under the influence of Descartes in particular, have subscribed to a rigid rationalism which led to the dismissal of the roles of tacit knowledge and of the emotions. So it was therefore for the classical models of the studies of economics. Reassessment of the role of tacit knowledge, lying fallow for decades is now under way in earnest in many disciplines. The confluence of experimentation in neuroscience, neurology, cognitive psychology and, in particular, the tragic but decisive partial traumatic prefrontal leucotomy of a railroad foreman, one Phineas gage located the neural effects of emotional responses.

Damasio's studies, employing the emerging MRI and PET cerebral scans with clinical correlation were the necessary catalyst which led to a theory of judgement which placed the 'fuzzy trace theory' linking emotions to decision making. One could say that that he signalled the beginning of the multidisciplinary new alliances of 'neuroeconomics'. The potential impact on medicine, public health and theories of judgement, not to mention the financial implications for research stakeholders has not even produced a tremor as yet, however a time of reckoning is likely to come soon. All of this almost frenetic progress has had surprisingly little overt impact so far on current beliefs in scientific circles. Still medical education remains doggedly focused on the 'basic sciences,' to the virtually total exclusion of the social sciences, psychology, cognitive neurosciences and humanities. And it shows!

One of the fundamental attitudes feeding into medicine's public and political woes has been the current view of clinical diagnosis as an analytical quantitative process which can be readily modelled mathematically. In fact it is an interpretive process even to the untutored eye, much closer to the orientations and hermeneutic methods of the humanities and qualitative sociology than to those of the natural sciences. It should have not been necessary to say so explicitly because surely this much is obvious. Indeed, there is a large body of evidence to support this contention that much of the foundational underpinning of doctor's judgement is tacit or intuitive.

Ironically, we have already discussed this research at some length, noting that to dispute this is to also fly in the face of much research in cognitive science, neuroscience, neurology and psychology which are currently moving into a postmodern paradigm which is producing important new insights, not only vis a vis the real nature of clinical judgements as above but also the important role of the emotions in medical decisions. The appropriately comprehensive paradigmatic changes required will come only with a substantial paradigm shift to a postmodern medical one, immersed in a comprehensive societal. We introduced the emerging discipline called neuroeconomics which aims to fuse the theories, methods, and principles of psychology, economics, and neuroscience into a single theory of choice.

Over hundreds of years, biomedical and recently empirical statistical science have impacted upon medicine to cast the current modern medical paradigm in the image of the natural sciences. From the methods of Hippocrates to clinical methods of today is a big jump. For all of science's great contributions, there has been a downside. 'Clinical research' has meant biomedical research even when centred at the bedside, or more recently the conduct of clinical trials. Practically none have been directed at much needed refinement of the art of medicine.

All of this change should elicit a response or at least some recognition. Yet all of this has had surprisingly little overt impact on current beliefs in scientific circles. The outcome has been like water on a duck's back. And medical education remains doggedly focused on the 'basic sciences', to the virtually total exclusion of the social sciences, psychology, cognitive neurosciences and humanities. Basically, society is moving relentlessly into a postmodern world as part of which medicine must now adapt to a changing public mandate. This implies some radical changes to catch up with the times. Movements seeking or demanding change on pragmatic grounds, such as patient-centred care, have emerged in substantial numbers while governments and some in the higher echelons of the medical profession are moving to narrow this dismal gap between public demands and the current realities of health care delivery.

What is also absolutely an unavoidable imperative is to face the music with respect to the nature of medical judgements, and to the profound implications for patient care, public health and political decision-making, not to mention science at large. One of the fundamental attitudes feeding into medicine's public and political woes has been the current view of clinical diagnosis as an analytical quantitative process which can be readily modelled mathematically. In fact it is an interpretive process even to the untutored eye, much closer to the orientations and hermeneutic methods of the humanities and qualitative sociology than to those of the natural sciences. It should have not been necessary to say so explicitly because surely this much is obvious.

Indeed, there is a large body of provocative evidence to support the contention that much of the foundational underpinning of doctor's judgement is tacit or intuitive. We have already discussed this research at some length, noting that to dispute this is to also fly in the face of much research in neuroeconomics cognitive science, neuroscience, neurology and psychology. All of these disciplines are currently moving to conform as part of a postmodern paradigm which is producing important new insights, not only vis a vis the real nature of clinical judgements as above but also the important role of the emotions in medical decisions. The appropriately comprehensive paradigmatic changes required will come only with a substantial paradigm shift to a postmodern medical one, constrained by an overarching societal paradigm.

To understand it, we have to plumb the deepest levels of our knowledge. For all of science's great contributions, there has been a downside. This implies some radical changes from current rationalistic policies to catch up with the times is also in progress a major Kuhnian paradigm shift which will force its intellectual resources – clinical care, education and academic orientation - to re-align and conform, along with its philosophical stance (McDonald 2013). What is also absolutely an unavoidable imperative is to face up to some basic misunderstandings with respect to the nature of medical judgements, and to the profound implications for patient care, public health and political decision-making, not to mention science at large.

This new comprehensive approach hopes to provide a broader framework for investigations into the process of decision-making. I hope that the reader will agree that to understand how doctors and patients think is much more than a casual intriguing project undertaken for interest. For all of science's great contributions, there has therefore been a downside. 'Clinical research' has meant biomedical research even when centred at the bedside, or more recently the conduct of clinical trials. Practically none have been directed at much needed refinement of the art of medicine. Moreover there is increasingly germane scientific information from disciplines which focuses on decision making but which has not been supported by relevant observations in the real world of clinical practice, especially in the context of the almost forgotten area of emotional influences on judgement, and abundant evidence from recent studies in neurological and related sciences about the real combined unconscious and conscious nature of that judgement. This has had surprisingly little overt impact on current beliefs in scientific circles. And medical education remains doggedly focused on the 'basic sciences', to the virtually total exclusion of the social sciences, psychology, cognitive neurosciences and humanities!

The appropriately comprehensive paradigmatic changes required will come only with a substantial paradigm shift to a postmodern philosophical medical one, immersed in a societal paradigm with which it must obviously seamlessly articulate. Basically, society is moving relentlessly into a postmodern world as part of which medicine must now adapt to a changing public mandate. This implies some radical changes to catch up with the times. Movements seeking or demanding change on pragmatic grounds, such as patient-centred care, have emerged in substantial numbers as previously noted.

What is also absolutely an unavoidable imperative is to face up to some basic misunderstandings with respect to the nature of medical judgements, and to the profound implications of that revolution must have for patient care, public health and political decision-making, not to mention science at large. One of the fundamental attitudes feeding into medicine's public and political woes has been the current view of clinical diagnosis as an analytical quantitative process which can be readily modelled mathematically. In fact it is an interpretive process. Indeed, there is a large body of provocative evidence to support the contention that most of the foundational underpinning of a doctor's judgement is tacit or intuitive. We have already discussed this research at some length, noting that to dispute this is to also fly in the face of so much research in cognitive science, neuroscience, neurology and psychology. All of these disciplines, largely in the form of the developing 'neuroeconomics' are currently moving to conform with a postmodern paradigm which is producing important new insights, not only vis a vis the real nature of clinical judgements as above but also the important role of both tacit knowledge and impact of the emotions in medical decisions, in health decisions more generally, and in science at large.

References

Balint M., The doctor, his patient and the illness. London: Tavistock Publications; 1957.

Brainerd, C. J., & Reyna, V. F., Gist is the grist: Fuzzy-trace theory and the new intuitionism. *Developmental Review, 10*, 3–47, 1990.

Cabot R., Quoted in: Harvey and Bordley. *Differential Diagnosis.* W. B. Saunders, Philadelphia, 1955.

Clark, H. H., & Clark, E. V., Psychology and language: *An introduction to psychology.*

Doubt M., Evidence in Science June 2, 2014 November 7, 2014.

Dreyfus H. L, Dreyfus S. E., Mind over Machine: The power of human intuition and expertise in the era of the computer. Basil Blackwell., Oxford, 1986.

Feinstein A. R., Clinical Judgment. Kreiger, Malabar, 1967.

Feinstein A. R., Clinical Judgment Revisited: The Distraction of Quantitative Models. *Ann Intern Med* 1994; 120(9): 799-805.

Feinstein A. R., Clinical Epidemiology: The Architecture of Clinical Research W. B. Saunders Philadelphia 1985.

Goldman G. M., The tacit dimension of clinical judgment. *Yale J Biol Med.;* 63(1):47-61 1990.

Greenhalgh T., Intuition and evidence *Br J Gen Pract. 2002 May; 52(478): 395–400.* 2002.

Hammond K.R., Hamm R.M., Grassia J., & Pearson T., Direct comparison of intuitive and analytical cognition in expert judgement. In Research on Judgement and Decision Making (Goldstein W. & Hogarth R.M., eds), Cambridge University Press, New York, pp. 144–180 1997.

Hay C., Weisner, D., Naihua S., Niedzinski E. J., and Kravitz R. L., Harnessing experience: exploring the gap between evidence-based medicine and clinical practice. *Journal of Evaluation of Clinical Experience*, 14:707–713; 2008.

Hunter K. M., Doctors' Stories: the narrative structure of medical knowledge. Princeton University Press, New Jersey, 1991, p. 27.

Hunter K. M., Doctors' Stories: the narrative structure of medical knowledge. Princeton University Press, New Jersey, 1991, Hunter 1991, p. 152.

Koch C., Biophysics of Computation. Information processing in single neurones. Oxford University Press, New York, 1999.

Lindblom C. E., The science of muddling through. Public Administration Review; 19: 79-88. 1968.

Norman G., Young M., Brooks L., Non-analytical models of clinical reasoning: the role of experience. *Med Educ.* 2007;41(12):1140–1145.

Patel V. L., Evans D. A., Groen G. J., Biomedical knowledge and clinical reasoning. In Evans DA, Patel VL eds Cognitive Science in Medicine. MIT Press, Cambridge Mass, 1989. 53-112.

Polanyi M., a Knowing and being. In Knowing and Being. Chicago, University of Chicago Press, 1969, pp. 123-137.

Polanyi M., The tacit dimension. Garden City, NY, Doubleday, 1967 b, pp. 3-25.

Polanyi M., The logic of tacit inference. In Knowing and Being. Chicago, University of Chicago Press, 1969, pp. 138-158.

Paul J. R., Clinical Epidemiology. *J Clin Investig* 17:539-541, 1938.

Reyna, V. R., A theory of medical decision making and health: Fuzzy trace theory.*Medical Decision Making, 28*, 850–865 2008.

Reyna, V. F., Estrada, S. M., DeMarinis, J. A., Myers, R. M., Stanisz, J. M., & Mills, B. A. Neurobiological and memory models of risky decision making in adolescents versus young adults. *Journal of Experimental Psychology: Learning, Memory, and Cognition, 37*, 1125–1142. 2011.

Reyna, V. F., & Lloyd, F. J. Physician decision making and cardiac risk: Effects of knowledge, risk perception, risk tolerance, and fuzzy Reyna, V. F., & Rivers, S. E. (2008). Current theories of risk and rational decision making. *Developmental Review, 28*, 1–11. 2006.

Reyna, V. F., *Intuitive and unconscious cognitive processes in fuzzy-trace theory: An advanced approach.* Paper presented at the 23rd Subjective Probability, Utility, and Decision Making Conference, Kingston upon Thames, United Kingdom 2011.

Rittel H., Systems analysis of the 'first and second generations.' In Laconte p, Gibson, J, Rapoport A eds. Human Energy Factors in Urban Planning. NATO Advanced Study institutes Series D. Behavioural and Social Sciences No. 12, Martinus Nijhoff, The Hague, 1982, 35-63.

Schon D. S., From technical rationality to reflection-in-action. In Dowie J, Elstein A eds. Professional Judgment: A Reader in Clinical Decision Making. Cambridge University press, Cambridge, pp. 60-77. 1988.

Snow C. P., The Two Cultures and a Second Look: an expanded version of The Two Cultures and the Scientific Revolution. Cambridge University Press, Cambridge, processing. *Journal of Experimental Psychology: Applied, 12*, 179–195. 1964.

Weber, E. U., Johnson, E. J., Milch, K., Chang, H., Brodscholl, J., & Goldstein, D. Asymmetric discounting in intertemporal choice: A query theory account. *Psychological Science, 18*, 516–523 2007.

Chapter 14

Evidence-Based Medicine -
The Clash with Clinical Medicine

About 25 years have elapsed since evidence-based medicine (EBM) began to move away from its parent clinical epidemiology, to establish a more separate identity as 'a new boy on the block' (Straus and McAlister 2009). Since then, it has been controversial in medicine, and more recently in other disciplines as 'evidence-based practice' (Hammersley 2007). Its chief problem in medicine has been that clinicians have objected to its dismissive attitude to clinical experience, said to be 'anecdotal.'. EBM has valorised the randomised trial as the gold standard of scientific evidence for clinical management decisions, despite a serious problem in that the 'hard' evidence, that is of high internal validity, from randomised trials, an epidemiologic adaption, has limited external validity to apply to clinical patient populations.

In any case, it seems quite obvious that a wide variety of personal, emotional, social, and contextual influences as well as a range of variables from other sources usually enter into any significant clinical management judgement and decision (Chapter 13). This is particularly so for functional symptoms related to personal and social variables important in patient management. To mistake these for evidence of organic disease can be serious, causing at best just an unhappy patient at worst an unnecessary intervention or lifelong anxiety, a life sentence. The usual unhappy outcome is to miss a patient's real reason for seeking the help of the doctor, or failure to elicit personal preferences. This is 'consultation failure' (McDonald 2013). This can result in a dissatisfied patient, impaired placebo effect, rejection of medical advice, doctor shopping, noncompliance with medication, failure to accept appropriate reassurance, defection from treatment, even litigation.

'Clinical epidemiology' represents the belated introduction of empirical statistical science into clinical research - the completion of the paradigm shift which began with C-P-A Louis at the beginning of the 19th century, and which was completed by Feinstein (1967) relatively recently. We have suggested previously that biomedical science impacted on medicine, beginning in late 18th century France and continuing its rise, gaining further impetus from its achievements in two World Wars. Osler, Peabody and Cabot felt that doctors had lost much of the human touch by the early part of the 19th century (McDonald 2013). This trend was later confirmed by physicians White and Barondess, and echoed by opinion polls at the time. Empirical statistical science, however, did not gain purchase in the clinical scene until the early 1960s in the form of clinic-al epidemiology and later, evidence-based medicine. An urgent task now facing medicine is to restore a balance between all kinds of clinical science and the art of medicine.

Where Is the Proof of the Pudding?

Unlike its parent, clinical epidemiology, evidence-based medicine has become a controversial element in health services research. Some clinicians are proponents of evidence-based medicine, others are vocal in their disapproval. Few would question that to gather the best empirical data is misguided. However, evidence-based medicine has been accused of being authoritarian, of privileging a narrow definition of evidence (Tonelli 2006), with promulgating a preoccupation with clinical trials and a dedication to numbers divorced from clinical context and social meaning, of denigrating clinical judgement, and of questioning the art of medicine, as well as epistemological and philosophical issues. Enthusiasm for an exciting mission has even been seen as arrogance, even a kind of fascism (Walsh 2012). There is also the question of a lack of accountability in that it has provided no proof of efficacy let alone superiority to traditional care. I can locate no controlled study of evidence-based medicine. A randomized trial seems impractical if used alone. In fact what is needed is a program of evaluation comprising multiple studies in order to address the sheer magnitude and complexity of such an evaluation (Chapter 14).

The Spectre of Political Hegemony in Health Services Research

Even worse, evidence-based medicine has been accused of supping with the devil of managed care, a party to clinical coercion and control (Ashmore 1989). Some clinicians have suspected that guidelines incorporating data from trials might be used coercively by health bureaucracies and managed care interests to promote covert rationing, thereby impinging on clinical autonomy and on patient's rights. In this chapter we review the roots of this important clash of paradigms. Another criticism has EBM accused of nurturing 'managerialism.' In this regard, there is debate about the proper place of treatment guidelines. This will require some soul searching by those concerned. Again this is for the health profession generally and political agencies to tackle. Another is the sheer volume of research results to be read and appraised. Again this is not a problem that EBM alone can solve. EBM must work with political agencies and the health professions to highlight the issue. Finally, some 'oversized' trials may produce statistically significant results but the actual clinical benefit may be marginal. A basic problem too is lack of generalisability to clinical populations. Nevertheless all parties would benefit if clinicians and EBM could be reconciled over the issue of clinical judgement and expertise in relation to empirical trial results.

Although we have concentrated on criticism, we suggest references which can balance the account. A wide ranging but rather intemperate critique of evidence based medicine has been undertaken by Charlton (2009). Straus and McAlister (2000) provide a balanced account, and Sackett et al. (2000) a comprehensive introduction. What evidence-medicine has achieved is to highlight the importance of sound design of clinical trials, and of the skills in 'clinical appraisal' needed to assess this epidemiological evidence.

Reactions to EBM

Much of current concern is a reaction to what many see as evidence-based medicine's promulgation of what is seen by many as a form of 'scientism' - privileging empirical statistical evidence with a diminished role for clinical experience, little attention to contextual influences, patients' wishes, preferences, values, contributions of family and friends, biomedical science, constraining social and political factors, even a reduced role for the clinical sciences. One means of contributing to both art and science is by achievement of a workable rapprochement between such movements and evidence-based medicine, thereby having the best of both worlds. A specific area of concern previously flagged is neglect of those 'soft variables' which are so important in management, especially as harbingers of functional illness (Feinstein 1967). Such variables may be rendered 'hard' using Feinstein's clinimetrics. In addition, they can be captured by thorough history-taking with sympathetic listening and close attention to the patient's narrative account of the illness and non-verbal clues.

Over the past 20 years, the call for restoration of medicine's more humanistic face has grown louder as evidenced by the appearance of a plethora of movements which have the basic aim of developing just such a humanistic renaissance (Kravetz 2008). I recently counted 58! To name but a few, these have included the biopsychosocial model, patient-centred clinical care, person-centred, narrative-based care, values-based care, integrative care, holistic medicine, humanistic medicine, evidence-informed health care, complexity-based medicine, interpretive medicine, patient and family-centred care. A continuing acrimonious debate instead of a cooperative attempt at understanding the issue will be harmful to good clinical research and efficient health care evaluation. A healthy debate predicated upon goodwill and a mutual objective of integrating clinical care has much to offer.

There is even controversy about the concept of the nature of the evidence used for a doctor's clinical decisions. Inappropriate restriction of appropriate interventions by EBM is an important criticism. Clinicians often fail to elicit important personal, relevant family and social contextual information. This sin can be traced to 'scientistic' thinking which has burgeoned during the 20th century rise of biomedical influence (Habermas 1978). In addition, EBM has included clinical experience with the 'soft' data, while results of randomised trials, as being science-based are defined as 'hard' (Feinstein 1987). The stance of 'evidence-based medicine' has been that data that doctors should use in diagnosis and treatment choices should come solely or predominantly from randomised clinical trials, the medical equivalent of the controlled laboratory experiment. In this context, clinical experience is also dismissed as of low quality even unscientific. Even evidence derived from biomedical sciences has been downgraded by evidence-based medicine. Not surprisingly, few clinicians would agree.

Should Evidence-Based Medicine Itself Be Evaluated? Can It Be?

Finally, evidence-based medicine promotes healthy scepticism about the efficacy of interventions. This has led critics to insist that it too is a technology which must be rigorously evaluated (Tobin 2008). That is, evidence-based medicine should be hoist by its own petard! If so, how is this to be done? Should it be evaluated according to its own criteria, hence be subjected to a randomised trial? We discuss the problems in chapter 14. There is a risk that, in such an adversarial atmosphere, evidence-based medicine could inadvertently cleave the paradigm of clinical medicine by widening the gulf between the art and the science of medicine, as well as by driving a wedge between public health and clinical practice at a crucial time when they need to work together. These are important issues. The critique to follow should therefore be seen as constructive, as a springboard for developing a broader more inclusive model of clinical practice and research for the next millennium, the outline of which we present in the last chapter.

Evidence-Based Everything

Nonetheless, when all is said and done, evidence-based' practice is surely the flavor of the month. Even the name has been labelled 'rhetorical' and the claim made that it has been used as a sales pitch. Practically every health discipline - clinical medicine and its specialties, allied health and nursing professions, education, dentistry, public health and health administration, veterinary science, even music therapy and medical chaplaincy have recently proclaimed that its practice is or should be 'evidence-based' (Hammersley 2007).

The definition of evidence-based medicine put forward by the proponents of evidence-based medicine is hardly controversial. It is 'the conscientious, explicit and judicious use of current best evidence in making decisions about the care of the individual patient.'(Sackett et al. 1997). The McMaster group has taken pains to point out that the addition of a 'science of the art of medicine' was not to be taken as a denigration of the art, so that the justification of clinical epidemiology 'stems from its ability to explain and to teach, not replace, the art of medicine' (Sackett et al. 1997). There has been some retreat from this rather radical point of view.

The problem is to have general agreement of what is to count as evidence, and how much weight each contributor to a judgement should be allocated. Also important is overlooking or denying the crucial role of Polyanyi's tacit knowledge (Polanyi 1958). As Schon (1983) the Dreyfus brothers (Dreyfus and Dreyfus 1986) and Patel (1989) have found, an obsessive belief that science is all about conscious analytical reasoning leaves no room for tacit knowledge or the art of a practice. Lay people, lawyers and doctors differ in the kind of evidence they seek and accept. While lay people are frequently swayed by professional expertise and status, the law pays more attention to the reliability of personal testimony, clinical medicine is much influenced by the authority of clinical experience, and empirical statistical scientific medicine is more inclined to accept evidence on the grounds of probability estimates. As Saunders (2000) put it: We easily forget that the consensus of the guideline writers is not itself "evidence" but, at best, the summary of practical wisdom.'

Clinical experience with its reliance on experience, extrapolation and the critical application of other ad hoc rules, must be applied to traverse the grey zones of practice. As Naylor (1995) said, 'the prudent application of the evaluative sciences will affirm rather than obviate the need for the art of medicine.'(Naylor 1995).

The Pros and Cons of the Randomised Trial

Central to the paradigm of evidence-based medicine is its emphasis on the randomised trial, the health services equivalent of the scientifically proven controlled laboratory experiment. The randomised trial is only one method used in health services research but it is central to our story because it became the linchpin of drug evaluation, surrounded by a seductive aura of high science, and its obvious importance for drug evaluation, especially to prevent the community risk of toxic effects. This makes any critique, or expression of concerns about when it and how should be applied, seem unreasonable. Moreover the focus on the randomised trial is what has distinguished the narrower agenda of evidence-based medicine from its more broadly based parent, clinical epidemiology.

Yet, in retrospect, despite the randomised controlled trial's great achievements, it may have also been inadvertently a party to misleading us. The relative ease of controlling the circumstances surrounding the administration and context of administration of an intervention as simple as a drug has had an unanticipated 'side-effect.'. It has made us complacent about evaluating much more socially immersed and complex interventions such as diagnostic tests, surgery, information technologies, evidence-based medicine or indeed the clinical process of clinical diagnosis and management itself (McDonald 2013)! A preoccupation with randomised controlled trials has been seen as inappropriately narrowing the focus of clinical epidemiology, distracting from the equally important tasks of studying and refining the processes of clinical examination, and more comprehensive evaluation of health interventions in their full social and cultural context.

Evidence from randomised controlled trials contributes to clinical decisions which relate to technological interventions. However physicians know intuitively that they base their judgements on a wide variety of individual pieces of evidence, hence they baulk if one form of evidence, specifically efficacy data from randomised controlled trials, is privileged above the rest (Tonelli 2006). It certainly is reasonable that we should first demonstrate the efficacy of an intervention - its performance in selected patients under ideal and controlled conditions of use in centres of excellence – its efficacy - as soon as possible after its introduction. If the intervention cannot be shown to work under such ideal conditions, then there is no point in introducing it into routine practice. But the demonstration of efficacy alone is not enough.

The Importance of Evaluating Effectiveness as Well as Efficacy

The conditions of randomised trials are artificially controlled, and the results are expressed as averages - which denies us access to the variety of outcomes observed in individual participants. In fact it flies in the face of the importance of Feinstein's range of multivariable patterns of disease manifestations, therapy and health outcome. Hence it is often difficult to predict the extent to which a particular patient is likely to benefit or to be warned that some rarely may even be harmed. This problem of lack of generalisability of trial results is even more troublesome in the case of intricate therapeutic interventions such as coronary angioplasty where operator skill and laboratory standards are major local variables, and for diagnostic tests where local quality of imaging and accuracy of interpretation can vary considerably from one institution to another.

What clinicians, consumers and policy-makers need for their routine decisions is information on the effectiveness of interventions where treatment is actually taking place which is crucially dependent upon local standards of quality of care and constitution of local populations. Indeed information on the performance of coronary angioplasty from the Mayo Clinic, or of magnetic resonance imaging from Hammersmith Hospital might well be misleading if accepted at face value by local clinicians, or if incorporated into calculations of cost-effectiveness for policy decisions. Thus clinicians considering referral of patients with angina for coronary angioplasty should know the local track record of effectiveness and patient satisfaction. Similarly clinicians who order echocardiograms for young people with heart murmurs must have information about the local quality of performance and interpretation; false positive or doubtful results can wreck a patient's employment prospects, even launch careers of illness.

Increasingly patients want such local information, and health policy makers, charged with the responsibility of monitoring quality of care should be able to access aggregated local effectiveness data of this kind for the institutions they control. Hence the testing of efficacy of interventions under controlled conditions in large multicentre randomised trials should be seen as no more than the 'first cut' in an ongoing program of evaluation, albeit an important one, which must be followed by a more extensive program of evaluation of effectiveness in relation to local variations of quality of care and composition of patient populations.

Thus to complement the efficacy research which confirms feasibility of clinical benefit established in highly controlled trials, we need effectiveness research to bridge the gap between ideal conditions of testing and those of local routine practice. Thus effectiveness of an intervention must vary from one clinical setting to another depending on selection of patients for an intervention, how appropriately the intervention is used, levels of clinical skill and experience, the disease spectrum under investigation, the quality of equipment and numerous other aspects of the standard of care. The local data needed for these judgements must come from smaller rigorous trials, both randomised and non-randomised, and from observation of patient cohorts with representative sampling of patients in individual hospitals and on a regional basis (Charlton 1997). Studies of cohorts of patients in the context of routine care can provide information which controlled trials cannot. This includes context of use, appropriateness of clinical patient selection, documentation of their preferences, expectations and satisfaction, impact of the intervention on patient functional status and quality of life, and documentation of complications and adverse events.

The capacity to accumulate experience in this way could provide access to high quality aggregated clinical experience especially valuable for quality assurance and health care planning. Production of the necessary data base has been greatly facilitated by advances in information technology. We have already asserted that, for example, by interrogating a data-base a clinician could, in the future, get direct assistance for disease diagnosis and for choice of treatment in an individual patient by a search for matching patterns of patient characteristics and presentation in this locally generated data. For rare conditions or those posing special treatment problems, the search might be extended to a national or international data-base. Clearly the local data on tests to guide policy would also be coded as part of such a facility.

Thus the demonstration of the efficacy is only the first step in the comprehensive iterative evaluation of an intervention. Study of its effectiveness in the battlefield of routine clinical practice must follow. Thus the randomised trial and the detailed information from a physician's pattern recognition, based upon tacit knowledge, yield complementary information! Anyone who studies clinical decision making has found that many variables clearly make a contribution to any clinical judgement. Moreover, they usually interact with one another in an intricate way. Much evidence has proved conclusively that tacit knowledge, storage of clinical information and of emotional responses can no longer be blithely ignored as determinants of decisions of all kinds including clinical judgements and health care decisions.

Is the Evidence-Based Movement in Crisis?

Serious conflict in health care does not augur well for cooperation needed for the progress of evaluation. Modern medicine has come in for criticism for cultivating rationalistic, technology dominated, hospital-centred clinical care. The 'science' referred to in the past in the context of the structure of health care has, until recently, been biomedical science, not empirical statistical science. Hence at the same time as it stands accused of being unscientific in the eyes of evidence-based medicine, medicine is also faced with the rise of narrative-based, person-centred clinical practice (Levenstein 1986). Nor has the recent rise to prominence of evidence-based medicine escaped some fundamental criticism. Greenhalgh et al. (2014) have identified factors suggesting the possibility of 'crisis' in evidence-based medicine. The most serious is the problem of the proportion of RCTs funded by pharmaceutical companies, and in some cases, fraudulent misconduct in withholding negative results or use of misleading statistics. Most large clinical trials are funded by big pharma. Furthermore doctors may not declare conflicts of interest. This is clearly a major ethical problem for the medical profession and for politicians.

Is It 'Unscientific' to Question EBM?

Is this difference of opinion at root inevitable or can we reconcile these two points of view which at first glance seem poles apart? In our culture, to question the assumptions of 'evidence-based practice' can be seen as unscientific even irrational. Even the name 'evidence-based medicine' itself has been used as a deliberate rhetorical device to inhibit argument. Gaining influence in medicine for over 20 years, during which time there has been a rapid spread of an analogous 'evidence-based practice' to many professional disciplines, as mentioned above. Virtually every activity has or plans to stake out a claim to be seen as evidence-based!

Is The Basic Problem Simply a Misunderstanding at Root?

If we stand back a little, we see that there is misunderstanding or lack of understanding at the root of this debate. In fact, there are two related misunderstandings. One uncomfortable but unavoidable fact is that many patients, especially in general practice and outpatients, present to the doctor with 'functional symptoms' related to personal stress or problems of living. Hence it is necessary to understand the true explanation for symptoms and their treatment preferences. These are quintessentially 'soft data' but we obviously have to use them in patient care! This is the first misunderstanding. The second concerns the concept of 'external validity,' the generalizability of evidence from a randomised trial to patients in a variety of clinical populations.

The 'Soft' Clinical Data Rendered Hard

It is important to note that to express diagnosis in scientific terms, and to devise appropriate grading scales for such variables as severity of pain and anxiety, will require us to scientifically operationalise the innumerable relevant variables comprising clinical patterns of illness. A valuable spin-off of the need to focus on the clinical patterns will be to turn the spotlight on the currently neglected personal and social variables, especially when the patient presents with 'functional symptoms.' The onus therefore rests squarely on physicians to fine tune their history-taking to include relevant 'soft data' as we have defined it. The role of the skills of clinical epidemiology and EBM is, as at present, to develop and operationalise such data so that it is suitable for computer storage of clinical patterns, and available for quantitative statistical analysis, as well as qualitative analysis or both as appropriate.

EBM and Clinimetrics

A few clinical variables are obviously already routinely expressed in quantitative form – to whit heart rate, blood pressure, respiratory rate, temperature, body weight, duration of illness. Nor have clinicians been entirely remiss with regard to developing the necessary definitions and ordinal grading scales which constitute 'clinimetrics.' Severity of pain is usually quantified according to the common 'mild, moderate, severe' scale, as would be expected and the same is true for symptoms such as limitation by angina of effort and intermittent claudication. Nevertheless, the quality of such instruments should be more stringently evaluated using psychometric indices of reliability and validity. Textbooks and research papers already contain many important definitions, classifications and grading scales. In 1939, Wagner and Keith produced a grading scale for severity of hypertensive retinopathy. Other well-known examples include the New York Heart Association grading scale for dyspnoea, the Apgar score for neonatal respiratory distress, grading of carcinoma (e.g., breast, colon) for prognosis and treatment, a classification of coronary events, the Glasgow Coma Scale widely used to express depth of unconsciousness and the Jones criteria for the diagnosis of rheumatic fever. No doubt many more clinimetrics could be developed for patient assessment. Quality assurance would also benefit from more precise data.

The Rise of Qualitative Research

Driven by our culture's preference for a 'scientific approach' to problem solving, widespread use of the randomised trial, the equivalent of a 'medical experiment,' simply eclipsed the Feinstein insight. Thus the EBM movement maintained that, when available, only the results of clinical trials, preferably randomised, should be used as the most reliable scientific evidence for patient management decisions - the 'level 1 evidence' of evidence-based medicine. Clinical judgement was first relegated to the lowest rung. (Guyatt 2008) Clinical expertise was later given a partial reprieve, along with biomedical evidence. Both remained still on the lowest grading of the current methodological league tables. But qualitative data analysis was initially spurned as an essential tool for clinical research (Guyatt 2008), however its potential contribution has been subsequently acknowledged (Giacomini 2001). However, we can be thankful that Feinstein's insights showed the way to reunite evidence-based medicine and clinical epidemiology, and to heal today's clinical schism between clinicians and the proponents of evidence-base medicine.

Clearly the skills of Feinstein's original broad definition of clinimetrics are central to this crucial task of rendering the 'soft data' possible to manipulate mathematically. In an ideal world, clinicians themselves should be able to operationalise the clinical data, armed to the teeth with knowledge of clinical epidemiology. Unfortunately such physicians are currently thin on the ground! Hence clinical researchers for the present need the cooperation of those clinicians versed in evidence-based medicine who do have the necessary depth of knowledge in clinical appraisal to do the job.

Given current educational arrangements, however, more and more clinicians should soon be able to participate. In fact, clinical epidemiology and evidence-based medicine will become an essential part of that store of conscious and unconscious tacit knowledge which provides that invisible framework which underpins their clinical reasoning – constituting just one of many disciplinary sources like physiology, anatomy, pathology and biochemistry have already done in the past. Thus it seems that clinicians to some extent shoulder the blame for not eliciting the important clinical variables in the first place.

Randomised Controlled Trials and the Validity of Clinical Evidence

To illustrate the problem, we shall consider two hypothetical 'experiments' - one an agricultural experiment and one a clinical randomised trial. The randomised controlled trial (RCT) had its modern beginnings in agriculture. Our first hypothetical experiment is to test the effect of an antifungal agent on leaf damage. The extent of leaf damage (defined) is the specified outcome variable. The experiment is conducted in a single hothouse in which temperature, humidity, hydration, soil and additives are held constant i.e., 'controlled.' Past experience and earlier research indicates that no other variable is likely to influence the outcome, hence they were left uncontrolled. Suppose that the intervention batch does have reduced leaf damage. The outcome is unequivocal as a difference which is highly unlikely on statistical grounds to be attributable to chance, say $p < 0.01$.

This result can assumed be to free of bias by dint of the control measures incorporated and random error set by statistical control - yielding high 'internal validity.' In addition, the result can also be safely extrapolated to similar farms which suggests that 'external validity' is also high because the experimental conditions are quite replicable. But there is a catch. An important contributor to this high external validity, however, once known possible confounding variables have been controlled, is that the plants can reasonably be regarded as identical in all important respects other than the intervention. Not so for our patients! As clinicians would have it – 'no two patients are the same.' Patients happen to live in a complex social and political context.

The structure of a clinical randomized clinical trial is similar to the agricultural one in many ways but differs in some crucial aspects. Unhappily, these differences have caused much controversy and misunderstanding. For example, the EBM concept of clinical 'levels of evidence' is flawed on these grounds since it is based upon the maximisation of 'internal validity' by randomization and control – but variables which are 'soft' but important to clinical management are not recorded. Therefore high internal validity has been achieved at the expense of una-voidable impairment of 'external validity.' A second related problem is that it hardly seems reasonable to reject information as central to patient care as patients' preferences, social conditions, clinical experience, pathology, physiology and biochemistry which frequently make a contribution to a management decision, a fact now conceded by the EBM movement (Tonelli 2006, Charles et al. 2011).

Two study populations for a clinical randomised controlled trial the impact of coronary artery surgery on mortality are selected by random (chance) allocation. This has the desired effect of producing two essentially identical populations - the 'intervention group' to receive a new treatment under test, and a 'control group' receiving previously standard treatment or none at all, as appropriate. Allocation of patients to treatment is 'blinded' to both experimenters and, where feasible, to patients, in order to avoid a common source of bias. Random allocation of patients also ensures that the control and intervention groups have the best chance of including equal proportions of potential 'confounding' variables such as the nature and quality of clinical care, known previous damage to heart muscle, high blood pressure, valvular disease, diabetes, age and gender. The success of randomisation in distributing these confounding variables can also be checked. But what of ethical issues, such as political implications and justice of decisions about equitable access to interventional technology such as the use of urgent coronary angioplasty in emerging myocardial infarction?

In addition, can the personal and social aspects of the functional symptoms which have resulted in patient seeking medical help be meaningfully quantified? This is a problem of external validity. If the study outcome is not statistically significantly different for the two groups, then the hypothesis is confirmed, and vice versa. Because of control measures and randomisation, we can claim high 'internal validity' brought about by maximal desired reduction of random error and bias. We can also claim reasonable external validity seeing that known potential confounding variables have been controlled. However, there remains the problem of heterogeneity of particular patient populations hence the difficulty which often occurs when attempting to apply the trial results to an individual patient. Another recent approach has been the appearance of 'mixed methods research' (Sandelowski et a.l 2006) which can be used to apply both quantitative and qualitative data analysis even to data from randomized trials.

Validity – Internal and External

Not surprisingly then, as a scientifically controlled experiment, the RCT has become the 'gold standard' for 'experimental validity' in health research. However we should really specify 'internal' validity. Equally important is 'external' validity, that ability to generalise the trial result to other populations, which means that those recruited for trials have been selected (Feinstein 1995). For one thing, trials are frequently multicentre – different in several respects from a clinical population to which we may wish to generalise or extrapolate the trial results. Unhappily, there are a large number of variables which can jeopardise external validity, and these have been documented is has been so for many studies in the past.

Some important challenges to external validity include: trial setting: (recruitment from primary, secondary, or tertiary care, selection of participating centres, eligibility criteria); characteristics of the randomised patients: (stage, severity of disease, comorbidity); intervention procedure (differences between trial protocol and routine practice, timing of treatment, adequacy of non-trial treatment); outcome measures and follow-up: (frequency and length of follow-up, adverse effects of treatment, completeness of reporting, rates of discontinuation of treatment, exclusion of patients at risk of complications) (Rothwell 2005).

Thus the randomised controlled trial for all its elegance, high internal validity and scientific appeal, cannot provide data on all of the illness variables constituting the clinical pattern required for the care of the individual. Instead we get an 'average' patient profile which cannot easily be generalized to apply to those infinitely variable patterns of clinical variables which represent individual patients in practice. 'Soft data' essential to management is missing. Even if information for clinical guidelines has been collected according to the recommendations of 'evidence based medicine,' i.e., using the methods of 'clinical appraisal,' the limitations of generalizability of randomized trials and lack of access to important personal and social influences on patient outcome cannot be entirely circumvented.

Despite these limitations, the randomised controlled trial nevertheless can provide high quality data on overall afficacy and indispensable evidence regarding the safety of treatments. However, rather than simply wringing our hands and bemoaning the deficiencies of clinical experience yielding 'soft' data, we could be constructive. First, it is incumbent on clinicians to make the first move by improving the comprehensiveness of their clinical history-taking to capture the often overlooked personal and social details. Indeed, the storage of the clinical patterns of illness would oblige clinicians to do just that in order to program the computer as we suggest below. Using a combination of methods, including data from clinical trials, a local and even an international data-base, data with high internal and external validity could thereby be on tap. Essentially, we would be combining bedside capture of refined expert clinical judgement by combining scientifically appraised clinical trial evidence with computer-based recognition of Feinstein's taxonomic clinical patterns.

A Complex Clinical Decision

An example of a management decision with a relatively small number of inputs is to terminate an attempted resuscitation of a patient with a cardiac arrest. Even then the decision to cease a patient's resuscitation attempt still poses a complex system of numerous interacting variables to be interpreted. These might include the patient's wishes, if known, those of the family, religious beliefs, scientific medical knowledge of the limits to resuscitation and past experience, risk of the patient's remaining life being on a respirator or with unacceptable complications such as irreversible brain damage, the duration of the arrest, number of countershocks, patient level of consciousness, the success of the attempt so far, especially the electrocardiographic heart rhythm, the cause of the arrest, time to commencement of resuscitation attempt, and comorbidity, especially lethal illness such as an incurable cancer. There may also be perhaps a sense of personal failure, and the anticipated negative response of some attending doctors and nurses to the decision, and sometimes even the prospect of litigation. Although the clinical scenario might seem extreme, it is a common enough occurrence in hospital practice.

Most treatment decisions do have a large number of mutually interacting determinants which have to be weighed up. In chronic disease, the problem is even worse. The number of variables determining a decision can be greater, and they can include ethical dilemmas. For instance a middle aged woman with angina on exertion and at rest had coronary artery bypass grafting recommended. The moral dilemma arose because she was a Jehovah's Witness. Following WW II, the Watchtower Society, introduced a ban on accepting blood transfusions, even in life-threatening situations. The religion forbade the administration of blood products. Coronary artery grafting with appropriate modifications to avoid the use of blood or products was recommended, and accepted but only after a protracted discussion about the morality of the intervention. We counted, in all, fifteen variables other than the moral and ethical influences which were significant contributors to the clinical decision.

Hence to automatically privilege the empirical statistical results of clinical trials for management seems rather unrealistic. Furthermore, the importance of each of these factors which feed into a clinical decision will vary. Obviously those factors carrying most weight in the judgement will depend on the specifics of the particular patient and illness. In addition, one should remember that, according to complexity theory, these many variables interact as part of a system in innumerable unpredictable ways. Note that some of the required information is clinical data, some scientific, some humanistic, some social and some practical. Small wonder that clinical judgement is so demanding, and that medical training takes so long!

Evidence-based medicine has focused attention on the importance of scientific rigour in gathering clinical evidence, and the need for clinicians to apply it. Clearly this should be applauded. But there can be no real resolution to conflict however until the importance of all of the clinical data, including the patient's narrative, is also acknowledged, together with encapsulated computer-based summaries of the personal and social context of illness of individual patients. Currently deemed 'soft,' such data is nonetheless complementary with that from clinical trials, provided that it can be properly operationalized and, when relevant, quantified. If physicians do respond to the call, perhaps advocates of EBM would accept the importance of clinical experience, the 'soft' clinical data diligently made 'hard' by clinimetrics, and the limitations of RCTs in individual patient management could be more clearly acknowledged.

The main bone of contention between EBM and clinicians could be removed by such a compromise which recognises the complementary nature of the two enterprises, according to each its appropriate place. The current counterproductive stand-off of evidence-based medicine with many clinicians should then cease. The likely outcome of some merger between the competing art and science of medicine seems certain to be a compromise with which neither will be entirely satisfied but with a foundation in scientifically informed decisions in a matrix of patient-centred care leading to a balanced delivery of medical care. Systems theory would predict just such an outcome when two potent subsystems engage in intellectual and political conflict. So too would a classical dialectical process of resolution according to Hegel. At a commonsense lay level, it would indeed seem inevitable!

Methodological Bias Causing a Distorted Clinical Research Agenda

The impact of empirical statistical science in the form of population epidemiology and evidence based medicine implies a commitment to numbers. Interpretive research in sociology and anthropology works with the spoken or written word, with narrative. If these camps committed to different intellectual paradigms work in isolation, this can have a blinkering effect which seriously distorts the agenda of clinical research. Thus there is a pervasive temptation to rely solely on familiar and favoured quantitative methods even if these are inappropriate for the problem at hand. Hence the randomised trial came to be seen as a methodological gold standard, its results automatically at the top of evidence-based medicine's hierarchy of evidence (Guyatt 2008). It is true that the randomised trial is best for testing an hypothesis - if the project is ethical, if the intervention is not a moving target, that is, still in the process of rapid technical evolution or changing clinical application, if the evaluation issue is efficacy, if suitable quantitative outcomes can be measured, if a study population can be recruited which is sufficiently representative of patients in practice, if the context and intervention can reasonably be controlled, and if adequate resources are available.

If, on the other hand, the question relates to understanding the motivations, judgements and behaviour of doctors and patients, an interpretive approach using interview and qualitative data analysis is the only appropriate method. Too much emphasis on surveys and trials will restrict the scope of health services research such that some of the most important and intractable problems of clinical care and of health care delivery, such as patient dissatisfaction, delay in seeking medical help, noncompliance and failure of reassurance, will simply be avoided or the research program will miss the core of the problem.

This is an implicit denial that studies sensitive to local context, usually non-randomised comparisons, will be essential for the study of local effectiveness, and that qualitative studies are necessary to decipher the meaning of numbers. There is also an implicit bias here towards the evaluation of technical effectiveness of therapeutic interventions, and against the very important personal and social contextual elements of clinical judgement. To increase the rationality of decision-making in health is a worthy goal. However, it is also clear that human beings will continue to be influenced by feelings and life circumstances in their day-to-day judgements whether they be seeking medical help or making medical or policy decisions. When considering the appropriateness of an intervention, an unduly sharp focus what clinicians call the 'clinical indications' can create the impression that other influences on the decision-making of doctor and patient are less real or less legitimate. Many patients limit the effectiveness of their treatment by not taking their medication as prescribed, delay seeking medical advice for serious problems, or worry about symptoms after being reassured on the basis of negative test results. In these areas, investigation by survey, trial and mathematical modelling alone has failed dismally to reveal the important determinants of these crucial patient judgements.

Evidence-based medicine can distort clinical research in a more immediate way than through methodological prejudice. Apart from the problem already discussed of the sponsorship and financial support of randomised trials in hospital departments by pharmaceutical companies poses a tempting research option for departments severely financially pinched and with increasingly restricted opportunities for clinical research. The downside is that trial protocols have been professionally constructed by the companies in line with regulatory requirements, so that there is little intellectual challenge for local clinicians and trainees. Research nurses often supervise the data collection for multicentre trials, and busy junior staff with little stake in the study may be tempted to cut corners. Limiting time devoted to the details of patient recruitment and protocol supervision can severely compromise rigour. This is bad training for staff as well. Financially lucrative participation in multiple randomised trials can also distract from the biomedical research which tends to the long term needs of both clinical practice and pharmaceutical research. Peripheral involvement in trials can be misleadingly construed as 'doing clinical epidemiology' or 'practising evidence-based research' - to the detriment of the broader program of real clinical epidemiology.

Warrants for a Clinical Decision and Clinimetrics

The legion of variables which can influence a clinical decision (warrants) is highly varied, Some of the required information is clinical data, some scientific, some humanistic, some social and some practical. In addition, one should remember that these many variables interact as part of a system in innumerable unpredictable ways which can result in millions of combinations and permutations for the outcome. Clinimetrics can perform a valuable service by providing a tool for operationalizing, i.e., 'hardening the soft data,' needed for the interpretation of clinical trials (Crowther-Heyck 2005). This is the basic hurdle facing evidence-based medicine and other quantitative methods, acknowledging their contribution as an important complementary one. It could allow room for compromise between evidence-based medicine and clinicians who tend to promote diametrically opposed views, a kind of stand-off between randomized clinical trials and clinical judgement. The analytic reductionistic approach of clinical epidemiology and evidence-based medicine to such awesome complexity is simply no match as a means of interpreting the outcome of such a complex dynamic system of mutually interacting clinical variables. It seems likely that for analyzing such a system in humans, cerebral pattern recognition based upon tacit knowledge is responsible (Polanyi 1958).

Small wonder that clinical judgement is so demanding, and that clinical expertise is critical in decision making! It is the narrow focus of 'the evidence,' the tendency to valorise quantitative scientific evidence over clinical observations experience, biomedical research, and contextual factors which has drawn most fire from general practice. Here the personal and social factors are so important, clinical trials are most difficult to conduct, clinical research hardest to conduct and to interpret. In fact, evidence obtained in hospital settings is potentially misleading if applied in general practice.

Evidence-Based Medicine, General Practice and Qualitative Analysis

General practice has led the way in recognising and studying problems of doctor-patient communication, an area where there is little scope for randomised trials. Clinical epidemiology and evidence-based medicine were developed and are now mainly deployed to study technological or drug interventions, the epitome of the teaching hospital Central Zone the high ground of clinical practice. Reliance on quantitative methods alone makes it difficult for evidence-based medicine to study the diagnosis of the ubiquitous symptoms in general and supportive patient care which are at a premium in the 'Peripheral Zone' of care. Here illness is often ill-defined, linked to problems of living and social context, often presenting in the form of a symptom complex rather than as clear cut organic disease.

Evidence, Clinical Judgement and Clinical Experience

A charge repeatedly levelled at clinical epidemiologists who espouse evidence-based medicine is that they do not adequately acknowledge the importance of clinical experience and of clinical judgement. Yet even randomised trial pioneer statistician Bradford Hill spoke of the need to incorporate highly skilled subjective clinical judgment into medical decisions (Matthews 1995). Even those protagonists of evidence-based medicine who are the butt of current criticisms have repeatedly stressed the complementary nature of good external evidence and clinical evidence in good clinical decision-making. Evidence based medicine set out to de-emphasize. However Sackett et al. state categorically that good practice 'means integrating individual clinical expertise with the best available external clinical evidence from systematic research,' emphasising that 'neither alone is enough' (Sackett 1995).

Sackett and coworkers also acknowledge the importance of the art of medicine: 'this additional basic science for clinical medicine must be applied with abundant humility, recognizing that much of its justification stems from its ability to explain and to teach, not replace, the art of medicine.' (Sackett et al. 1991). Nonetheless this position is implicitly denied when randomised trial evidence is weighted at the top of the grading scale for evidence and clinical evidence at the bottom, and when mathematical models such as decision analysis are proposed for decisions at the bedside.

Evidence-Based Medicine – The Art of Medicine Cannot Be Replaced

The danger, seen from the clinical perspective, is that the art of medicine is much more difficult to articulate, to transmit and to defend than is an appeal to science, rationality and mathematical models. Hence it can be ignored, factored out in controlled studies, denigrated as unscientific or condemned as a cloak for ignorance, relegated to the status of 'practice style' (Wennberg 1984), or simply banished from clinical thinking - but it cannot be replaced. Cohen et al. (2004) have nicely summarized the criticisms of evidence-based medicine. We believe that the most important relate to not acknowledging the shere complexity of clinical judgement, and the disparagement or neglect of qualitative method. More generally, there is a narrow focus on quantitative method, especially on the randomized controlled trial with lack of attention to that wide spectrum of evidence needed in clinical practice research. This is reinforced by a similar emphasis on quantitative methods in research funding and in ethics committees.

A Basic Clash - Epidemiological Averages versus Clinical Individuals

The strong commitment of the paradigms of clinical epidemiology and evidence-based medicine to empirical methods and the statistical average represents a fundamental clash with the clinical paradigm's commitment to the individual. As physicians see it, 'each patient is different.' This is epitomised by the difficulty clinicians have encountered applying results of trials for groups of patients to their own patients - an echo of the 19th century debate when the numerical method was the centre of controversy. Objecting to Quetelet's concept of the 'average man,' Double, a clinician, likened its effect on diagnosis to: 'a shoemaker who after measuring the feet of a thousand people persisted in fitting everyone on the basis of an imaginary model' (Matthews 1995).

Louis himself, who had sparked these debates, claimed that 'it is not sufficient to count,' since the clinician must also pay attention to 'distinguishing factors of age, sex and patient history' - that is to the individuality of the patient (Matthews 1995). Bernard, a physiologist, saw statistics in human affairs as 'designed to strip away the individuality in man.' Even the inventor of the concept of the average man, statistician Quetelet, expressed concern about loss of the individuality of the patient when he referred to: 'the abuse of statistics - when doctors slavishly treated all patients the same way without considering their constitution, their age, or their sex.' (Matthews 1995). Shades of the modern concern over the generalisability of the results of randomised trials which is still at the heart of the debate over evidence-based medicine!

Should Evidence-Based Medicine Be Evaluated?

Given the calls for evidence-based policy-making decisions, the importance of evidence-based medicine as a policy tool, and the problems we have just discussed, the answer must be - of course! Potent health policy interventions can have adverse effects as well as benefits, and on a grander scale that any clinical technology! Surely what is good for the clinical goose is good for the policy gander. Evidence-based medicine must indeed be evaluated - but how? Some of its proponents have taken the surprising position that its evaluation is not possible or not needed: 'The proof of the pudding of evidence-based medicine lies in whether patients cared for in this fashion enjoy better health. This proof is no more achievable under the new paradigm than it is for the old, for no long term randomized trials of traditional and evidence-based medical education are likely to be carried out.' (Evidence-based Medicine Working Group 1991). This stand has also been justified on the a priori grounds that evidence-based medicine could not have adverse effects (Ghali et al. 1999). This is not a reasonable claim either. A flawed literature search instead of a consultant opinion could harm a patient, distortion of the research agenda has a potentially serious toxic effect on the delivery of health care, and so does providing ammunition which allows managed care interests to inappropriately restrict clinical autonomy and patient rights. We also must consider the rift which has developed between clinicians and evidence-based medicine.

The most ambitious suggestion to date has been to insist on randomised trials of impact on patient outcomes (Dearlove et al. 1995). Trials of its educational potential have been conducted, but randomised trials with patient outcome as the end-point seem unlikely to be undertaken for logistical, methodological and ethical reasons. A non-randomised study of the impact of scientific evidence from the literature on clinical decisions and, by inference, likely patient health outcome would be feasible. But, as we have maintained, such should be seen as but one step in a comprehensive program of iterative evaluation which is needed for any complex technology. Can care by a nonspecialist physician who relies on evidence in the literature, as opposed to obtaining a specialist consultant opinion, have an adverse impact on patient health? I submit that the answer is yes. Both well informed student and experienced clinician can be aware of the best available treatment but obviously this cannot replace good judgement on whether to apply it to the care of this individual patient.

Information from individual randomized trials can be pooled, using the statistical technique of meta-analysis. However, there is need for more methodological research such as study of the strengths and limitations of statistical meta-analysis (Eysenck 1994, Feinstein 1995). Important issues for study include the magnitude of the problem of generalising results from megatrials to patients, the place of non-randomised studies to test the effectiveness of interventions, how to synthesise subjects in which there is need to access the 'grey literature' such as reports from consumer groups and policy documents (Naylor 1995). Other issues which warrant a lot more scrutiny are the best way to utilise local clinical data-bases as well as repositories of centralised data-collection such as the Cochrane Library, the form in which clinicians want their information, the impediments to the diffusion of evidence-based medicine into practice, patient requirements for information, and attitudes to its provision. Whether or not a randomised trial of the impact of evidence-based medicine on clinical practice is feasible or desirable, it is surely necessary to subject this technology to an ongoing program of research needed to evaluate any complex intervention in clinical care and health care delivery. This will be a program of studies which must be iterative and eclectic and include both quantitative and qualitative methods.

The Problem of Politics

Until the emergence of evidence-based medicine, controversy surrounding clinical epidemiology had been low key. Despite its initial distinctively clinical focus, evidence-based medicine has now become the key stone of health services research, closely allied with public health and with health economics in the evaluation of the cost-effectiveness of clinical care. In contrast, evidence-based medicine therefore quickly became embroiled in political controversy which has important implications. The injection of the skills and application of the methods of evidence-based medicine into health services research has been welcomed, and particularly enthusiastically supported by managed care organisations and by health bureaucracies committed to managed competition and cost constraint. Evidence-based medicine therefore uncomfortably straddles the political divide.

Evidence-based medicine has brought clinical medicine closer to public health but not in a way that all clinicians applaud. Kerr White tried to heal the schism between clinical medicine and public health by engaging the interest of clinicians through clinical epidemiology (White 1991). The project was funded by the Rockefeller Institute. That is, we have already observed that the discipline was used as a kind of Trojan Horse in the hope that clinicians could be induced to take a more panoramic view of the health system and to engage their active support in research into its problems. They never looked like doing so. Unfortunately, the role of public health in the managerial revolution in health care, linked to economic rationalist policies, has alienated many clinicians. The emergence of evidence-based medicine as an authorised source of clinical evidence informing clinical guidelines has been seen by some within the profession and outside as a stick with which to beat clinicians. Hence the increased power accruing to public health may again widen the schism.

Clinical Guidelines

One of the most versatile tools at the disposal of the bureaucratic agenda of health services research and reform is the clinical guideline which can be used to standardise clinical interventions. Their promotion is a key element which managed care organisations and health bureaucracies use to control costs and as part of their quality assurance activities. There has been a strong move away from guidelines based on expert opinion towards those which are 'evidence-based.' As Gray, a public health physician has put it: 'the development of managed care does, however, offer important opportunities in the introduction of evidence-based health care.' (Gray 1997) Such guidelines can, however, be used to reinforce an approved orthodoxy, to reinforce the position of managed care or health bureaucracy as a means of achieving control over doctors in the interests of cost-containment and in the name of quality assurance. In truth, in a study mounted in a managed care organization, only 3.3% of deviations from local guidelines were considered 'inappropriate' by consensus. Horwitz and Feinstein (1997) framed the dilemma of evidence-based medicine succinctly: 'The threat of official, corporate, or private abuse will always remain, however when any collection of information has been prominently heralded as the "best available evidence.'. A new form of dogmatic authoritarianism may then be revived in modern medicine, but the pronouncements will come from Cochranian Oxford rather than from Galenic Rome. Thus health bureaucracies and managed care, by encouraging evidence-based medicine as a natural ally have bestowed upon it the privileged status of officially approved information.' (Horwitz and Feinstein 1997).

Many worry that clinical guidelines based primarily on randomised trial and meta-analysis results can be used by health bureaucracies and managed care interests to restrict access to interventions - an assault on clinical autonomy and curtailment of patient rights. They fear that guidelines will be used to constrict their legitimate autonomy in decision-making, hence narrow patients' options, at worst introducing a form of rationing by the back door. Evidence-based medicine can then be seen as primarily a tool to contain costs, 'a springboard for the introduction of the American concept of managed care' (Fairfield and Williams 1996).

Health care can become a commodity, and evidence-based medicine can be used to justify a list of treatments 'shown to be effective' when no such list really exists (Kassirer 1995). Were these fears to be realised, managerial dominance would be substituted for the old and much criticised medical dominance since: '(t)hey see your beloved evidence based medicine as a means to shackle the doctors and bend them to their will.' (Grahame-Smith 1995). Clinicians are not alone in viewing evidence-based medicine and outcomes research as a technology for political power, a response to a lack of trust in the medical profession. Evidence-based guidelines and protocols can be generated as policy rules to change and control the behaviour of clinicians and institutions. Tanenbaum (1994), a political scientist, has seen it this way and views the health outcomes movement as 'a flight from the real inadequacies of health care.' Not surprisingly then, there is some worry that evidence-based medicine is a threat to medical professionalism, a means of empowering the health services research community.

Numbers and Power

Our cultural reverence for science therefore allows governments in Western countries to emphasise solutions based on 'objective hard data,' thereby imposing technical solutions as a quick and less controversial fix for vexing problems of health care than is an attempt to gain consensus. Health services research can therefore be interpreted as an example of the 'instrumental rationality' in society that Weber feared (Kallberg 1980). The technical solution, implemented with the authority of the scientific expert, can be used to truncate public debate, that very political problem addressed by Jurgen Habermas' critical theory (Habermas 1976). The power of the technical solution is further reinforced by the use of numbers.

Clinical epidemiology and evidence-based medicine deal in numbers. Numbers can be used to sidestep invoking expert opinion which might be contaminated by vested interests. 'By covering opinion with a veneer of objectivity, we replace judgement by computation.'(Hacking 1990). Porter has made a strong argument that quantitative modelling has primarily functioned as a device to impose objectivity 'where elites are weak, where private negotiation is suspect, where trust is in short supply.' (Porter 1995). Reliance on professional judgment seems undemocratic unless it comes from a representative consensus so that 'mere judgement, with all of its gaps and idiosyncracies, seems almost to disappear.' (Porter 1995).

Dreyfus and Dreyfus (1986,) agree that: 'since wisdom and judgment proved too hard to defend, information, decontextualized facts, and contrived numerical certainties are substituted..' Hacking's view of the early use of statistics in medicine is even more explicit: 'When the numbers were used, it was more out of professional jealousy than in a quest for objective knowledge.' (Hacking 1990). 'In a culture still in awe of science and mathematics, at a time of instability, numbers can be used as a tool for sidelining professional judgement, seen as inevitably biased, and in the case of a powerful profession like medicine, unwaveringly self interested.' This argument clothes C.P. Snow's Two Cultures (1964) and the intellectual paradigms in a political garment, and reinforces the feeling of some clinicians that clinical epidemiology and evidence-based medicine are aiding and abetting this process of control.

There has been some response to these political concerns by the evidence-based medicine movement. Thus Sackett has acknowledged that '(s)ome fear that evidenced-based medicine will be hijacked by purchasers and managers to cut the costs of health care.' (Sackett 1996). They defend evidence-based medicine by claiming that identifying the most 'efficacious' interventions 'may raise rather than lower the cost of their care..' In the long haul, it is true that only better clinical decision-making is likely to substantially lower the cost of care (Southon and McDonald 1997). Moreover clinicians have a moral responsibility to support appropriate research aimed at improving the efficiency of clinical care (McDonald 1996).

On the other hand to simply categorise the use of evidence-based medicine as a tool for inappropriate cost containment as 'misuse' (Sackett 1996) does not refute the charge nor absolve the clinical researcher from responsibility for the consequences. Thus Frankford states that 'the regulatory ideal for this research, even if not the scientists' intent, places biomedicine's practices of diagnosis and treatment in the service of an overarching goal of technical efficiency' (1994). He went so far as to describe information technology and statistical modelling (meta-analysis) as 'a new form of Taylorism driven by technology with researchers claiming that they are not responsible for the social ramifications of their work..' Health services researchers, especially the clinicians involved, have to be alert to possible abuse of their project, an ethical lesson learned so painfully by scientists during the Second World War.

The issue of standardisation and micromanagenment of clinical care has struck a raw nerve by directly challenging clinical autonomy and professional independence. Increasing bureaucratic management of clinical medicine in such countries as the U.S., Britain and New Zealand are unevaluated experiments in health care intervention. As one physician saw it, health services research is currently in political ascendancy whereby it can question clinical judgment and skill, individual variation of patient needs and clinical circumstance, the uncertainty and contingency of practice, is a form of 'scientism' (Belkin 1997). When medicine itself promotes such research in an attempt to initiate reform from within, it ironically courts its own corporatization. In the face of such a paradigm which threatens to replace the clinical: 'physicians should seriously articulate and defend the nature of their enterprise' (Belkin 1997).

Conclusion

In light of this pressure for re-alignment of fundamental beliefs, it is not at all surprising that there has been a paradigmatic clash with clinical medicine and resistance to evidence-based medicine. This is inevitable as a reflection of tension between premodern clinical practices honed as a craft skill and their recent scientific reinterpretation. There is a risk, nonetheless, that the baby will go out with the bathwater. Some of this resistance is no doubt a knee jerk conservative response to threats to the aura of science, cherished beliefs, intimidation by quantitative calculation and challenges to clinical autonomy. But some do result from an important mismatch between what empirical statistical science is offering and the realities of clinical care. Given the deep traditional roots put down by medical socialisation, these paradigmatic issues are difficult to discuss openly, so that the debate generates more heat than light. Surely the trick will be to bring these competing paradigms into balance.

Prior to the birth of 'scientific medicine,' the validity of knowledge shifted from reliance on textual authority to a new concept of probability based upon external evidence. The new paradigm, whereby evidence was a matter of belief justified by appeal to empirical observation rather than upon approval by respected authorities, shaped the intellectual climate in which Louis, in post-Revolutionary made his abortive attempt to introduce empirical statistical science into medical research. This historical confrontation of clinical experience and authority versus justification from scientific evidence is of great importance for understanding the current responses of clinicians.

Evidence-based medicine relies on numerical results of randomised controlled trials, an excessively narrow focus for most clinical evidence. The complexity of the clinical management decision we have emphasized in a system of many variables and copious interaction between variables which defy a reductionist analytical approach. The pervasive use of numbers to guide clinical practice and bureaucratic policy can be interpreted as an instrument to replace professional judgement and circumvent public debate. This is reflected in the current emphasis on performance indicators, on quantitative methods in health services research, and on the randomised trial in the case of evidence-based medicine.

In a climate of uncertainty this preoccupation with numbers and 'evidence-based' clinical guidelines has been seen as a tactic of health bureaucracies under political hegemony, and of managed care tied to the corporate sector, a way of winding back medical autonomy by providing an objective substitute for clinical judgement. Thus evidence-based medicine has become a political issue in a way that the original clinical epidemiology never was. It is vital that these differences be settled since they have the potential to derail a cooperative multidisciplinary program of clinical practice research which might otherwise be supported by clinicians with intimate knowledge of the territory.

In the last two chapters we have devoted to the methodological resources currently available for the evaluation of clinical care. In the next chapter, we consider the likely shape of clinical medicine in the decades to come. Over this time, attempts at prediction are reasonably safe. In the final chapter, we predict the cultivation of a comprehensive program of clinical research, supported by a centre for the study of clinical practice which will guide the evolution of the medical paradigm into currently unknown waters. This will likely mean continuation of the early trends, but will also undoubtedly be accompanied by unpredictable shifts of a complex system which will lead into postmodern medicine in ways quite unexpected at present but for which we must be prepared.

References

Ashmore M., Mulkay M., Pinch T., Health and Efficiency. Open University Press, Milton Keynes, 1989, p. 160-3.

Balint M., The other part of medicine. *The Lancet;* 1:40. 61.

Belkin G. S., The technocratic wish: making sense and finding power in the 'managed' medical market place. *J Health Politics;* 22: 509-32. 1997.

C. Weisner D., Naihua S., Niedzinski E. J., and Kravitz R. L., Harnessing experience: exploring the gap between evidence-based medicine and clinical practice. *Journal of Evaluation of Clinical Experience,* 14:707–713; 2008.

Cohen A. M., Stavri P. Z., Hersch W. R., A categorization and analysis of the criticisms of evidence-based medicine. *International Journal of health informatics.* 73; 35-43, 2004.

Charles C., Gafni A., Freeman E., The evidence-based medicine model of clinical practice: scientific teaching or belief-based preaching? *J Eval Clin Pract.* 2011;17(4):597-605.

Charlton B. G., The PACE (population-adjusted clinical epidemiology) strategy: a new approach to multi-centred clinical research. *Quart J Med;* 90:147-51. 1997.

Charlton B. G., Zombie science of evidence-based medicine. A personal perspective. *J evaluation in clinical practice.* 15: 930-934, 2009.

Crowther-Heyck H., *Herbert A. Simon: The Bounds of Reason in Modern America,* JHU Press 2005, p. 65.

Dearlove O., Sharples A., O'Brien K. et al., Letter to the editor. *BMJ;* 311:258, 1995.

Dreyfus H. L., Dreyfus S. E., Mind over Machine: The power of human intuition and expertise in the era of the computer. Basil Blackwell., Oxford, 1986.

Evidence-based medicine Working Group, Evidence-based medicine: a new approach to teaching the practice of medicine. *JAMA;* 268: 2420-5. 1991.

Eysenck H. J., Meta-analysis or best-evidence synthesis? *J Evaluation in Clinical practice;* 1:29-36. 1995.

Fairfield G., Williams R., Clinical guidelines in the independent health care sector. *BMJ;* 312: 1554-5. 1996.

Feinstein A. R., Clinical Epidemiology: The Architecture of Clinical Research W.B. Saunders Philadelphia 1985.

Feinstein A. R., Clinical Judgment. Baltimore, Williams and Wilkins Co., 1967. Clinical Judgment. Baltimore, Williams and Wilkins Co., 1967.

Feinstein A. R., Clinimetrics Yale U P New Haven and London 1987.

Feinstein A. R., Statistical alchemy for the 21st century. *J Clin Epidemiol* 1995;48: 71-79.

Frankford D. M., Scientism and economism in the regulation of health care. *J Health Politics;* 19: 773-811. 1994.

Ghali W. A., Saitz R., Sargious P. M., Hershman W. Y., Evidence-based medicine and the real world: understanding the controversy. *Evaluation in clinical practice;* 5:133-8. 1999.

Giacomini M. K., The rocky road: qualitative research as evidence. *Evid Based Med* 2001;6:4-6.

Goldman G. M., The Tacit Dimension Of Clinical Judgment, *The Yale Journal of Biology And Medicine* 63 (1990), 47-61.

Grahame-Smith D., Evidence based medicine: Socratic dissent. *BMJ;* 310: 1126-7. 1995.

Gray JAM., Evidence-based Healthcare. Churchill Livingstone, New York, 1997.

Gray JAM., Evidence-based Healthcare. Churchill Livingstone, New York, 1997, p. 256.

Guyatt et al. for the GRADE Working Group., Rating quality of evidence and strength of recommendations GRADE: an emerging consensus on rating quality of evidence and strength of recommendations. *BMJ;* 336:924-926; 2008.

Greenhalgh T., Jeremy Howick., Neal Maskrey., Evidence based medicine: a movement in crisis? *BMJ.* 348: g37252014.

Habermas J., Legitimation Crisis. *Polity press,* Cambridge, 1976.

Habermas J., "The Idea of the Theory of Knowledge as a Social Theory." In *Knowledge and Human Interests.* 2nd ed. Translated by Jeremy J. Shapiro. London: Heinemann Educational 1978.

Hacking I., The Taming of Chance. Cambridge University Press. Cambridge, 1990, p. 4.

Hacking I., The Taming of Chance. Cambridge University Press. Cambridge, 1990, p. 83.

Hamm R. M., Clinical intuition and clinical analysis: expertise and the cognitive continuum. In Dowie J, Elstein A, editors. *Professional judgement: a reader in clinical decision making.* Cambridge: Cambridge University Press, 1988:87.

Hay Hammersley M., Educational Research and Evidence based Practice SAGE Publications 2007.

Horwitz R., Feinstein A. R., Problems in the 'evidence' of evidence of 'evidence based medicine.' *Amer J Med;* 103;529-35. 1997.

Kallberg S., Max Weber's types of rationality: cornerstones for the analysis of rationalization processes in history. Amer J Sociol;85:1145-79. 1980.

Kassirer J., The Next Transformation in the Delivery of Health Care. *N Engl J Med* 1995; 332:52-54.

Kravetz R. E., Spiro., Medical Humanism: Aphorisms from the Bedside Teachings & Writings of Howard M. Spiro, M.D. Yale: Yale University School of Medicine, 2008.

Levenstein J. H., McCracken E. C., McWhinney I. R., Stewart M. A., Brown J. B., The patientcentered clinical method: I. A model for the doctor-patient interaction in family medicine. *Fam Pract* 1986;3:24–30.

Matthews J. R., Quantification and the Quest for Medical Certainty. Princeton University Press, Princeton, 1995.

Matthews J. R., Quantification and the Quest for Medical Certainty. Princeton University Press, Princeton, 1995, p. 29.

Matthews J. R., Quantification and the Quest for Medical Certainty. Princeton University Press, Princeton, 1995:p. 63.

Matthews J. R., Quantification and the Quest for Medical Certainty. Princeton University Press, Princeton, 1995, p. 68.

McDonald I. G., Controversy in Contemporary Medicine and the Rise of the Reflective Physician. Nova Science, New York, 2013.

Medawar P., Pluto's Republic. Oxford university press, Oxford, 1984.

Naylor C., *Grey zones* of clinical practice: some limits to evidence-based medicine. *Lancet.* 1995; 345(8953):840-2.

Patel V. L., Evans D. A., Kaufman D. R., A cognitive framework for doctor-patient interaction. In Evans DA, Patel VL eds Cognitive Science in Medicine. *MIT Press,* Cambridge Mass, 1989. 257-312.

Polanyi M., *Personal Knowledge.* Chicago: University of Chicago Press, 1958.

Porter T. M., Trust in Numbers. The pursuit of objectivity in science and public life. Princeton University Press, New Jersey, 1995.

Porter T. M., Trust in Numbers. The pursuit of objectivity in science and public life. Princeton University Press, New Jersey, 1995 p. 7.

Rothwell P. M., To whom do these results apply? *Lancet;* 365:82-93, 2005.

Sackett D., Evidence-based medicine: what it is and isn't. *BMJ:* 711-2; 312: 312, 1996.

Sackett D. L., Haynes R. B., Guyatt G. H., Tugwell P., Clinical Epidemiology: A Basic Science for Clinical Medicine. 2nd edition. Little Brown, Boston, 1991.

Sackett D. L., Haynes R. B., Guyatt G. H., Tugwell P., Clinical Epidemiology: A Basic Science for Clinical Medicine. 2nd edition. Little Brown, Boston, 1991. p. 46.

Sackett D. L., Richardson W. S., Rosenberg W., Haynes R. B., Evidence-based Medicine: How to Practice and Teach EBM. Churchill Livingstone, New York, 1997, p. 213.

Sackett D. L., Richardson W. S., Rosenberg W., Haynes R. B., Evidence-based Medicine: How to Practice and Teach EBM. Churchill Livingstone, New York, 1997, p. xv.

Sackett D. L., Richardson W. S., Rosenberg W., Haynes R. B., Evidence-based Medicine: How to Practice and Teach EBM. Churchill Livingstone, New York, 1997.

Sandelowski M., Barroso J., Voils C. I., Defining and Designing Mixed Research Synthesis Studies *Res Sch. Spring;* 13(1): 29, 2006.

Saunders J., The Practice of medicine as an art and as a science. *Med Humanities* 26:18-22, 2000.

Schön D., Educating the Reflective Practitioner, San Francisco: Jossey-Bass 1987.

Southon F. G., McDonald I. G., Challenges for the quality movement. *J Qual Clin Practice* 17:137-45; 199.

Straus S. E., and McAlister F. A., Evidence-based medicine: past, present and future. *Annals of the Royal College of Physicians andSurgeons of Canada*, 32: 260–264; 1999.

Tanenbaum S., Knowing and acting in medical practice: the epistemological politics of outcomes research. *J Health Politics* 19: 27-44; 1994.

Tobin M. J., Counterpoint: Evidence-based medicine lacks a sound scientific base. *CHEST,* 133:1071-104. 2008.

Tonelli M. R., Integrating evidence into clinical practice: an alternative approach to evidence-based approaches. *J Eval Clin Pract* 12(3): 257–59. 2006.

Walsh B., A Post-structuralist viewpoint on evidence-based medicine. Submitted for the degree of Doctor of Philosophy University of Otago 2012.

Wennberg J. E., Professional uncertainty and the problem of supplier-induced demand. *Soc Sci Med* 16:811-24;1982.

White K. W., Healing the Schism: epidemiology, medicine, and the public's health. *Springer-Verlag,* New York, 1991.

Chapter 15

Postmodern Medicine

It has been said that prediction is difficult especially when it involves the future. So it is with clinical medicine. It is not too difficult to spot present trends which will continue to operate in the foreseeable future. These we can readily document in this chapter. But we can surely expect unpredictability as an accompaniment of a paradigm shift involving a social system as complex as clinical medicine, imbedded in and subject to forces for change with the health care system, and in society more generally. Some of this change will occur as the result of concatenation of cultural and political pressures. However a system in transition will offer many opportunities for planned modifications of clinical care. In the future the direction of such changes will be guided by the results of a program of continuous clinical practice research. To consider what such a program might look like is the next mission.

Continuous Clinical Practice Research

Continuous quality improvement, or quality assurance, is an iterative evaluation of clinical procedures and protocols, the results of which are fed back to continuously improve and refine the processes of routine clinical procedures. What we propose is a parallel system of clinical practice research, conducted by individual doctors or health care investigators or multidisciplinary teams, coordinated by reflective physicians and supported by the centre for the study of clinical practice, including the social sciences and humanities as appropriate. The results of this research, using both quantitative and qualitative methods, will be similarly fed back to improve clinical practice. Revolutionary changes will continue as a result of quality assurance activities under the rubric of continuous quality improvement. This will occur at local level and as a result of formal attempts to restructure clinical practice which have been initiated in the U.S. and in Britain. There will undoubtedly be unanticipated opportunities at times as a result of more revolutionary changes in the paradigm of clinical care.

We cannot hope to predict the shape of practice in the postmodern paradigm of medicine. The most we can hope to do is to use science and humanistic skills in an attempt to mould it to the desired shape as if on a potter's wheel. However we can at least get a feel for what we face, and how to address the task, by carefully considering the case of evaluation of information technology in the clinical environment, the task of this chapter. First we will scrutinise the evaluation of information technology, arguably the second most difficult to evaluate after the process of clinical diagnosis and management itself. Both require an iterative evaluation process such as befits any truly complex technology, including evidence-based medicine. This cannot be done for clinical practice without the assistance of clinicians, clinical epidemiologists, economists and sociologists in particular. Clinical practice will no doubt continue to respond to the changing culture and paradigmatic forces.

Introduction of I T as a Bellwether of the Problems of Changing Clinical Practice

The most important catalyst for a paradigm shift in medicine will, in fact, be the inroads of information technology which is relentlessly imposing pressures for integration by facilitating communication between the elements of the health care system, helping, almost forcing them to cooperate. We will see in this chapter that the development of a technology in clinical medicine and health care system cannot be divorced from the evaluation process which must guide it at every step. The establishment and evaluation of information technology therefore provides us with an invaluable instructive exemplar of such clinical innovation and research. Such an evaluation requires an iterative process to adequately address its complexity.

All of this change will be guided by a bottom up program of 'continuous clinical practice research,' the currently underdeveloped clinical counterpart of top down health services research. The belated arrival of empirical statistical science in clinical medicine has brought undeniable benefits. But new constellations of thought and belief have inevitably collided with the old to create tensions. These paradigmatic tensions can subtly undermine the interdisciplinary research agenda which is required, both by creating conflict and by distorting the direction of the research program. What is needed is a step back, to allow reflection on how a balance of paradigms can be re-established, allowing us to retain what is good in the traditional and adopt what is better in the new. We have argued that the focus of clinical epidemiology and evidence-based medicine - on the scientific evaluation of the technical intervention, mainly in the hospital setting - is too narrow as a sole source of the information required for clinical research about patient management. There has to be interpretive qualitative research as well. This provision of on-line evaluation of practice should be led by the 'reflective practitioners' specifically trained for such interdisciplinary clinical practice research by the centre for the study of clinical practice, backed up by social sciences and humanistic skills.

Medicine evolved as an ancient craft. Under the classical paradigm of clinical medicine its methods were traditional – consisted of simply talking to the patient and kin, taking a careful history, and the examination as general inspection of the patient, as master observers, looking at the tongue, taking the pulse and examining the urine. These were methods dating back to Hippocrates in Ancient Greece. Galen in ancient Rome synthesized the knowledge of his time. Case studies were collected. Then followed the Dark Ages. Not until the 18th century could we say that science had impacted on the physical examination. First there were the anatomical and pathological observations such as the anatomical dissections of Vesalius and Morgagni, and the discovery of the empirical patterns of illness by Sydenham, 17th century precursor of Feinstein in the 19th century. Auenbrugger introduced percussion and Corvisart popularized it. Laennec contributed much to utilization of the autopsy, and Louis the notion of the experimental method in the clinical evaluation of treatment (Porter TM. 1988). There followed the introduction of numerous 'scopes for and examining internal organs via various orifices. It was Feinstein, we have observed, who was the critic who noted the lack of even rudimentary science such as a taxonomy of presentations, course and treatment of illness as practised by Sydenham, or the use of quantitative methods as pioneered by Louis. The second half of the 19th century saw the invention of the imaging technologies which today can provide a 'living autopsy.'

The Systems Review

The contribution of the new science to the modern clinical history was to add a questionnaire, comprising a short list of questions pertaining to the pathology of the organ systems – a kind of aide memoire for patient and doctor based upon extensive collective pathological knowledge. Information on the social background, a short account of past illnesses and a summary of smoking and drinking habits concluded the account. The patient's opinion of the nature of the illness was not considered relevant to the doctor. A detailed recounting of the bulk of the history of the present illness provides nearly all of the required information. A free account of the illness is today sought with a minimum of physician interjection, with particular care to avoid the bias of leading questions. This clearly involves a form of qualitative analysis, a hermeneutic process allowing interpretation of the meaning of symptoms and events.

Indeed, a moment's reflection reveals that the clinical interview is what a social scientist would call a semi-structured interview! However the social sciences have not made any contribution to medical history taking. This is because it would require acknowledging the medical interview to be a form of qualitative interpretive analysis belonging to the subjugated hermeneutic interpretive tradition of sociology and the humanities. We have discussed how we can provide access for the social sciences and humanities. The 'go between' could be a member of the centre for the study of clinical practice who should welcome their contribution and the learning opportunity. It is in this way that a theory of clinical practice can continuously evolve and made available to practising doctors. All clinicians would benefit and so too would their patients. This research should be coordinated with quality assurance activities which have similar aims while focussed on paraclinical procedures instead of the processes of clinical care itself.

Improving the Delivery of Clinical Care

Before tackling the iterative process of evaluating information technology, we briefly review changes in practice arrangements already suggested. The pragmatic concept of continuous quality improvement is based upon systems thinking and the concept of the dialectical evaluation loop (Chapter 4). It aims to optimize patient care. Constant incremental improvement is the aim. Hence what is studied and improved cannot be easily anticipated.

Nonetheless the process can also be focused in areas of particular need by major cooperative quality assurance research activities sponsored by private health bureaucracies such as managed care organisations or a national health service. We will consider examples of such initiatives in the U.S. and in Britain. Given the key place occupied by information technology, its introduction into clinical practice is a matter of the highest importance to clinicians. They must ensure that they exploit its offerings to the full and face up to the complexity of its evaluation.

Indeed we believe that the impact of information technology will act as a catalyst for the reshaping of the health care system, perhaps acting as the most powerful single influence. On the other hand the development of information technology must be skillfully guided by clinicians so that it delivers what they need. Given its pervasive influence and its great importance, the evaluation of information technology on-line is one of the key challenges facing clinician investigators. For this reason we will consider the problems of its introduction and its evaluation in detail as prime example of the process of and difficulties confronting the evaluation of clinical practice itself which is of comparable or even greater complexity.

Clinical Care Prototypes

The really difficult problems of clinical practice, the most damaging clashes of paradigm, are to be found in the Peripheral Zone of care, comprising ambulant care in particular, especially the chronically ill and the 'worried well.' This is not to be taken as meaning that better supportive care is not necessary in the Central Zone, concentrated in hospital practice. Nevertheless radical reorganisation of ambulant care, general practice, office practice, care of chronic illness and management of the 'worried well' must be a top priority. The most ambitious attempt to predict the immediate future of such practice has been the work of the Committee on Quality of Health Care (2001), a group of health experts sponsored by the Institute of Medicine in the United States. They have produced 'a vision of how health care could be delivered in the 21st century' based on the principle of continuous quality improvement which has the necessary iterative approach. An important feature of this work is that it was based on systems thinking. Thus its limited predictions were based upon explicit aims, on formulation of a set of rules, and were essentially extrapolations of existing trends. The Committee saw the reasons for currently inadequate quality of care as the growing complexity of health science and technology, the increase in proportion of care of the chronically ill, and a poorly organised delivery system. In addition the simple set of rules there was need of good vision, of space for emergent innovation. The unpredictability of the outcome in detail and over time was recognised.

The clinical care system is seen as a 'learning organisation.' The basic aims of reform are that clinical care should be safe, effective, patient-centred, timely, efficient and equitable. 'Safe' means avoidance of error leading to adverse events. This is to be achieved by redesigning the delivery system so that there is transparency and a culture of continuous quality improvement rather than individual blame. 'Effectiveness' means basing evidence-based care on systematically acquired evidence to ensure that intervention results in better health outcomes than alternatives. The evidence, both quantitative and qualitative, will be applied together with clinical expertise, with the objective of eliminating inappropriate variations in management. Important sources of information will be the Cochrane Collaboration and the American Health Research and Quality Evidence-based Practice Centers.

'Patient centredness' implies a focus on the patient's experience of illness and treatment, incorporating the ideals of empathy, and responsiveness to patient needs, values and preferences. 'Efficiency' means minimising waste, not simply reducing the cost of care. 'Timeliness' means reducing patient waiting, and provision of continuous access to care by exploiting new information technology such as e-mail. In addition to the individual personal consultation, patients may attend in groups, be contacted by e-mail or via a teleconsultation. 'Equity' means excluding bias on any characteristic such as age, gender, or ethnicity. The committee recognised that there are immense barriers of custom and culture involved which will mean homeostatic resistance of the health system to change. A continuous effort and much organisational support will be required. Of particular importance are to align payment incentives with the aims of continuous quality improvement, and to prepare the workforce by promoting major changes in the education of health professionals.

The objective is a continuous healing relationship with the patient in control in so far as is possible and desired. In place of physician autonomy is care customised for the individual patient. Information, including that in the patient record, is shared as a resource for patients as well as carers. Clinical decisions are based upon scientific evidence, such as is the objective of evidence-based medicine, as well as upon the clinician's experience. The system of delivery has built in checks to enhance safety. The traditional secrecy surrounding care, characteristic of the current medical paradigm, is replaced by transparency which facilitates patients' choices. The system does not simply react to events. There is anticipation of need and prevention of illness or complications.

Professional demarcations are replaced by team cooperation. Commoner chronic illnesses which comprise a major burden of illness, and where there is scope for major improvement and reduction of cost, are to be targeted in the first instance. Guidelines are to be evidence-based incorporating the principles of best practice, and applied with clinical experience. The whole enterprise will exploit information technology to synthesise evidence, improve communication and facilitate the coordination of care. Other initiatives in the U.S with similar objectives are currently involved in implementing and evaluating changes in ambulant care. These are the Institute of Health Improvement's 'Idealized Design of Clinical Office Practice' (2001) and the Robert Wood Johnson Foundation's 'Improving the Care of the Chronically Ill in the U.S..'

While some important incremental change can be brought about by local continuous quality improvement activities, more fundamental change requires active and radical redesign of the delivery of clinical care. This is the motive of the Institute for Health Improvement in the U.S. which has studied clinical office practice by applying the familiar methods of continuous quality improvement loop. Thus a problem is identified, studied by applying scientific methods as far as possible, then the results are used to improve existing practice. The basic objectives of the scheme are to improve clinical outcomes, enhance patient and staff satisfaction, and to deliver good financial performance. The framework for improvement focuses upon easy access for patients to clinical care and information, minimal waiting time, coordination of care involving teamwork, high quality of doctor-patient relationship, knowledge-based care, allowing for patient control as desired. Clinical management is linked to community health, monitored with real-time data, and conducted in a satisfying work environment.

The project is guided by four themes - access, interaction, reliability and vitality. 'Access' refers to health information, support and reassurance, and to treatment via face-to-face visits, paper or electronic communication including e-mail. Use is made of open access scheduling, group visits, and support is provided for self help. The method of 'interaction' includes customised methods of communication of information with shared decision-making as desired, patient preparation for visits, patient control over decisions, exploration of self-care alternatives, involvement of family and friends, attention to comfort, and privacy and provision of organisational memory. 'Reliability' refers to evidence-based practice, based also on knowledge of the individual's personal, social and cultural background, and improved by comparison with best practice. 'Vitality' aims for a learning organisation in which it is a pleasure to work, developing innovative plans, undertaking research and development, including innovative payment systems, providing for staff development and for strategic alliances. There is already evidence that these objectives are achievable. We note that successful implementation of such a model of care would vastly improve patient care in the Peripheral Zone of care.

A national program of the Robert Wood Johnson Foundation in the U.S., Improving Chronic Illness Care, aims to convert the care of the chronically ill from a reactive approach to a pro-active one (2001). The elements of the model are utilising the health system, self management support, delivery system design, decision support and clinical information systems. The objective is to make appropriate use of existing community programs such as exercise programs for the elderly, and to use department of health facilities. Patients are encouraged to play an active role in their own health care, working in collaboration with providers, and trained to use methods for minimising complications, symptoms and disability. Patients are also provided with evidence-based guidelines as part of continuing education. Primary care physicians are kept informed in the event of specialist referral. Clinical information systems can be used to develop disease registries which establish treatment guidelines, to check treatment conformity, to measure outcomes and to issue appointment reminders. A program such as this would also do much to overcome the problems of managing chronic disease in the Peripheral Zone of clinical care.

Britain has an advantage over the U.S in implementing quality improvement by virtue of possessing a National Health Service. Much of the effort has, as in the U.S., been directed at the reform of ambulant care, in this case general practice. General practice in the U.K. has many of the features needed for good primary care practice (Smith 2001). These include an emphasis on good doctor-patient interaction, a focus on patient expectations and needs, a registered population, practice teams with nurses running chronic disease clinics, electronic patient records and disease registers. The N.H.S. now operates under the principle of 'clinical governance.' Clinical governance is defined as 'a framework through which NHS organisations are accountable for continually improving the quality of their services and safeguarding high standards of care by creating an environment in which excellence in clinical care will flourish.'(Scally and Donaldson 2001).

'New rules' for practice include patients seeing their own doctor, help to prepare for the visit, improved access, group visits, phone and electronic communication and capacity increased by elimination of waste and improved efficiency. The NHS Plan's modernisation agency provides practical assistance for trusts and health authorities to reduce waiting time.

Its National Primary Care Development Team also works to improve access to primary care, and to improve linkage to secondary and tertiary care.

Information Technology Systems

Health telematics is the application of information technology in the health sector. This includes the connection and integration of health services within and between institutions such as hospitals, clinical practices and social services. Thus we have electronic medical records which can also incorporate treatment guidelines, communication with patients and transfer of test results by e-mail, linkage of hospitals allowing transmission of clinical summaries and test results, and making of appointments, linkage of social welfare services, and facilities for teleconsultation even for surgery at a distance (Institute of Medicine 1996). Patients can also directly access health information and guidance on management of symptoms through a health kiosk or pharmacy. Information technology enterprises are likely to improve the efficiency of practice and enhance patient satisfaction in many ways.

The introduction of information technology into clinical practice provides an excellent example of evaluation and reform in action in a highly complex system. We have asserted that it can be seen as analogous to evaluating clinical practice itself which, after all, is our ultimate goal, using the new and evolving methods of clinical practice research. Indeed, as arguably the most complex area of medical technology it provides, not simply a model for the evaluation and continuous quality improvement of clinical practice, but one also one for the evaluation of all other complex technologies. For this reason we examine the process and the problems in more detail. So pervasive and complex will be the impact of new information technology on health system communication that the task is like introducing and evaluating a new language! Information technology, for example telemedicine, has already made inroads into clinical practice providing a means of providing services at a distance and of better integrating services.

High Cost of Failure and Choice of Evaluation Methods

Although greater efficiency and reduced cost is the long term goal of such telematics programs, individual projects have proved costly, and failure has been common. Governments and managed care interests are frequently demanding a business plan with evidence for effectiveness as a condition of support. It is clear that evaluation has to take place on-line with each project. Thus the evaluation of telehealth initiatives must begin before the establishment of the service. Indeed evaluation of plans, including a business case, must often begin before each project since such initiatives are expensive. But evaluation is proving difficult. Conventional methods of technology assessment which place stress on controlled trials and cost-effectiveness analysis are not versatile enough for the job (McDonald 2000).

Telematics projects require preliminary demonstration of feasibility and of likely cost-effectiveness. This will initially exploit the on-line methods of quality assurance to demonstrate anticipated trends, and to warn of impending problems which can be investigated by simple audit. This information, aggregated and analysed, is fed upwards to guide planning and policy-making. From above comes administrative and policy guidance. These bottom-up and top-down links form an iterative feedback loop which links the clinical coal-face quality assurance activities to health bureaucracy.

Evaluation is fundamentally a learning process. Once the plateau of the learning curve has been reached, formal evaluation of a stable information technology application is then possible using the familiar customary methods of technology assessment. Thus the evaluation of a technology as complex as information technology must be iterative which involves a feed-back loop between bottom-up quality assurance activities and top-down commissioned formal evaluation studies. Premature evaluation of cost-effectiveness may be misleading. The iterative process of evaluation must be allowed to evolve. It can be planned in advance to a limited extent only. The program should prioritise problems for solution and choose the best study designs, qualitative and quantitative, to solve these. The choice of research method should never be on the basis of methodological prejudice. All stakeholder perspectives must be represented, technical support must be excellent and, for clinical projects, recruitment of enthusiastic physician 'drivers' is mandatory.

The lack of evaluation of information technologies has been stressed. Governments are anxious for information on which to base policy, and managed care interests need to justify their investments (Yellowlees1998). Somehow our usual methods of evaluation seem to have let us down. In particular, there is confusion over which methods should be used. On the other hand, I will argue that the problems of evaluation posed by information technology have actually done us a favour. Information technology has exposed the conventional corner cutting which has characterised the evaluation of health technologies, forcing us to acknowledge important difficulties which we have managed to side-step in the past by concentrating on top-down methods and summative outcome oriented evaluation. If we are to develop a program for the evaluation of the process of clinical practice itself, we must take heed of these issues.

The notion of a one-of assessment of the effectiveness and cost of an established or 'mature' technology, using the methods successfully used for evaluation of drugs, such as the randomized controlled trial, has proved to be simplistic and naive. Drug evaluation emerged in the 1950s as a response to serious adverse events, in particular the thalidomide disaster (Matthews 1995). Medical technology assessment arose in response to early perceptions of the need for cost constraint, seen from the perspective of the health policy maker (Foote 1987). Its focus was on the high unit cost 'big ticket items,' its methods mainly formal studies of efficacy such as clinical trials and economic studies such as cost-utility analyses, and syntheses of such studies (Banta and Luce 1993). We see that many research programs, including liver transplantation, have neglected the sociological perspective, and there has been a predictable over-emphasis on analytical quantitative studies. There also have been large data-bases established, including one by the Cochrane Collaboration. However, these approaches were never intended to assess the feasibility of a technology before it was introduced or to monitor its early development and progress - both crucial to clinical and administrative aspects of the evaluation of a new information technology project.

The manifest success of the randomised controlled trial in the evaluation of drugs has misled us by suggesting that such a controlled reductionist approach could be used to evaluate any health technology, and that it alone provided 'level 1 evidence.' What we argue then is that the unique difficulty of evaluating telematics initiatives in health has exposed the limitations and the shortcomings of these earlier approaches to the assessment of medical interventions in general. What is the basis of this unique difficulty? Unfortunately, the evaluation of a drug is unusual in that a randomised trial can be undertaken almost entirely free from concerns about context of administration or user perspective, using a definitive end-point, usually life or death. The context has been 'factored out' in the interests of control. Even the evaluation of diagnostic interventions, of expensive imaging tests like magnetic resonance imaging and positron emission tomography, is much more complex than that of drugs. In these cases, complexity has simply been side-stepped by confining assessment to image quality and diagnostic accuracy, thereby ducking the real challenges of measuring impact on patient health outcome, psychological and social effects, and appropriateness of use!

Mutual Re-Engineering

In the case of information technology, what has to be evaluated is no less than a change in our basic system of symbolic communication in that most complex of all human environments - the health system of clinical practice and delivery of care! Not surprisingly, attention to human and social variables is an integral part of such an evaluation process (McDonald et al. 1998). Instead of having a technology which has been engineered in the factory to have a particular effect, what is required for in the case of information technology is a process of 'mutual re-engineering' - the iterative moulding of the developing technology to user needs on the one hand, and reciprocal accommodation of professional work practices to the changes introduced by the technology on the other. Absolutely essential, therefore, is continuous dialogue between developers and users in the course of a difficult adaptive learning process.

Another fundamental difference between the evaluation of information technology and that of therapeutic and diagnostic technologies is that development of the latter have been initiatives of practising doctors and industry, supported even applauded by clinician colleagues. A new clinical technology was not an imposition or an unwanted challenge. Its introduction was a happy event not a contentious external intervention. In the case of information technology, instead of being the prime movers, most clinicians are on the receiving end, so that the technology may not be perceived as meeting a clinical need, as making their job easier. To have available clinicians willing and able to drive the introduction and evaluation of an information technology project is a key requirement for its success. Otherwise they may be too busy to cooperate, reluctant to change their practice habits, and in some cases suspicious of the use of the technology as a means of reducing their autonomy.

Finally there is a basic Catch 22. Information from evaluation of a technology is at a premium during the planning and developmental stages when it is constantly moving target, rather than later when it is already well established and stable. Necessary protection against an unwise investment requires information before funds are allocated. But in order to keep the project on track from the outset, we need to have the capacity to monitor progress on-line and to react to unanticipated problems as they arise. On the other hand, there is a fundamental paradox here since a communication technology can be expected to achieve maximum efficiency only when it is imbedded in supportive matrix. Hence to formally study the cost-effectiveness of a data-base or telemedicine system before it is embedded as part of such a supportive communications network runs the risk of obtaining a misleading false negative result. Yet it is equally clear that information technology, a late starter in health care, is now moving fast, so that it will become established over a fairly short time whether it has been properly evaluated or not.

So cunningly has the real complexity of evaluation of information technology been concealed that its introduction has often been poorly planned, inadequately supported and not properly assessed. All too often the equipment gathers dust in a storeroom, or its availability drives inappropriate or unnecessary use. Even if evaluation is planned, it has often not been appreciated that information technology projects are much too complex for evaluation using only the clinical trials and cost-effectiveness studies conventionally applied by medical technology assessment. Indeed the evidence-based medicine approach, which relies almost exclusively on randomised trials, is seriously hampered by its lack of access to interpretive, qualitative methods of evaluation which can study the human dimension, to handle those social and the organisational problems which are so often the major threat to the success of a project.

The Answer to Complexity - Iterative Evaluation

Formal controlled evaluation was designed for the summative (outcome) evaluation of mature technologies, and chiefly for studies of efficacy - their performance under ideal circumstances of use in centres of excellence. Such studies are often in the format of cost-effectiveness evaluations. Studies of an information technology project, on the other hand, are local events. They begin with demonstration of feasibility, including a business plan, and early monitoring of their early progress requires on-line formative (process) methods of evaluation such as tracking trends, using indicator statistics to flag problem areas, mapping processes using flow charts, obtaining feedback from staff, arising from use and solving specific problems using local audit studies. These assessment activities, mainly formative and initially no more than commonsense and really, in essence, essentially early quality assurance studies, grow organically into the routine activities of quality assurance. The prime movers in evaluation at this early stage are therefore the local staff, and evaluation is conceptually simple and ongoing.

Much of the mystery surrounding the process of evaluation of a complex technology is dispelled if we see it as an extension of normal activity, such as we all constantly engage in when planning our daily lives, but spiced up by an injection of science and scholarship. In the last chapter, we will explore further the notion that the case of information technology is an exemplar which can be used to illustrate how that highly complex technology we know as 'clinical practice' can be improved by a process of guided evolution and systems thinking, exploiting the unexpected opportunities thrown up by paradigm shifts (Chapter 4). The basic elements are the same as for all rational and explicit human inquiry, whether it be scientific research, scholarship in the humanities, interpretive sociological inquiry or a clinical consultation.

Hegel's Dialectic

As we have seen, interpretation, understanding or a model of the system is built up by the process of iterative synthesis at attributed to the philosopher Hegel in the 19th century (Taylor 1975). The idea of the 'quality circle' or 'evaluation loop' is no more than a reinvention of this basic process in special circumstances. Our current state of knowledge, our extant working model of how things are now, Hegel called the 'thesis.' We then encounter or seek out additional information by evaluation and experimentation, exploring especially what does and does not fit into the current model. This information, the 'antithesis,' fills gaps and explains apparent contradictions, leading to a more refined model which incorporates this new knowledge. This updated model or 'synthesis' then becomes the thesis for another iteration and so on to yet another synthesis. The process constitutes a dialectic which incorporates an iterative feedback loop which generates an increasingly accurate and refined appraisal of what we are evaluating or researching. The formal top-down evaluation 'ends' with 'saturation,' that is when the major issues have been successfully addressed. The bottom-up evaluation continues as continuous quality improvement.

Moreover, the procedure can, and must continue as an ongoing program of evaluation, merging with routine quality assurance measures. If we provide this loop with a time axis, we have a 'spiral staircase' of knowledge accrual. In addition, all evaluation is a process of learning, so that the spiral follows the well known S-shaped learning curve with early slow progress, rapid learning then a plateau representing diminishing returns. However, this kind of argumentation has been used from ancient time as a form of debate, known as as a 'dialectic.' Recently, use of this same iterative structure as a basic method of quality assurance has been referred to as the 'evaluation loop.' As we claimed earlier, no truly complex medical technology can be evaluated over time except by using this dialectical iterative method, and this applies to the evaluation of clinical practice itself, using ongoing clinical practice research and evaluation (Chapter 16).

Linking Bottom-Up to Top-Down Evaluation

Unlike the introduction of new treatments and tests in the past, the great majority of information technology projects have required external financial assistance, hence there is usually a bureaucratic structure responsible for their support and its evaluation. Thus a typical health system involved in a telematics project often consists of an area of professional practice, an institutional practice setting, commonly a hospital, and one or more health bureaucracies. The iterative loop as described above is set up to connect evaluation activities at the clinical coal face to supervising bureaucracy and to policy-makers (McDonald et al. 1996). Initially this data will be confined to that related to quality assurance, including such basic indicators as those of technical success (good image quality, minimum down-time), progress (increasing referrals, costs as predicted), user satisfaction (inventory of complaints), obvious benefits or problems for patients (convenience, cost).

This kind of basic information will not only be applied as a basis for local improvement, it will be aggregated, further analysed, combined with information from coordinating meetings and site visits, and fed upwards to inform administrative planning and policy formulation. Thus intelligence fed bottom-up from the clinical front line, generated by the techniques of quality assurance, provides crucial on-line feedback data on quality and effectiveness. The top-down arm of the loop from the bureaucracy meanwhile must constantly provide policy guidance which incorporates the system objectives, local and political.

Maturity – Shift from Bottom-Up to Top-Down Focus of Evaluation

As the project approaches maturity, that is when it reaches the top or plateau of the S-shaped learning curve, the evolution of the evaluation project is approaching a steady state. Quality will continue to be monitored on a routine basis as long as the project continues but the focus of evaluation can then shift towards the addition of formal summative studies of effectiveness and efficiency. In many information technology projects, this will involve studies conducted across multiple sites. Likely questions are overall evidence of effectiveness and cost, specific problems targeted by early experience, and perceived obstacles to progress. Such studies are often contracted out. However, methodological experts will be commissioned to work closely with the end users and administrators to produce the evaluation 'snapshots' provided by more formal methods of study. Such an iterative process with feed-back loops must be applied to any complex clinical technology. Information technology therefore provides us with a model of clinical evaluation of an important technology as we have suggested.

The very complexity of information technology has therefore exposed the need to integrate two complementary forms of evaluation when assessing any complex medical technology, including the daunting task of clinical practice research. Day to day monitoring and formative evaluation of quality and progress applies the methodological toolbox of quality assurance. The formal techniques of technology assessment, which are needed later for the summative evaluation used for questions related to policy, draw upon an armamentarium of techniques borrowed from epidemiology and economics, especially surveys, randomised trials and cost-effectiveness modelling. For most medical technologies, the methods of technology assessment have been used for formal one shot assessments only after the technology had reached maturity.

In the pioneer departments much valuable clinical information has been obtained early during a rapid learning phase. This information ranged over such issues as extent of patient benefit and early warning of possible harm, technique of use and protocols of examination, selection of patients and contexts of clinical use, likely clinical demand, compatibility with existing practice, comparison with other tests, impact on their use, and projections of likely cost implications. However, in the past, this day to day exploratory learning process in clinical practice was largely wasted. Such relatively simple but important information was rarely published probably because it was deemed to be 'unscientific.' These valuable lessons were often passed at specialist meetings over a drink at the bar or in the course of a visit to pioneer centres. Such a haphazard, disjointed and inefficient process would hardly be acceptable for a new information technology project. It should not be tolerated for any clinical technology.

Lessons for the Iterative Evaluation of Clinical Practice

A systematic program of evaluation in the clinical field must be an iterative one which follows opportunities and responds to the emerging problems. Hence it follows that such a strategy cannot be planned far in advance. Rather it must be allowed to evolve as a chain of studies in response to priorities and to problems as they arise in the local context, and to provide answers to the questions raised by earlier studies. The notion of a long-term fixed strategy of evaluation using summative methods is therefore a misleading myth. The key to successful evaluation is to skillfully control and guide the evolution on-line, acting in response to emergent trends or unexpected shifts of thinking. The crucial issues are the appropriate prioritisation of evaluation questions and the choice of the 'right' research methods with which to answer them.

In order to address problems ranging from technical to cultural, it is essential to have access to the full gamut of quantitative and qualitative research methods. Numerical indicators are obviously invaluable to monitor demand, surveys essential to measure client satisfaction. However, when exploring the nuances of process or when seeking serious obstacles to success such as sources of clinician resistance, formal interview of key players with qualitative data analysis will be important (Cusack and Poon 2007). Hence evaluation must be driven by problems, not by methods. Among the consequences of inappropriate research methods are distortion of questions to fit a familiar or favoured research method, addressing the wrong problems, and systematic neglect of whole areas of research because of methodological prejudice. The choice of study design must be flexible, open-minded and eclectic - a case of 'have problem find method,' not 'have method will travel.' To access the toolbox of methods needed will often mean interdisciplinary cooperation (Daly and McDonald 1992). It is one of the contributions to be made by a centre for the study of clinical practice.

Similarly, the logical way to choose research methods is straightforward. Once again, Confucius may well have had some advice to offer about going out through the door. Choice of a research method to address a particular problem is logically a process of triangulation which must simultaneously satisfy three requirements - (a) to match the precise nature of the question prioritised for study, (b) to maintain a commitment to optimum intellectual rigour while (c) facing up to inevitable constraints posed by the context of the evaluation, including ethical concerns. With respect to the nature of questions - obviously those which are a matter of how big, how much, how many or how different (including hypothesis testing) require quantitative methods with statistical analysis, while questions which involve meaning in social context or human motivation will require qualitative methods and interpretive analysis. Given that the reason for lack or failure of evaluation of information technology always involve human, social and organisational factors, qualitative research is obviously essential to successful evaluation.

Our objective may be to get an overview of a field, a low power view as it were, or to obtain a detailed view of a small area, a high power view. We may wish to undertake an empirical study or to synthesise existing information. Maximum rigour in a quantitative study means a design which minimises bias and puts statistical limits on random error, seeks to be as generalisable as possible, and uses valid statistical methods for the analysis. Maximum rigour in a qualitative study means good scholarship - collecting high quality evidence, developing a narrative argument using tight reasoning and accessing appropriate theory, considering threats to validity of analysis and exploring alternative interpretations in an open-minded way. The constraints to be addressed are likely to include practical difficulties in collecting data in a busy clinical environment, professional issues such as obtaining cooperation from health professionals, limitations of resources available in terms of skills, finance and time, and ethical barriers (McDonald et al. 1998).

When questions, standards of rigour and constraints have been triangulated in this way, the best method to a large extent chooses itself - as a kind of 'vector' resultant as it were. Once we have solved the simultaneous equations of question, rigour and constraints, we have actually calculated the basic study design, so that only fine tuning of methodological detail is left. Again this sounds like so much commonsense. The method must absolutely not be chosen on the basis of familiarity to the investigator, nor must the questions be chosen to accommodate the method. Why is it then that this is not usually the way that things are done? One important reason is that a dominant worldview which privileges quantitative methods and objective analysis has led to a schism between science and the humanities.

The use of quantitative methods as an exclusive means of studying social institutions has a long history of failure. Unless we want to re-invent the wheel for the evaluation of information technology, we must recognise that, in order to study the social, cultural and organisational issues involved, we will need to employ as well research methods unfamiliar to most scientists and doctors. In particular, we will have to invoke the cooperation of sociology to design interpretive methods based upon field observation and interview and qualitative data analysis. We have noted that the term 'wicked problem' was coined to describe evaluation of a social institution or service (Rittel 1982), as opposed to a 'tame problem' which could be solved by reductionist methods. Wicked problems were essentially defined by their immersion in a changing social context, and by their intractability if using only quantitative methods such as those of operations research. The evaluation of an innovation like information technology is most assuredly a wicked problem!

When it comes to the formal summative evaluation, a rigid insistence on the primacy of randomised trials as a gold standard, and on cost-utility analysis as a financial bottom line will totally miss the fact that important outcomes may simply not be measurable in quantitative terms, and that such methods are quite inappropriate for the basic task of interpretation of human motivation and crucial responses in the early decisions and transactions of health care. Ideological commitment to the discredited idea that science is value free can also lead to naive denial of the social and political dimensions of evaluation. Thus the evaluation of applications of complex technologies in clinical medicine from the top-down community perspective by health bureaucracy or managed care interests may have overtones of control in the interests of containing health expenditure, even of covert rationing. These considerations apply also, only more so, to the iterative evaluation of clinical practice itself, where the social element is so dominant.

Evaluation Program Adapted to Context

Although it is not possible to predict in advance how a program of evaluation will unfold, it is often clear from the nature of the technology and context where the emphasis will lie. We illustrate this by reference to two common areas of information technology which have posed very different problems (McDonald et al. 1998). Teleradiology moved quickly through evaluation to general acceptance. For a start, many of the issues are technical ones related to image quality. Many of the technical problems of image resolution, compression and transmission had already been solved by radiologists from earlier experience with computerised tomography and magnetic resonance imaging, and from experience with image transmission and storage within hospitals (Patient Archiving and Communication Systems). User acceptance was facilitated by the technical inclinations of many radiologists, evaluation by their 50 year tradition of testing the accuracy of their imaging tests. Since the imaging test is a technical procedure with a minimum of human interaction, problems of the doctor-patient relationship did not have to be confronted. Off-line (store-and-forward) transmission of compressed image data is used so that the problems of videoconferencing are also avoided. The foci of evaluation have therefore been on demonstration that standards of image quality have been maintained so as not to increase clinical error, and on cost-effectiveness of providing such a service.

In striking contrast is the teleconsultation. We refer here to the performance of a standard medical consultation using videoconferencing. In some specialist areas like psychiatry and renal dialysis, clinical conferences involving patient, medical and non-medical providers have proved to be of great value for providing services to a remote area (Yellowlees 1997). The use of videoconferencing for routine general practice and specialist consultations, the backbone of clinical practice, is another kettle of fish. There is risk of impairment of the art of medicine, in particular a loss of quality of supportive care. Patients may be prepared to trade off personal contact for convenience and lower cost, especially for follow-up interviews. However many general medical and specialist consultations hinge on the patient's willingness to reveal, and the doctor's ability to discern the central importance of the social context to the illness. Symptoms, as we have seen, are very often related to 'problems of living' rather than to organic disease.

The extent of the trade-off in diagnostic accuracy and patient satisfaction in this most important area is not yet clear. Also relevant are compromises in the physical examination associated with transmission of low frame rate or poor resolution images, problems with the use of peripheral devices such as the electronic stethoscope, or in having a surrogate perform the physical examination. The involvement of remote consultants in large teaching hospitals could also lead to over-investigation with its attendant problems of false positive diagnosis anxiety, iatrogenic illness and escalating cost. Then there are practical but important issues for evaluation such as the difficulties of scheduling doctors to attend a central location for a real-time consultation, and possible lack of cooperation because of fears of loss of practice to outside consultants. In many situations, it is much easier to use telecommunications for off-line transmission of information using the store-and-forward off-line method.

The Complexity of the Evaluation of Clinical Patient Care

The evaluation of information technology in its clinical applications is both urgent and difficult. The conventional approach of technology assessment, which awaits 'maturity' of development, then uses formal methods such as trials and mathematical models, cannot possibly do the job alone. These methods must be linked to those of quality assurance. Both disciplines must contribute their complementary skills to an ongoing, iterative, multidisciplinary, problem-driven program of evaluation. Qualitative as well as quantitative methods, including formative evaluation, must be used as appropriate if the program is to address the human, social and organisational issues which are often the major determinants of success or failure (Cusack et al. 2009). The objectives and perspectives of all of the stakeholders must be factored into the evaluation if the right questions are to be asked, if the needs of patients and their families, doctors, administrators, bureaucrats and politicians are to be addressed, and the full cooperation of all players enjoyed.

The evaluation of clinical care is a task of similar complexity. The basic Hegelian iterative investigative strategy of thesis, antithesis and synthesis cannot be avoided for information technology, nor can it be for clinical practice itself which, remarkably, has never been subjected to any form of scholarly evaluation! The reason is the impossibility of using only quantitative summative methods. This process has hardly begun. There is a need for a great deal of empirical statistical science. Clinical epidemiology, evidence based medicine and quality assurance have the scientific evaluative tools for that job. For example, we are still ignorant of the diagnostic accuracy of most symptoms and signs. The same is true of, for example, the sensitivity, specificity and predictive values of evidence from our imaging tests.

The Journal of Evaluation of Clinical Practice lists its scope as 'evidence-based medicine, clinical practice guidelines, clinical decision analysis, clinical services organization, implementation and delivery, health economic evaluation, health process, outcome measurement and new and improved methods (conceptual and statistical) for systematic enquiry into clinical practice.'. The emphasis on the quantitative and analytical, summative evaluation and health policy perspective is evident, as is the absence of the interpretive, qualitative and clinical orientation. I should not have to labour the point about issues which are squarely in the court of the social sciences and humanities. We shall consider their place in more detail in the final chapter.

Conclusion

There is general agreement on the major deficiencies of clinical care such as we have outlined. It is also clear what kind of innovations are required in principle to overcome most of these barriers to high quality clinical care. Efforts are underway to implement such changes in health care delivery. We have discussed examples in the U.S. and in Britain. Information technology will be a key player in changing clinical practice to its postmodern form, not surprisingly in the Age of Information. Its major role is as a source of pressure for change, for more integrated care and for changes in clinical practice. This will loosen the hold of older and less efficient practices and clear the way for change. Considering the case of information technology has other benefits. Its intricacy is such, the pressure for change so compelling and the cost of failure so great that we have had to view the process of iterative evaluation of a clinical technology in its full complexity.

Evaluation is surely an intrinsic part of daily life, and has always been with us in our work. What is different now is that evaluation of health care is financially and politically driven, and much more formal and compelling. It is important to see clearly that there are distinctive levels, each with a unique focus, different methods adapted to its specific task, and with a characteristic view of the world. At one end is technology assessment which adopts a community perspective on techniques of heath care, using summative methods; at the other is quality assurance which has its emphasis on local standards of delivery of clinical care using mainly formative methods. Both are linked dialectically, and are currently pursuing their respective mandates. But surely the most basic unit of health care is the clinical transaction between a doctor and his or her patient.

Traditional techniques of patient evaluation developed thousands of years ago, and have survived as the art of medicine but buttressed now by a strong commitment to biological science. However, these methods of patient assessment have remained almost entirely unevaluated. What is required is a process of continuous quality improvement at the clinical end, with technology assessment and related activities representing the bureaucratic perspective linked to it in a feed-back loop. This is actually a model for the evaluation of clinical care in general. Organising and supporting this venture is a basic task for centres for the study of clinical practice supported by multidisciplinary research which must include input from continuing bedside biomedical research, from clinical epidemiology and evidence-based medicine, from sociology and anthropology, and from any other body of appropriate knowledge.

References

Banta H. D., Luce B. R., Health Care Technology and its Assessment: An International Perspective. Oxford University Press, Oxford, 1993.

Committee on Quality of Health Care, Crossing the Quality Chasm. Institute of Medicine, 2001.

Conrad L. I., Neve M., Nutton V., Porter R., Wear A., Eds., The Western Medical Tradition 800 BC to 1800 AD. Cambridge University Press, Cambridge, 1995.

Cusack C., Byrne C. M., Hook J. M., McGowan J., Poon E., Zafar A., Health information technology toolkit. Agency for Healthcare Research and Quality. ACHQ National Resource Center for Health Information Technology. 2009.

Cusack C. M., Poon E. G., Health care evaluation toolkit. AHRQ National Resource Centre for Information Technology. Agency for Healthcare Research and Quality. 2007.

Daly J., McDonald I. G., Introduction: the problem as we saw it. In Researching health care; designs, dilemmas, disciplines. London, Routledge 1-11;1992.

Foote S. B., Assessing medical technology assessment; past present and future. The Milbank Quarterly 65:59-80; 1987.

Foucault M., The Birth of the Clinic: an archaeology of medical perception. Tavistock, London, 1976.

Guba E. G., Lincoln Y. S., Fourth Generation Evaluation. Newbury Park Sage, 1989, p. 35.

Gutting G., Michel Foucault's Archaeology of Scientific Reason. Cambridge University Press, Cambridge.

Haynes B., Can it work? Does it work? Is it worth it?: the testing of health care interventions is evolving. *BMJ* 319:652-3;1999.

Institute for Health Improvement, Idealized Design of Clinical Office Practices. 2001.

(IOM) Institute of Medicine, Committee on Evaluating Clinical Applications of Telemedicine. *Telemedicine*: a guide to assessing telecommunications in health care. Washington DC, National Academy Press, 1996.

Jewson N., The disappearance of the sick man from medical cosmology, 1770-1870. *Sociology* 10:225-44; 1976.

Kuhn T., The Structure of Scientific Revolutions. University of Chicago Press, Chicago, 1970.

Lindblom C. E., The science of muddling through. *Public Administration Review;* 19:79-88; 1968

Matthews J R., *Quantification and the Quest for Medical Certainty*. Princeton University Press, Princeton, 1995.

McDonald I., Hill S., Daly J., Crowe B., Evaluating Telemedicine in Victoria: a generic framework. Acute Health Division, Victorian Government Department of Human Services, 1998.

McDonald I. G., Daly J., Research methods in health care - a summing up. *In Researching health care: designs, dilemmas, disciplines*. Daly J, McDonald IG, Willis E eds. Routledge, London, 1992, 209-16.

McDonald I. G., Telemedicine as a challenge to evaluation: a blessing in disguise? *Telehealth International* 2000; 211-28.

Porter T. M., *The Rise of Statistical Thinking, 1820-1900*. Princeton University Press. 1988.

Porter T. M., Trust in Numbers: The Pursuit of Objectivity in Science and Public Life. Princeton University Press, Princeton, 1995.

Rittel H., Systems analysis of the 'first and second generations.' In Laconte P, Gibson, J, Rapoport A eds. Human Energy Factors in Urban Planning. NATO Advanced Study institutes Series D. Behavioural and Social Sciences No. 12, Martinus Nijhoff, The Hague, 1982, 35-63.

Scally G., Donaldson L. J., Clinical governance and the drive for quality improvement in the new NHS in England. *BMJ* 317: 61-65; 2001.

Schon D. S., From technical rationality to reflection-in-action. In Dowie J, Elstein A eds. *Professional Judgment*: a reader in clinical decision making. Cambridge University Press, Cambridge, 1988, 60-77.

Smith J., Redesigning health care. *BMJ* 322: 1257-1258; 2001.

Snow C., The Two Cultures and A Second Look: an expanded version of the two cultures and the scientific revolution. Cambridge University press, Cambridge, 1964.

Smith J., Redesigning health care. *BMJ* 322:1257-1258; 2001.

Taylor C., Hegel. Cambridge University Press, London, 1975 www.improvingchroniccare.org Improving Chronic Illness Care.

Yellowlees P., Successful development of telemedicine systems - seven core principles. *J Telemedicine and Telecare* 3:215-222;1997.

Yellowlees P., Practical evaluation of telemedicine systems in the real world. *J Telemedicine and Telecare:* 4, Suppl 1, 56-7. 1998.

Chapter 16

The Reflective Physician, Continuous Clinical Practice Research and the Centre for the Study of Clinical Practice

The time has come for us to pull the threads of our argument together. These threads represent three major concepts - (a) the 'reflective physician,' whom we will define as, above all, a lifelong learner, the notion of the continuous improvement of clinical care which is underpinned by what we call (b) 'continuous clinical practice research,' and (c) 'the centre for the study of clinical practice' which is responsible for training the former and coordinating the latter. The major functions of the centre, directed towards bringing together university teachers and clinicians together, we see as to train reflective physicians, acting as a forum for interdisciplinary and interdepartmental discussion and debate, to provide a repository of research skills relevant to clinical practice and statistical assistance for hospital staff, to provide graduate and undergraduate training in research method and statistics, and to supervise a computer base of clinical patterns of illness such as we will describe. It would be run by an expert in research method theory and practice, and be responsible to a steering committee with the appropriate representation. A particularly important objective would be to complement the university's continuing encouragement of the involvement of the social sciences and humanities in the medical curriculum, and to recruit these disciplines for interdisciplinary clinical practice research. This would be tantamount to aiding the effort to broaden the medical paradigm's curriculum from its modern to its postmodern form. We begin with concept of the reflective physician because we will use it frequently in our subsequent discussion.

Training the Reflective Physician

We believe that training the reflective practitioner is the most important single function of the centre for the study of clinical practice. The role of this postmodern 'reflective practitioner' is to participate in and coordinate the evaluation of clinical care itself, the clinical practice research program which has as its objective the continuous improvement of clinical care. We could say that clinical diagnosis and management are medicine's ultimate technology and certainly it offers the greatest challenge to evaluation. The practice of medicine is about making interpretations called clinical judgements and executing management decisions. If these judgements are unsound then the quality of care must suffer. This process of judgement is largely subconscious but is subject to conscious editing. This is true of the reflective practitioner who practices largely subconsciously and consciously critiques the process. The issues contributing to a clinical judgement, apart from purely diagnostic information, are usually numerous, commonly including a personal philosophy, attitudes to patients, various psychological quirks, under the influence of cultural forces and moulded by education both general and professional.

However, the modern scientific paradigm of medicine tends to constrain the clinician's reflection to the manifestations and cause of organic disease or to the social context to the extent that this can be addressed by traditional clinical tenets picked up informally at the bedside. Physicians working in specialized areas generally have an informal, intuitive grasp of the accuracy and relevance of important symptoms and physical signs from their own experience. Missing however is a scientific or scholarly critique of evidence or of clinical methods of patient examination.

This narrow biomedical and clinical focus can also lead to neglect of the psychosocial dimension of illness, leading to conflict with patients, clinical errors and other problems as we have seen. As we see it, the dominance of the scientific analytical paradigm of science in clinical research has limited the scope for a deeper understanding of illness, and also blocked scholarly refinement of the techniques of the clinical examination itself. Schon (1983) has taken a similar view of problems afflicting professional practice and education more generally. Certainly the evaluation of clinical practice must depend to a large extent on techniques of qualitative as well as quantitative data analysis.

Professional Thinking-in-Action

It is clear enough that clinical reasoning is not 'science reasoning' (Waymack 2009). But what then is it? We have argued that it is, to a large extent, hermeneutic or interpretive in nature. However we should start at the beginning and ask what is known about human judgement and decision making. In truth, the mode of thinking of humans when problem solving is still poorly understood. Hence we should start with common sense. Observing an experienced and expert physician in action it is quite obvious that they sometimes make conclusions and even some diagnoses without recourse to conscious thought – the 'spot diagnosis.' They do not usually enjoy discussing this 'global' or intuitive act. Many regard it as they would a paranormal process - not to be explored or even discussed. Yet it is the very essence of their expert problem solving as we have seen!

When considering the roles of the 'reflective physician,' the key concept is that of 'reflection.' The concept was pioneered by educationist Dewey (1910), and was elaborated by Schon (1983), another educationist. One method of Schon's 'reflection' occurs during a professional's daily practice. This form of knowledge accrues with experience and is the basis of the expertise and the art of practice. Schon called the process of acquisition of such knowledge 'reflection-in-action.' Explicit knowledge gained from conscious rumination during or after a period of professional activity he called 'reflection-on-action.' This process we consider in more detail below. The truth is that little is known about human judgement as a neurological event, except that it seems to be the same basic process for non-professionals. It seems that both forms of reflection somehow operate in parallel; it is like using a neural network computer for the unconscious work, when the knowledge resides in the connections between nodes - analogous to tacit knowledge - and a conventional computer for conscious rational thinking, editing and theorizing, when the knowledge is symbolic, propositional or explicit.

Recall that Polanyi (2009) – a physical chemist and later a sociologist and philosopher - made a brilliant move which we discussed in Chapter 13. He dichotomized knowledge into 'explicit' and 'tacit' forms. This is the basis of Schon's classification of reflection. Reflection-in-action generates tacit knowledge while reflection-on-action involves conscious knowledge. Explicit knowledge can be recalled and manipulated by reasoning processes of which we are fully aware. Tacit knowledge cannot be verbalized by definition because the process is performed unconsciously. It is of crucial importance to understand that unconscious knowledge is the main basis of expertise and judgement. Epstein (2008) has written a review of the process of reflection in medical education. Most attention is devoted to a conscious process which seems to correspond to Schon's reflection-on-action. Only a paragraph covered unconscious reflection, that is Schon's reflection-in-action. To teach reflection-in-action which generates the tacit knowledge which comprises clinical experience requires often hours spent working in the field. These concepts apply to all thought, and certainly to professional thinking, including medical. We concluded that it is well established by now that the bulk of the expert's knowledge is tacit and beyond conscious reach. Therefore they do not have to work consciously with guidelines as much as the non-expert is obliged to do. To understand the idea, it is necessary to reflect upon the nature of human judgement in general, and of professional judgement in particular.

Schon provided illustrations of the phenomenon of knowing-in-action by reference to such disciplines as architecture, town planning and clinical psychiatry. In each case, he was able to demonstrate that systematic thinking-in-action was, to some extent at least, a feature of the practice of some elite individuals, the 'unusual practitioners,' but that awareness of existence of reflection-in-action can be appreciated and cultivated. Operating in parallel is conscious reasoning. The more familiar the problem, the greater the expertise, the less is conscious reasoning invoked, at least initially. Under these circumstances, knowing cannot be separated from action. This why Schon (1996) refers to 'knowing-in-action.' We could therefore think of problem-solving thought as invariably comprising (a) unconscious reflection-in-action and (b) conscious editing, refining and testing process known as reflection-on-action.

Thus reflection-in-action seen in this way is simply an extension of our normal problem solving armamentarium. Surprisingly we cannot visualize or verbalise this phenomenon which is occurring in our own heads. Schon (1996) has provided helpful analogies. Speaking about jazz musicians improvising, he described their 'feel for the music,' as a manifestation of reflection-in-action: 'we need not suppose that they reflect-in-action in the medium of words..' Most likely an expression of the same phenomenon is what Albert Einstein once said: 'I rarely think in words at all. These thoughts did not come in any formal formulation. A thought comes and I may try to express it in words afterward.'. This too is entirely consistent with Polanyi's concept of 'tacit knowledge.'. Furthermore, Schon (1996) observes that '(m)uch reflection-in-action hinges on the experience of surprise. When intuitive, spontaneous performance yields nothing more than the results expected, then we tend not to think about it. But when intuitive performance leads to surprises, pleasing and promising or unwanted, we may respond by reflecting-in-action..'

We can extend the idea further if we assume that some professionals, at least, do consciously reflect over the course of days even weeks over their entire careers, progressively broadening their self-understanding and grasp of the nature of the problems that they face, occasionally innovating and improving professional practice. This practice of systematic self learning Schon dubbed 'reflection-on-action.' Reflection-in-action is an unconscious process but clearly there is transfer of knowledge from the realm of the individual unconscious to the conscious during rumination during and after a patient interview. This knowledge can then be not only be subject to conscious editing, but can also be discussed with colleagues.

The Influence of Positivism

Schon applies the concept of 'instrumental rationality,' which pioneer sociologist Max Weber (1904) saw as leading to a damaging reductionist, rationalist influence on societal thought generally. This can also be seen as the legacy of the discredited creed of 'positivism.' This philosophy of science, developed by Auguste Comte in the 18th century, claims that in the social sciences, the only authentic data is that derived from sensory data and the logical and mathematical manipulation of same. It is therefore chiefly characterized by a narrow minded overemphasis on the scientific analytical paradigm of enquiry and rejection of the hermeneutic qualitative tradition. This has been much criticized of recent years but is alive and well in community attitudes to science versus the humanities, and certainly in medicine and health care. This narrow view of the world is at the root of the Two Cultures problem pointed out by CP Snow (Snow 1963). The reflective physician will be a kind of 'medical research generalist' comfortable with the methods of both quantitative and qualitative intellectual paradigms.

The concept of unconscious tacit knowledge as the basis of judgement, including clinical judgement is similarly rooted in the same process. These closely related concepts we discussed in detail in Chapter 13. The opposing process is the basis of Weber's 'instrumental rationality' which consists of instrumental problem solving which we have outlined as characteristic of the scientific analytical paradigm. His fear was that society would be constrained be an 'iron cage' of bureaucracy. This model is therefore deeply imbedded in the institutional practice of professional life and curriculum of the professional school, the heritage of positivism which has been the dominant philosophy in the modern Western cultural paradigm.

Thus science has tended to supplant craft and artistry in the professional education and attitudes. This has led to discrediting of craft skills in general and of expert clinical judgement in particular. Recognition of the importance of positivism of this kind as the basis of a clash of paradigms in professional education has led to a crisis in professional practice, and in public acceptance of the legitimacy of professional activities. We have seen how even the way professionals really think has been distorted by implicitly casting it as an entirely conscious rational activity, contaminated, as it were, by global judgements which are opaque hence irrational and not to be trusted (Chapter 13). The dilemma, however, is that such global judgements are the very essence of professional expertise! Many of the professions, medicine for one, have embraced the scientific analytical intellectual paradigm to the extent of denying the way that they actually do think and conduct their daily work. They long to be seen as 'scientific' when, in truth, clinical diagnosis is conducted quintessentially according to the humanistic interpretive (hermeneutic) paradigm, albeit with some scientific refinement.

The artistry, a crucial element of professional expertise itself, is even denigrated, seen as lacking in rigour or as mysterious, beyond rational study (Schon 1996). The emphasis in management of problems is instead on science's separation of means from ends, and neglect of the importance of professional skill in problem setting as well as problem solving. One important outcome of this dominance of positivist thinking in the social sphere has been the inappropriate application of operations research developed for war time use to the attempted solution of complex social problems such as town planning and educational planning. Here the operations research approach has been a spectacular failure yet continues to have a life of its own. This is a classical example of paradigmatic blinkering.

Similar has been the push for the introduction of decision analysis and cost-utility analysis in clinical medicine. These simplistic models been generally rejected by clinicians who may not be knowlegable about the nuances of the process of diagnosis but they can usually quickly recognize an impostor. A key element in countering this distortion of professional practice and education is to encourage professionals to examine their own thought processes and the judgements which enderpin their everyday decisions and actions. Through such reflection-in-action, the working professional becomes a life-long learner since he 'can surface and criticize the tacit understandings that have grown up around the repetitive experiences of a specialized practice, and can make new sense of situations of uncertainty or uniqueness which he may allow himself to experience' (Schon 1983). The capacity to do this is characteristic of the 'reflective practitioner' who can thereby recognise and overcome the conflicts and limitations of paradigmatic differences between disciplines. This, we will argue, is the function of the postmodern reflective clinician.

Schon proposes that the process of a professional using reflection-in-action to make a global judgement be accepted as 'knowing-in-action,' and that the rational deliberation during and between professional transactions be consciously encouraged as 'reflection-on-action.' Recent research has shown that there is every reason to believe that these basic principles apply to all professional thought and, in fact to all human problem solving. In this chapter we will consider the proposition that Schon's conceptualisation is directly applicable to medical education and practice. Indeed we will argue that this same clash of paradigms, largely unrecognized, is at the very root of many of the most serious problems of health care. Recognition of this problem and a commitment to understanding postmodern medicine as well as for the comprehensive program of clinical research which will increasingly guide the practising physician.

Thus the alert physician can become aware of the influence of subtle but damaging tacit paradigmatic influences on a diagnosis or even on the relationship with a patient. This recognition would be a giant step towards getting to the roots of 'clinical inefficiency' which causes so much distress in the health system and which costs so much. Hence some of the most occult of influences may become evident, reinforce the memory and increase awareness of just how prevalent and pernicious these can be. The process begins as reflection-in-action but is reinforced by reflection-on-action. Moreover, there is no a priori reason why this skill cannot be taught in the training of the reflective physician in the case of reflection-on-action.

There is evidence that the unconscious and conscious processes operate together so that use of both processes can be cultivated in the education of the reflective practitioner. Obviously discussion of these processes between physicians would dramatically improve the acceptance and appreciation of the complexity and beauty of a process either rejected as 'spooky' or, worse, taken for granted.

It is the storage of this know-what and know-how knowledge which allows the reflective physician to eventually accrue 30 years of experience instead of thirty times one year's! There is also a social process of spreading knowledge by example – like osmosis. This means collective learning by our reflective practitioners. It is our fervent hope that by virtue of establishing centres for the study of clinical practice, we can foster this much needed study of clinical practice. What is intended by Schon and urgently required in the training of all kinds of professionals is to go further and to encourage this process by connecting it to the academic study of professional practice itself.

Currently realistic academic studies of the way in which professionals, including doctors, make their decisions is in short supply. Moreover studies have been mainly in the scientific analytical paradigm which does not include the introspective interpretive methods needed for detailed study of clinical practice or other professional decision-making in the field. We recall that for the influential 'cognitive continuum theory,' intuitive thinking processes are at one pole, analytical thinking at the other, with most thinking, dubbed 'quasi-rationality' exploiting both approaches. It is intriguing that the accrual of clinical experience and its application as clinical judgement both culminate in the same constructions of Polanyi, Schon and Brainerd and Reya (Chapter 13) respectively. This should not be so surprising, given that both rest upon similar theoretical bases and both underlie knowledge, judgement and decision making as supported by a formidable weight of evidence.

What is needed then is the reform of professional education and practice methods such that the hermeneutic and interpretive nature of professional diagnosis and action is acknowledged, thus joining the study of the science of the diagnostic process to the scholarly study of the art. Scientific and humanistic rigour can then be applied to the refinement of practice techniques. Reflection-in-action of this kind can call upon the rigour of both the scientific analytical and humanistic interpretative intellectual paradigms, both further refined in the 19th century, as an ongoing program of research in practice with a feedback loop into practice through the reflective physicians. There should therefore be an increasing number of clinicians who can undertake and teach clinical practice research using both quantitative and qualitative methods.

More recently, others have invoked a similar principle of the reflective practitioner and of reflection-in-action to apply to the work of the clinician. Thus Novack et al. (1997) discussed the effects of physicians' experience, values, attitudes and biases on communication with patients. They defined 'physician personal awareness' as 'insight into how one's life experiences and emotional make-up affect one's interactions with patients and other professionals.'. This is a broader concept than clinical judgement. People have core beliefs seldom fully articulated and sometimes organized into their own personal philosophy about life. These affect how physicians interact with patients. Potentially dysfunctional beliefs can include: physicians' beliefs and attitudes, including family influences, gender issues, sociocultural influences, physicians' feelings and emotional responses about love, caring, conflict and anger, challenging clinical situations such as difficult patients, dying patients, medical mistakes, and physician self-care, including managing stress. Physicians must also resolve their 'philosophy,' a kind of 'personal paradigm' as it were, with those of other members of the health care team. Hence there is a need for the study of behavioural science, and for keeping up with its literature.

Working along similar lines, Epstein (1999) described 'mindful practitioners (who) attend in a non-judgmental way to ordinary physical and mental processes during ordinary, everyday tasks. This self-reflection enables physicians to listen attentively to patients' accounts of illness, to recognize their own errors, refine their technical skills, make evidence-based decisions, and clarify their values so that so that they can act with compassion, technical competence, presence and insight.'. This is just what we expect of our reflective physicians. 'Mindfulness' is therefore a wider manifestation of reflective practice which goes beyond active observation of oneself, the patient and the problem, extending as far as examining the affective domains and involves critical reflection on action in clinical practice, teaching and research.

The objective of this book is to go further still, and affirm that there must be increased awareness by doctors of the role of the basic professional paradigmatic beliefs and attitudes on the routine judgements, decisions and actions of patient management and personal interactions with others in the health care system. This is especially so as the paradigm of medicine is constantly changing. Better understanding of the paradigms of health care is crucial not only to good quality patient care, but also to the smooth functioning of a system dependent on the goodwill and cooperation of many kinds of health professionals. We can only hope that 'the pen is mightier than the sword.'(Bulwer-Lytton 1839).

Clinical Practice Research –
The Way to Continuous Improvement

Closely connected with the idea of continuous clinical practice research is its coordination, the key function of reflective physicians under the auspices and with the support of the centre for the study of clinical practice. The idea of evaluating medical practice would have seemed strange to ancient and even to early modern physicians. The old idea of the doctor and patient bound by filial piety and committed to their common mission of helping the patient to regain good health now seems rather quaint. Today, patients and governments are intent on ensuring that health care stands up to external scrutiny, and want evidence to prove it. Clinical practice research can also be seen as locating then addressing the problems of 'clinical inefficiency' and 'consultation failure.'

We argue that what is required is a program of clinical practice research which is of an iterative kind, similar in principle to that used to evaluate the introduction of information technology. Such a process with its emphasis on feedback ensuring continuous improvement of clinical care and improved patient outcomes. A prime example of scientific clinical research of great importance arising from 'bedside' observations is Doctor Kate Campbell's discovery (1951) that 100% oxygen caused blindness (retrolental fibroplasia) in neonates. Another was the discovery by Professor E.J.M. Campbell (1967) that too high an oxygen concentration caused carbon dioxide narcosis and coma in patients with serious lung disease. Cooperative studies involving clinicians and biomedical scientists are relatively commonplace. Similar studies involving sociology and anthropology have been very much less common, and will often require the support of a centre for the study of clinical practice when interdisciplinary skills are required. Such social sciences studies led by a doctor are almost non-existent. Thus our research study of failure of patient reassurance McDonald et al. (1996) arose directly from an event in our clinical practice, and required an interdisciplinary study with sociology providing the qualitative analysis required. Because clinicians had very limited knowledge of reassurance failure, we felt that the study was important.

There are two basic requirements for clinical practice research. The first is to have analytical statistical science applied to evaluate the technical procedures and technologies of patient care. The second is to have an injection of scholarship by the social sciences and humanities to inform the humanistic aspect. What kind of science do we need? Biomedical science scarcely needs justification in the modern era; we have all partaken of its benefits. Empirical statistical science has made a late start after a false dawn represented by Louis' early evaluation of bloodletting in revolutionary France. But it is now firmly ensconced in the form of clinical epidemiology and biostatistics, and evidence based medicine. The science of taxonomy, the classification of patterns of illness, has been indispensable in biology. It should also be a crucial contributor to clinical diagnosis and prognostication as Feinstein (1967) insisted, but it has not yet caught on.

Given the grateful acceptance of biomedical science by the community, dissatisfaction with medicine centres largely on the doctor-patient relationship. Since the manifold errors of clinical inefficiency are not obvious to patients, it mainly the consultation which concerns us. Hence we settle on problems of communication as a primary target for reform. These require hermeneutic interpretive studies of the social sciences and humanities to provide the research basis and theoretical foundations for refinement of the art. As we shall see, these have been largely left out of clinical research where biomedical science is dominant and clinical epidemiology, empirical science, is gaining a substantial foothold. However, as yet, these 'humanistic' disciplines, 'basic knowledge' for the art of medicine, scarcely feature in the undergraduate curriculum. We should all be aware of the consequences of this distortion.

The Evaluation of Drugs – Empirical Statistical Science at Work

Drug evaluation was born of public concern about side-effects. The first randomized controlled trial, in the 1940s, was of streptomycin for tuberculosis (1948). Now randomized trials are the gold standard for evaluation of drugs. The randomized controlled trial is the clinical equivalent of the controlled laboratory experiment. Its methods are rigorous, its statistical interpretation is beyond question, hence it has maximum credibility. This can lead to its exponents seeing it as the only wheel in town. Is it? If randomisation is ethical, if variables can and should be controlled, if the project is practical and financially viable, if quantitative outcomes are required, and results are likely to be generalisable in clinical practice – then the answer can be yes. It is then the gold standard, 'level 1' evidence in the parlance afficianados of evidence based medicine. But if any of the above conditions cannot be met, then this is not so. For example, if evaluation's objective is to find out why a substantial proportion of patients thought to have been 'reassured' after exclusion of serious disease by appropriate investigation, are not reassured at all, the initial study must involve interview of patients and their doctors with qualitative, interpretative data analysis. In other words this would constitute 'Level 1' evidence under these circumstances.

In one sense, despite its magnificent contributions, the ready application of the randomized trial to drug evaluation has also done us something of a disservice! Drugs are the only interventions the evaluation of which is largely independent of a complex context. For example a patient can hardly be blinded to the fact that he or she has had a coronary graft operation. This is especially so since persistence or recurrence of chest pain can mean that the pain did not come from the heart in the first place, and that the period of relief was due to the placebo effect of the intervention. This is not an uncommon occurrence, and it is important to recognize.

The Evaluation of Diagnostic Tests – Clinical Epidemiology at Work

Investigations, particularly imaging tests are widely employed. The context is complex and evaluation correspondingly difficult. In particular, they are frequently used to rule out disease, hence to allay patient anxiety, often due to the complex interplay of personal influences. Randomisation can rarely be employed as a tactic. Moreover, few studies have measured their impact even on patient plan of management; as we have seen impact on patient anxiety has been anything but reassuring. As a result, most evaluation is confined to image quality and diagnostic accuracy (sensitivity and specificity). These indices were developed by radiologists in the 1940s (Birkelo et al. 1947, Garland 1949), but their use is more common among clinical epidemiologists, certainly not by clinicians who ultimately utilize the evidence. There is much work to be done. It is possible to use a combined quantitative and qualitative research design. In this way we can document impact of test results on a doctor's diagnosis and plan of management, and attempt, based on the literature and our clinical experience to estimate the likely effect on the patient. Important for some uses of a test, for example for reassurance, we can also document any impact on patient anxiety (McDonald 1995). Hopefully reflective physicians will lead the way in implementing this kind of detailed study of currently neglected but clinically important patient outcomes.

The Evaluation of Clinical Symptoms and Signs

This is a sad story. Clinicians have certainly not been at work here evaluating the evidence which is basic to their day-to-decisions, with the rare exceptions of research oriented clinical epidemiologists (Simmel 2008). Louis in early 19th century Paris used autopsy as the gold standard for studying clinical evidence but this initiative lapsed. McGee (2005) has reviewed the limited information in the literature and collected a large number of references. Joshua et al. (2005) and Simel (2005) have also reviewed the subject. The case of patient symptoms and signs is urgent, since they have been subjected to almost no evaluation at all some 200 years into the modern era. The end result is that clinicians develop their own tacit impressions of accuracy, informally linked by experience to impact on management and health outcome. We do not have much idea of the accuracy of a history of chest pain as common and important as it is. Nor do we know the accuracy of a claim of feeling an enlarged liver or spleen, or a claim of reduced ankle jerks, even when we are the claimant. Hence the urgency of the need for a process of continuous clinical practice research promoted and assisted by the centre for the study of clinical practice.

One of the contributions of biomedical science to clinical history taking has been the development of a check list of common symptoms of organ damage, an aide memoire for patient and doctor, another initiative of C-P-A Louis. Biomedical science has also underpinned the physical examination, mainly through applying knowledge of pathology. The urgent need is for clinical practice research for the appraisal of evidence from the clinical transaction, led by reflective clinicians well versed in clinical epidemiology and biostatistics, and coordinated by the centre for the study of clinical practice. So even the empirical statistical movement has not yet impacted much as yet on the real basics of clinical assessment. The evaluation of symptoms and signs is undeniably difficult but this is hardly a valid excuse for its blatant neglect.

Take, for example, the evaluation of the accuracy and reproducibility of the jugular venous pressure in the neck. It is often crucial to accurate diagnosis in a critically ill patient. Say we are examining a patient in shock shortly after abdominal surgery. We must quickly distinguish between intra-abdominal bleeding for which blood and perhaps reoperation at high risk may be required, and pulmonary embolism for which clot-busting medication may be required but with a higher risk of aggravation of bleeding if the latter happened to be the correct diagnosis. The most important sign is a low venous pressure in the case of haemorrhage, raised in severe pulmonary embolism. This vital physical sign cannot be considered in isolation however. The likelihood of pulmonary embolism is determined by a multiplicity of other interacting pieces of evidence which are relevant to the diagnosis, ranging from varicose veins to obesity. Even more confusing is that obesity may render the venous pressure hard to measure, especially in an emergency under difficult conditions for such an observation. Moreover it can aggravate breathlessness to boot perhaps incorrectly suggesting pulmonary embolism. So too can post-operative lung collapse.

To evaluate the accuracy of clinical venous pressure means that we must structure a research study which takes account of these important modifying factors or the conclusions would likely be misleading. Very important are the experience of the examiner, hence time since graduation and subsequent clinical experience. This is a 'wicked problem,' if ever there was one, and not an isolated example. Then consider the sheer number of symptoms and signs which need evaluation. As we shall see, the textbooks of bedside diagnosis lack information of this kind, and so does the medical literature which should be constantly feeding results of clinical epidemiological evaluation of such signs to the textbooks.

The Taxonomic Imperative

We have already discussed the importance of taxonomy, the classification of living things. It is crucial to the science of clinical medicine. This was recognized by Sydenham in the 17th century and much later, by Feinstein in the 20th. An insight before its time is, however, prone to founder. So it has been for the science of taxonomy in medicine. This defect in the clinician's armory was clearly detected by Feinstein (1967) who noted that the patterns of clinical manifestations exhibited by ill patients could be expressed as Venn diagrams with overlapping circles representing the variables, as used in set theory. He acknowledged that Sydenham had previously described such patterns of illness manifestations. It is also is fair to say that doctors have communicated intuitively using these patterns at least since Hippocrates.

A masterstroke was that the idea was revived by French physicians who saw the resemblance of these patterns of illness manifestations to the laws of combinatorial probability, and also an analogy with the structure of molecules and the nature of chemical compounds. The basic idea is that these clusters of variables could be related to age gender, diagnosis, prognosis, treatment response, test results, health outcome, patient characteristics, patient satisfaction and social class and context. Moreover, the clinical profile can be extended to include attitudes to risk, record of compliance with treatment and available social support. They are therefore succinct yet comprehensive summaries of patient illness, personal attributes and attitudes, and social context of illness. The idea did founder but did not sink without a trace as we shall see; the computer may still come to the rescue if clinicians care to lay the foundations. The problem is not so much technological as trying to match clinical manifestations with best treatment.

Will Clinicians Rise to the 'Soft Data' Challenge?

Imagine that these patterns, summaries of illness in personal and social context, could be incorporated into, say, a bar code as in a supermarket. They could then be made available as silent consultants to clinicians everywhere. A clinician with a difficult patient could then consult the computer to tap into his own career experience, as well as conducting a search - city, state or country wide - seeking a match for a problem patient. The procedure would be supported at the bedside and in the clinic by voice recognition capability and computer storage of the medical records of this or other patients, even at distant sites. A reflective physician could supervise the use and conduct research on this computer. So far so good. However Feinstein warned that unless clinicians had previously designed classifications, other 'clinimetrics,' and grading scales, they would not be able to either interrogate or program the computer. Moreover, there would be nobody who could instruct them so that they would be effectively hamstrung. His prediction has come true, and very few physicians have the clinical epidemiologic qualifications for the job.

As only Feinstein could put it: 'After another 20 years of development without careful supervision, the accumulated abuses of an unregulated computer technology will be so immense and obfuscating that a young clinician may not be able to find his way through the confusion. Moreover, the medical student from now may have no suitable teachers to give him an appropriate background to understand clinical problems.' (Feinstein 1967). Feinstein pointed also to the chaos which would ensue if clinicians did not provide the necessary clinical classifications and grading scales. In fact that is precisely what they have done! What the computer represents is no more than what doctors have done for centuries, to collect information unconsciously, and presumably some have reflected upon it. They obviously have textbooks, access to the medical literature, case reports and series, and in some cases to computer algorithms.

The computer storage of raw collective clinical experience in the way Feinstein suggested is a compelling idea the time of which has come. The notion is potentially more attractive with the development of the notion of 'fuzzy set' theory, a concept related to probability, which more closely represents the indistinct margins of disease entities used by clinicians which facilitates their manipulation when considering differential diagnosis (Zadeh 1965). A way to use scientifically appraised sanitized clinical data, expressed as 'clinimetrics,' collected and stored for future routine use has been described as 'evidence farming' (Hay et al. 2008), as we have seen previously.

Even sadder than the lack of evaluation of the art skills of clinical care is the story of the behavioral and social sciences, and of the humanities, once a fellow traveller with medicine. In chapters 10 and 11, we have discussed the all too common problem of 'consultation failure.' Just as sociologist Mills (2000) called for a 'sociological imagination' to link political problems to patient problems, we need a corresponding skill, say a 'clinical imagination,' to link consultation failure to the problems of patients and of the health care system.

Flexner's Legacy - Distortion of The Modern Medical Curriculum

When Abraham Flexner was commissioned to report to the Carnegie Foundation on the state of medical education in the U.S.A. and Canada (Flexner 1910), he was dismayed at what he found. Not only were the standards of medical education poor, but so too was the standard of students, and entrance requirements were minimal. In some cases students could graduate without ever having examined a patient. In addition, many medical schools were putting profit before professionalism. He travelled widely in the United States, Canada and Europe. Flexner was most impressed by standards of medical science taught in Prussia where many Americans were studying; he also admired the clinical standards in France, birth place of modern medicine, and in Britain. Another influence on his thinking was the excellent quality of instruction at Johns Hopkins University and a handful of other U.S. institutions, where science was taught before clinical instruction. He therefore recommended a 4 year curriculum, the first 2 years at university devoted to scientific training and 2 years subsequently for clinical instruction in hospital. There was just one problem – the social sciences and humanities had fallen through the cracks!

Flexner expressed regret at this wrong turn just 15 years after his report: 'scientific medicine in America - young, vigorous and positivistic – is today sadly deficient in cultural and philosophic background' (Flexner 1925). There have been numerous committees of enquiry but very little to show for them. This poses a challenge for us - to illustrate the magnitude of the problem of distortion of medical education, which must be held responsible for the frequent lack of 'humanism,' in a sufficiently objective way without deviating too far off course. Hence we include a summary of the results of a comprehensive statement by the committee which is in the form of a series of areas of behavioral and social science, and humanities, posited as topics to be included in the medical curriculum (American Academy of

Sciences, Cuff and Vanselow eds. 2009). We could not find a better or more authoritative statement in the literature. Indeed, it would be difficult task to mount an argument against any of their recommendations. Those gradings in the document represent a view reached by a formal consensus method by the committee. This committee rated 26 issues as 'high priority' for any medical curriculum, 9 'medium priority' and the remainder 'low priority'; the last category they did not consider further. In fact, for our purposes, we decided that it was sufficient to list only the high priority group in order to get our point across. We hope that this list is sufficient to make the point that there were an extraordinary range of highly relevant issues to which most medical students are not generally exposed.

The authors' table 3.1 we have taken the liberty of reproducing in text form as follows - Mind-body interaction in health and disease: biologic mediators between biological and social factors and health; behavioral, social and psychological factors in chronic disease; psychological and social factors in human development that influence disease and illness; psychosocial aspects of pain. Patient behavior: health risk behaviors; principles of behavior change; impact of psychosocial stressors and psychiatric disorders on manifestations of other disorders and on health behavior. Physician role and behavior: ethical guidelines for physician behavior; personal biases, attitudes and values as they influence patient care; physician well-being; social accountability and responsibility; work in health care teams and organizations; use of and linkage with community resources to enhance health care. Physician-patient interactions: basic communication skills; complex communication skills; context of patient's social and economic situation; capacity for self-care, and ability to participate in shared decision making; management of difficult or problematic physician-patient interactions. Social and cultural issues in health care: impact of social inequalities in health care and the social factors that influence health outcomes; cultural competency; role of complementary and alternative medicine. Health policy and economics: overview of the U.S. health care system; economic incentives affecting patients' health-related behaviors; costs, cost-effectiveness, and physician responses to financial incentives.

The unfavorable outcome, the almost total neglect of the social sciences and humanities, was apparently not anticipated by Flexner. But just how damaging this lesion was to prove for the medical curriculum we shall contemplate below. This was particularly so because the effect of Flexner's report, enthusiastically received in Europe, was to set the medical curriculum in concrete worldwide for the rest of the 20th and part of the 21st century! Generations of medical students have been deprived of an important input to their studies as a result. At the time, the science was moving towards ascendancy, especially in Germany where it dominated the clinical thinking, and in France where Claude Bernard was convinced that scientific medicine would eventually prevail over clinical medicine. As a result of these influences, biomedical science did dominate the medical landscape, effectively exerting a negative influence on the art of medicine and eventually on clinicians' teaching time due to prioritization of biomedical, especially laboratory research.

A moment's reflection reveals that this formidable list paints a depressing picture of 'paradigmatic blinkering'. Those planning such deficient medical curricula have demonstrated the manner in which the social and behavioral sciences, and the humanities have been sidelined. This represents a terrible indictment of many medical curricula. To say this certainly in no way overstates the case for reform! When curricular reform is mooted, the faculty wagons are sometimes drawn into a circle and conservative forces emerge which successfully limit change. To be fair, protection of curricular time and paradigmatic prejudice are not the only issues. Meeting managed care requirements, the priority allotted to research, and the distraction of private practice eat into faculty time for teaching as well, so that experienced clinical teachers are simply less available than they used be.

The plethora of enquiries into medical education in the U.S. since Flexner's landmark report (1910) makes depressing reading. Bloom, a sociologist, summed up the response to this barrage of good advice as 'reform without change' (Bloom 1995). It is unlikely that such a complex issue would have a single simple 'cause.' We have targeted the influence of the dominant scientific paradigm as a basic factor. Bloom has proposed another with which others concur, the financial conflicts facing universities. Finally, paradigmatic commitment translates into power which is readily mobilized to meet a challenge such as threatened curricular change.

A Teaching Role for Reflective Physicians

To bridge the gap, the social and behavioral, sciences and the humanities must find their niche in the curriculum and in the minds of students and medical teachers. Here the reflective physician and the centre for the study of clinical practice can play an important linkage role between university preclinical teaching and hospital clinical instruction. Here the intellectual bridges are few. Moreover, the connection could be such as to promote better understanding between science on the one hand and the, social, behavioral sciences and humanities - the 'humanism camp,' on the other.

Not only that, they could address a specific problem that many students find it difficult to relate what they may learn in, say social theory as part of a reformed curriculum, in the preclinical years when confronted by clinical reality. It would be feasible to have reflective physicians teach in the 'humanism' area together with staff from appropriate university departments. This could be done as a form of problem-based learning, or bedside teaching, perhaps supplemented by seminars. These initiatives could be part of both preclinical and clinical instruction. For example, our reflective physicians could also teach some preparatory clinically oriented material in the preclinical curriculum using the same approach.

Such a teaching commitment would become a responsibility of the centre for the study of clinical practice, as a skill to be cultivated by reflective clinicians. This activity could be seen as a close relative of clinical practice research. Our reflective physicians will be encouraged to join with university members in clinical practice research projects which should lubricate such a process. In this way, not only could the current deficiencies in teaching of the social sciences and humanities be remedied in a way which does not unduly threaten the biomedical sciences, but also space could be created for the eventual emergence of the broader postmodern paradigm of medicine for clinical practice and research to which we have referred.

There is no sense in which hospital-based centres for the study of clinical practice should be seen as in competition with evolutionary curricular reform in the university. What this offers also to these university investigators is much valued access, otherwise denied, to patients for their own studies or for interdisciplinary research. As we suggest, the representatives of the two institutions could be brought into closer contact which in itself might do much to bridge the present gap. In any case, it hopefully sends a clear message to students. A reflective physician's spin-off might include shared journal clubs to help them keep abreast of the literature. All in all, this would be useful consciousness raising exercise for all concerned. The reflective physician is clearly well placed to participate and to coordinate this effort.

Reflective Physicians and the Centre for the Study of Clinical Practice

The structure of the medical paradigm and the educational curriculum have been shaped in the crucible of the forces of the broader social paradigm. A number of important changes have been made mainly over the last 50 years. Among these have been the casting of medicine in the form of a postgraduate degree with credit given for humanities and social science subjects in the selection process. There has been increasing emphasis on earlier patient contact both in hospital and primary care. But all of this change is nowhere near enough.

The basic need is to use some imaginative planning to unite hospital and university in a program of clinical practice research, and to provide the training of reflective practitioners and resources necessary for them to do so. We will now outline what further developments are required to unite humanities and social sciences with science under the umbrella of a broader paradigm of medicine. To make an attempt to shift the paradigm of health in the direction of increased 'humanism' involves links with hospital and university departments and links to undergraduate and postgraduate education, as well as government bodies as appropriate, such as when evaluating medical technology.

A centre for the study of clinical practice which has functioned for 8 years at St Vincent's Hospital, Melbourne, has aimed in a broad sense to aid the necessary transition from a modern to a postmodern paradigm. The structure which we describe is specific to the intellectual environment and practical requirements of a university hospital. Undoubtedly similar structures could be designed for other kinds of environment; this could be in general practice where the norm has become some form of group practice sometimes with associated laboratory facilities. In any case this experimental model has worked at one site. The centre has, so far, been painted as a hospital and university resource. However, we believe that its potential for training the reflective practitioners required for grass roots research into the problems of clinical practice and the spin-off on the doctor, the student, nursing and allied health personnel will be its major contribution to health care. It could also provide sociology and anthropology much needed access to patients with the guidance of clinicians with depth of bedside experience – to the advantage of both. The problems facing are many and serious as we have seen. Yet research has scarcely begun to address them. So the need is urgent.

Reflection-in-Action in Postmodern Medicine

The concepts of paradigm and reflection-in-action are closely intertwined. Thus the prevailing clinical paradigm will shape doctors' attitude to the clinical process of diagnosis, specifically whether or not they respect the subtlety of the art and their own global judgements. It will determine also whether or not they systematically engage in reflection. More importantly, it will also determine what they are able reflect upon. The postmodern paradigm of medicine which will therefore both encourage and guide reflection-in-action which will consider many more determinants of clinical judgements derived from a variety of disciplines. Indeed, by reflecting-in-action, the practitioner will be expected to be able to dissect out or deconstruct clinical judgements and decisions, exposing the many interacting vectors of which the decision is the resultant. Thus the clinical communication will be analyzed according to personal and collective clinical experience, biomedical knowledge and in light of the reflective doctor's knowledge of himself or herself. However, unlike the traditional clinical paradigm, relevant knowledge from the social sciences and insights from the humanities can now also be factored in. So will issues such as the soundness of clinical techniques, reliability of results, relevant evidence from epidemiological studies on prognosis and treatment which will be the contribution of clinical epidemiology and evidence-based medicine. Patient values and social and other constraints on possible treatment must obviously be taken into account.

Thus, in making a decision about the diagnosis and treatment of chest pain, there may be conscious reflection upon the nature and course of the pain, its precipitants, aggravants, the family predicament, the pain's response to treatment, results of treatment interventions so far, relevant clinical evidence from the medical literature and hopefully from the local institutional computer data-base. This diagnostic aid, described above, can add information regarding the effects of such intervention on prognosis and treatment; also included are personal knowledge of the patient's likely responses and wishes, understanding of family reactions, knowledge of behaviour of people drawn from the literature, the quality of doctor-patient communication buttressed by sociological and anthropological insights, the literature on patient compliance with medication, its possible determinants in the present situation and often many more. The process of reflection-in-action will not only be a central part of the postmodern paradigm, but also the scope of the variables seen, on reflection, as contributing to judgements will be greatly extended.

Weber, one of the pioneers of sociology, warned last century that the emerging society in Europe was spawning a technocratic culture; he saw people constrained in an 'iron cage of bureaucracy' (Weber 1904). The medical education system can be seen as a microcosm, a professional paradigm nested within the modern paradigm of society. The postmodern paradigm of medicine will be much broader. This broadening, already under way, will involve a wider range of academic disciplines feeding into the tacit framework of belief which is the clinical paradigm, and similarly supporting the process of reflection-in-action. Thus the new paradigm of medicine will not only specifically encourage reflection-in-action, it will allow a much greater range of judgemental issues to be reflected upon. Ad hoc adjustments to the modern paradigm have already attempted to broaden its scope. For example, the incorporation of epidemiological thinking into the clinical paradigm has already had a substantial impact in the form of clinical epidemiology. This movement in medicine has evolved as a belated effort to inject epidemiological science into clinical care, side by side with biomedical science. Subdisciplines already absorbed into clinical knowledge in this way in past generations include clinical anatomy, clinical physiology and clinical biochemistry. In this way were laid the bricks for building the practice of medicine.

To add clinical epidemiology is a worthy expansion of the scientific component of the paradigm which encourages the application of accuracy measures applied to diagnosis, and information from randomized trials to complement the clinical and biomedical data. Evidence-based medicine has enjoyed considerable success, in line with its compatibility with the continuing strong influence of the scientific paradigm in medicine. Yet, even here, the inappropriate influence of the scientific analytical paradigm has somewhat distorting effect. Originally conceived as 'clinical epidemiology,' the introduction of epidemiological thinking promised to be on a broad front which encompassed most clinical activities, ranging from the varying spectrum of presentation of disease and implications for the treatment of the individual, to the errors inherent in technological diagnosis and their ill-effects. Evidence-based medicine is a kind of stripped down 'more scientific' reductionist version with its emphasis on the randomized controlled trial as a controlled scientific experiment and the implications of results for the treatment of organic diseases.

Much more slowly moving, however, is the trend to include sociology and the humanities in the medical paradigm. This would lead to a valuable broadening of the base of skills which the practitioner needs for reflection-in-action. We noted earlier that many clinicians early in the 20th century, specifically Osler, Cabot, and Peabody in the U.S. were aware of and concerned about the potentially damaging effects of medical science on the art of medicine. They were concerned that attention to the personal and social context of the patient would be diminished by what we are calling the technological emphasis of the burgeoning scientific analytical component of the clinical paradigm. Later, White and Barondess opined about the excessive emphasis on technology is patient care centred on organic disease in the modern hospital. We also documented an adverse effect on the public image of medicine.

What was needed was a balanced view: 'Cabot was by turns a prominent advocate for and an incisive critic of the new technology of early twentieth century medicine' (Crenner 2005). Osler put it pithily when he said: 'It is much more important to know what sort of patient has a disease than what sort of disease a patient has.'. In a landmark paper, Peabody (1927) remarked: 'The most common criticism made by older physicians, at present is that young graduates have been taught a great deal about the mechanism of disease, but very little about the practice of medicine or, to put it more bluntly, they are too " scientific" and do not know how to take care of patients.'. Clinician Engel (1977) was more explicit when he called for 'a more inclusive scientific model for medicine, one that extends the scientific method to the human domain.' This he dubbed the 'biopsychosocial model' (Engel 1987). This could be seen as an early attempt to consciously extend the clinical paradigm (model) by incorporation of the social sciences and humanities to refine the art of medicine just as clinical epidemiology has done for the empirical statistical handling of clinical evaluation, and to apply the results to practice. What is still required is a multidisciplinary method of studying clinical care which can merge the psychosocial component with the biomedical which is the basic aim of clinical practice research.

Clinical Reflection-in-Action under the Modern Scientific Paradigm

Having considered the important role that reflection-in-action plays in clinical decision making, we need to ask what clinicians should be expected to reflect about in the course of their daily work. This is precisely what is so powerfully determined by the prevailing medical and social paradigms. In the 18th century, before the paradigm shift to modern scientific medicine, the healer's thought processes must have been tacitly moulded and guided by the old Hippocratic paradigm of medicine based upon the balance of humours, disturbance of which was thought of as underlying disease. When they reflected on their judgements, say in a difficult case or when explaining to a client, we can assume that they must have pondered the problems in terms of a disease brought about by this disturbance of humoral balance. Thus the paradigmatic framework shaped their observations and interpretations. If they experienced difficulty handling a patient, they had little else to go on but their own clinical experience and what they were taught by apprenticeship as students.

Under the modern paradigm of medicine, the art and science of medicine co-exist in an uneasy alliance. But the influence of the old paradigm lives on - the art is seen as craft to be learned at the bedside and properly so. The science has, however, been taught first in an effort to produce doctors who are, or least see themselves as solely applied scientists. Such is the mental compartmentalization of the scientific and interpretive paradigms that the skills required for the clinical examination itself have been subjected to remarkable little critical scientific appraisal, let alone been subjected to systematic scholarly study. Nor have the skills required for understanding the psychosocial context of the medical encounter been refined by the application of insights from behavioral science, sociology, and the humanities as one might have expected, since these disciplines do not share the respect accorded to the medical sciences. There is a merger required between clinical knowledge of the traditional kind, and the clinical and the many potential academic and practical offerings of social sciences and humanities.

Hence, when the modern medical practitioner does reflect upon findings in the course of a clinical examination, especially when confronted by the atypical or difficult case, when writing a report, when communicating with consultants and patients, when teaching students, when presenting at grand rounds, what is likely to be considered is in the province is of disease aetiology or pathological mechanism, that is, the biomedical science with which they feel most comfortable. Thus an obscure case of jaundice may, on reflection, be seen as likely to be allergic liver damage due to sensitivity to a drug rather than an obstructing gallstone. Alternatively a problem of interaction with a patient will still be seen from a traditional clinical perspective. Hence if the patient does not take medication, he or she will be branded as 'failing to comply with medical orders,' a 'problem patient' rather than as a frightened person alienated from the doctor by a lack of communication. The issue is all too often the 'problem doctor.' What the clinician under the modern paradigm is not at all equipped to do is to reflect upon the way in which basic paradigmatic forces influence attitudes and beliefs to the extent that they may influence or determine any decision, whether it involve the care of the patient, bedside clinical research or an administrative matter.

A Forum for Interdisciplinary Discussion and Debate

Next we will consider some of the potential contributions of the centre for the study of clinical practice to practical concerns and to promoting and guiding intellectual debate, particularly as it concerns underlying issues of research methods and assumptions. What we see as the most crucial contribution is the training, support and supervision of undergraduate and postgraduate students. Hopefully, interested physicians, willing to become reflective physicians, with help and encouragement, will be welcome additions to a multidisciplinary clinical research team studying their patients and those of other interested physicians. The centre is an ideal locale for interdisciplinary debate concerning methods, theoretical assumptions, patient oriented case studies and problem-based learning. Interested hospital and university staff would have the opportunity to introduce debate on subjects of mutual interest, especially concerning research methods and assumptions. The vexed question, that old chestnut of quantitative versus qualitative methods should be high on the agenda. Perhaps some rapprochement or at least a truce could be declared on this topic.

Debate should be rigorous but participants should be respectful and mindful of the possible impact of challenging, even threatening views put forward by a researcher from an 'alien' discipline. Such seminars should include nursing and other allied health workers. Ongoing contact between disciplines would have some hope of cultivating the conviction needed to change rigid views or respect needed to relinquish cherished beliefs. Often applicable is the dictum 'convince a man against his will, he is of the same opinion still.' Obviously these contacts would also be an ideal way in which to recruit coworkers for multidisciplinary studies to the benefit of both parties. This dialogue between disciplines could be initiated by the director of the centre or another reflective physician, perhaps a registrar to the centre. Over time this could do much to overcome methodological prejudice and enrich research training.

Links to Other Hospital Departments

Another important function of the centre is to articulate with other hospital departments according to their needs and mutual interests. Firstly there is quality assurance. At St Vincent's Hospital, this department was run separately for good historical reasons. However, under different circumstances, the two units have so much in common that they could well be closely coordinated, or quality assurance run as part of the centre. Both units have a strong focus on clinical epidemiology and evidence-based medicine. In the future, both departments will require a very wide armamentarium of research methods in order to tackle difficult clinical problems. In fact many problems of bedside medicine and many outpatient evaluations could be included under the broader rubric of clinical practice research. Such research should be coordinated by the centre, and interdisciplinary as required and desired. Similarly research methodogical advice can be made available to any group requiring such help. Assistance with more advanced statistical methods, in particular logistic regression analysis, could be arranged. In-house courses in research methods and instruction on their underlying theoretical justifications and assumptions would be on offer. Doctors will obviously taught the variety of practical and academic skills with attention paid to local needs.

Evaluation Research

Evaluation research, especially medical technology assessment, is grist for the mill for the centre for the study of clinical practice. Under this heading, for example, the following studies have been undertaken by the Centre at St Vincent's Hospital: Commonwealth Government lithotripsy program (including a social and economic evaluation):

- radiological patient archiving (PACS),
- magnetic resonance imaging
- laparoscopic cholecystectomy
- percutaneous coronary angioplasty and chest pain
- review of patient delay in seeking medical assistance for chest pain analysis of the declining hospital mortality for patients with myocardial infarction digital radiological assessment of lung lesions
- brachytherapy for carcinoma
- diagnostic value of the rotating vestibular chair for vertigo
- clinical value and indications for echocardiography
- study of failure of a normal test and reassurance to allay patient anxiety
- evaluation of the public health implications of senile calcific aortic stenosis,
- assessment of Traditional Chinese Medicine
- evaluation of Victoria's telemedicine program
- evaluation of trends in the diagnosis and management of appendicitis
- evaluation of gallstone lithotripsy.

Technology assessment has, therefore, formed the largest proportion of the work of this new centre. However this emphasis is likely to change over time. Hopefully the education and support of reflective physicians engaged in clinical practice research will occupy a larger proportion of time, as we discuss below. When the centre was operating, the director was a member of the National Health Technology Advisory Panel, the mandate of which was to advise the Commonwealth Minister for Health. This explains the primary focus on the assessment of medical technology. He was also a member of the hospital research ethics committee.

Other activities of the centre included conducting a statistics course, involvement in research projects including the use of Doppler ultrasound for the measurement of the severity of mitral valve regurgitation (with the hospital physics department), development of a protocol for assessing the clinical contribution of percutaneous retrograde cholangiography in the diagnosis of suspected biliary disease, a plan for the structure of investigation units in relation to clinical units. From what has been said, it should be apparent that the director has needed to be expert in wide range of research methods, and literate in statistics. Indeed, the centre should be a repository of research methods for the hospital. He or she must also contribute to a range of hospital committees, including technology assessment, quality assurance and research ethics committees. There is need for a full time statistician to meet the needs of the centre and of hospital departments requiring assistance.

The Steering Committee

The activities of the centre for the study of clinical practice should be guided by a steering committee which should include the director of clinical services, chairman of the senior medical staff, representative of state and commonwealth governments who commission and fund studies such as technology evaluations, a representative of appropriate hospital departments, representation of university departments, and a representative of the quality assurance department. Experts in other fields should be seconded as appropriate. When the size warrants, a rotating registrar position should be established to assist organization and promote the educational function of the centre. A representative of students should be considered so that they have a stake in clinical practice research, hence exposure to their role as reflective practitioners of the future.

Institutions of Reflective Practice

It is not enough to recognize the importance of training reflective practitioners. The practice must not only be built into professional education but also into the institutions in which they practice. Frankford et al. (2000) point out that few graduates will practice as individuals in the future, so the task of the medical school includes institution building, concern for community values as responsive professionalism which strives for mutual interdependence with patients and society, responding to and partially creating social values, as part of the public good and organized collegially. Professional competence involves reflection-in-action and reflection-on-action over a lifetime. Professionals must work in teams so activities must be undertaken in groups, helping one another to understand others' background and experience, shaping current actions, actions and values. Institutional reflective enquiry brings education into practice and practice into education. Specifically, clinical practice research should be a top priority for the new practice arrangements that we have discussed in Chapter 14.

The 'Ecumenical' Role of a Centre for the Study of Clinical Practice

Journal clubs could be open to students who could also be invited to interdisciplinary seminars. In this way, not only could the current deficiencies in teaching of the social sciences and humanities be remedied in a way which does not unduly threaten the biomedical sciences, but also creates space for the eventual emergence of the broader paradigm of medicine to which we have referred. There is no sense in which hospital-based centres for the study of clinical practice should be seen as in competition with evolutionary curricular reform in the university. The two developments are clearly complementary. In fact, the spin-off should bring the two parties closer with respect to the clinical half of the medical course.

The recognition of the importance of the concepts of paradigm and reflective practitioner is the major justification for the development of a structure such as our centre for the study of clinical practice represents in the hospital setting. This book attempts to justify the importance of these ideas and to establish the importance an educational and research support structure to ensure that all medical practitioners become reflective clinicians. The doctor, educated in both scientific analytical and 'humanistic' paradigms, and given to reflect upon personal attitudes and feelings towards patients and their basis in past experience, including possible family influences, can reflect upon a wide range of specific determinants of clinical diagnosis and practice problems.

Thus the range of problems which the clinician can address both globally and intuitively and upon conscious reflection is greatly enhanced and likely to be that much more effective. As a corollary, the study of clinical care itself then will then be accepted as a legitimate form of professional knowing, and the basis of continuous quality improvement of clinical care. In the hospital setting, we envisage the centre liaising with university and promoting reflective practice, encouraging clinicians to engage in quality assurance and clinical research, facilitating multidisciplinary contact and research - a means of greatly extending the scope of research in the clinical field, and of broadening the clinical paradigm on which reflection and research must rest.

A representative of the centre should be a part of any clinical practice research project with two aims. One is to act as a go-between to access methodological assistance. The other is to gain additional experience. It is anticipated that studies should be published as appropriate. Members of the centre would be obvious persons to conduct a journal club. This should monitor the sociological, medical humanities and behavioral science literature as well as the biomedical. This should have the effect of underlining the multidisciplinary remit of the centre. A journal club should clear the way for getting to know and for enlisting candidates for interdisciplinary research projects, and also for making presentations. In particular, members of other centres could be enlisted to lecture or conduct seminars. Linkage of centres at other hospitals could be encouraged by regular meetings. Another good reason to meet would be to discuss computer downloads of the patterns of patient illness - in fulfillment of Feinstein's dream of an empirical approach to clinical practice (Feinstein 1967). These kinds of mutual learning we might refer to as activities of the greater centre for the study of clinical practice or perhaps as 'Feinstein projects.'

Teaching Function in the Community

Such a centre has considerable teaching potential for medical students and graduates. Obviously, presentations on research methods and its theoretical underpinning could partly overcome the prejudices which have already established themselves in our technocratic society. A popular development has been the notion of self-help. This has been the only form of health care available to most people until recent years. There is no problem for 'wise folk' handling most minor illness. However the big problem arises when the problem is apparently minor. An episode of 'indigestion' in a middle-aged man may, in fact, be the onset of a heart attack. Since the use of a coronary stent or fibrinolytic or 'clot busting' treatment can be life-saving, time taken to reach hospital often determines whether or not the patient survives, and, if so whether or not they are subsequently disabled by heart failure. This does not exclude the possibility of using physician extenders and nurse practitioners as a lower cost triage method; this solution to the dilemma will undoubtedly become more common.

The gulf between people with limited medical training, working in a community health centre, and the use of paramedical personnel could be bridged. There is also a precedent created by the use of specially trained triage community nurses by telephone. Even before this development, resident medical officers knew that experienced senior night nurses had little difficulty in sorting out most of these problems to everyone's satisfaction, otherwise the poor resident would get little sleep. There is another way in which reflective physicians could be of use. They would be ideally suited to training lay people to discern the basic manifestations of more severe illness, especially those mimicking a less serious problem, and convincing sufferers to seek medical assistance as appropriate. Reflective physicians could also give lessons in cardiopulmonary resuscitation and first aid. In addition, there is a place for community members to have a place on appropriate hospital and centre committees, to inject a dose of public attitudes into discussions.

It is becoming accepted that physician assistants, usually trained nurses, can play an important role, especially in the Peripheral Zone of medical practice as a major contributor to the solution of problems such as difficulties with compliance, failure of reassurance, with continuing anxiety after a health clearance, management of functional symptoms especially those of somatization. Certainly is this a large component of practice with which many doctors are not comfortable where the assistance of a physician extender might often be welcomed. This could be a valuable concept in hospital outpatient practice to more efficiently link a specialist with a referring general practitioner under difficult circumstances.

Such nurse practitioners could also be included in clinical practice research, supporting greater sociological and humanistic input, sometimes greater patient satisfaction, and the advantages which that can bring, including enhancement of the placebo effect.. Even in a high technology unit such as coronary care or renal dialysis when patient support is at a premium, doctors and specially trained nurses generally work well together. So they do in the management of diabetes which poses serious challenges such as a high rate of noncompliance, and need for a high level of patient understanding of the disease and of its complications and of treatment requirements. As the roles of physician assistant, nurse practitioner and physician extender become better defined, understood and accepted, the training of such workers will become a major issue. Reflective physicians could play an important role in this training-.

Conclusion

Our mission has been to create a structure which contributes to tying the teaching of university and hospital more closely together, with a particular emphasis on the teaching of behavioral and social sciences and medical humanities in the medical curriculum. The basic elements are the reflective physician, clinical practice research, the objective of which is continuous quality improvement of clinical practice, and centre for the study of clinical practice which trains the former and supports and coordinates the latter. Alvin Toffler's 'Third Wave' (1970) is well and truly breaking over medicine right now. Whether we can surf it to our advantage or have it simply break over our heads, or if physicians accept 'rescue' by managed care interests with cash registers, or public health evaluators armed with clip-boards and clinical guidelines, will depend on how skillfully physicians and others in the health care system meet the challenge. Santayana has observed that 'those who cannot remember the past are condemned to repeat it.'.

The Chinese word for crisis' is 'wei ji.' The first character represents 'danger' and the second 'opportunity'- an apt descriptor for a paradigm shift such as those in medicine are experiencing. History will not look kindly on those who cannot or will not recognize the need for these two faces of medicine to merge within the medical paradigm. There was only one snake on the staff of Aesculapius, not two. Those who seize the moment to balance the medical paradigm's commitment to science and to humanistic interpretive disciplines, and those doctors who habitually reflect, hence further hone their clinical skills and who contribute to clinical practice research, will have the honour of being accoucheurs, assisting at the birth of postmodern medicine.

References

Birkelo C. C., et al., Tuberculosis case finding. *JAMA* 143: 359-66, 1947.

Bloom S. W., Reform without change: Look beyond the curriculum. *Amer J Pub Hlth* 285: 907-8;1995.

Bulwer-Lytton., Richelieu; a play in five acts. London 1839.

Campbell E. J. M., The J Burns Amberson Lecture. The management of acute respiratory failure in chronic bronchitis and emph ysema. *Amer Rev Respir Dis* 96: 626-29: 1967.

Campbell K., Intensive oxygen therapy s a possible cause of retrolental fibroplasia. A clinical approach. *Med J Aust* 1951: 48-50.

Crenner C., Private practice. Johns Hopkins University. 2005.

Cuff P. A., Vanselow N. A., Editors. Improving medical education: Enhancing the behavioral and social science content of medical curricula. Institute of Medicine (US). Committee on behavioral and social sciences in medical curricula: Washington DC. National Academies Press (US) 2004.

Dewey J. How we think. DC Heath and Co. 1910.

Epstein R. M., Mindful practice. *JAMA* 282: 833-9, 1999.

Epstein R. M., Perception, reflection and the acquisition of wisdom. *Medical Education* 42: 1048-1050, 208.

Feinstein A. R., Clinical Judgment. *Williams and Wilkins,* Baltimore, 1967.

Flexner A. Medical Education in the United States and Canada. A report to the Carnegie Foundation for the Advancement of Learning. Bulletin no. 4 (1910).

Garland L. H., On the evaluation of diagnostic procedures. *Radiology,* 52: 309-328, 1949.

Hay C. Weisner T. S., Subramanian S., Duan N., Niedzinski E. J., Kravitz R. L., Harnessing experience: exploring the gap between evidence-based medicine and clinical practicem *Journal of Evaluation in Clinical Practice;* 14: 707–713 2008.

Joshua A. M., Celermajer D. S., Stockler M. R., Beauty is in the eye of the examiner: reaching agreement about physical signs and their value. *Intern Med J:* 35, 178-187. 2005.

McDonald I. G., et al., Opening Pandora's Box. The unpredictability of reassurance by a normal test result. *BMJ* 313: 329-322. 1996.

Medical Research Council, Streptomycin treatment of pulmonary tuberculosis: A report of council. *BMJ* 2: 769-782. 1948.

Mills C., W., The sociological imagination. Oxford University Press, Oxford, 2000.

Novack R. M., et al., Calibrating the physician. Personal awareness and effective patient care. Working group on promoting physician awareness. American Academy on Physician and Patient. *JAMA* 278: 502-9, 1997.

Peabody F. W., The care of the patient. *JAMA;* 88: 877-82, 1927.

Polanyi M. The tacit dimension. Routledge, The University of Chicago Press, London, 2009 (reprint).

Santayana G., Reason in commonsense. The life of reason. *Charles Scribner's Sons*, 1905, p. 284.

Schon D., The reflective practitioner: How professionals think in action. *Temple Smith,* London, 1983.

Schon D., From technical rationality to reflection-in-action. The Open University. Ch1 in Boundaries in adult learning. Routledge, London and New York, 1996.

Simel D. L., Rennie D., The rational clinical examination. Evidence-based clinical examination.. *Mc Graw-Hill Medical*. 2009.

Toffler A., Future Shock. *Bantam Books,* 1970.

Waymack M. H., Yearning for certainty and the critique of medicine as 'science.' *Theor Med Bioeth* 30: 25, 2009.

Weber M., The protestant ethic and the spirit of capitalism. *T. Parsons trans.* Routledge, London, 1905.

Zadeh L. A., Fuzzy sets. *Information and control*. 338-353. 1965.

Author's Contact Information

Dr. Ian McDonald
Email: ianmcdonald2012@hotmail.com

Index

D

E

F